C000318700

To My Parents

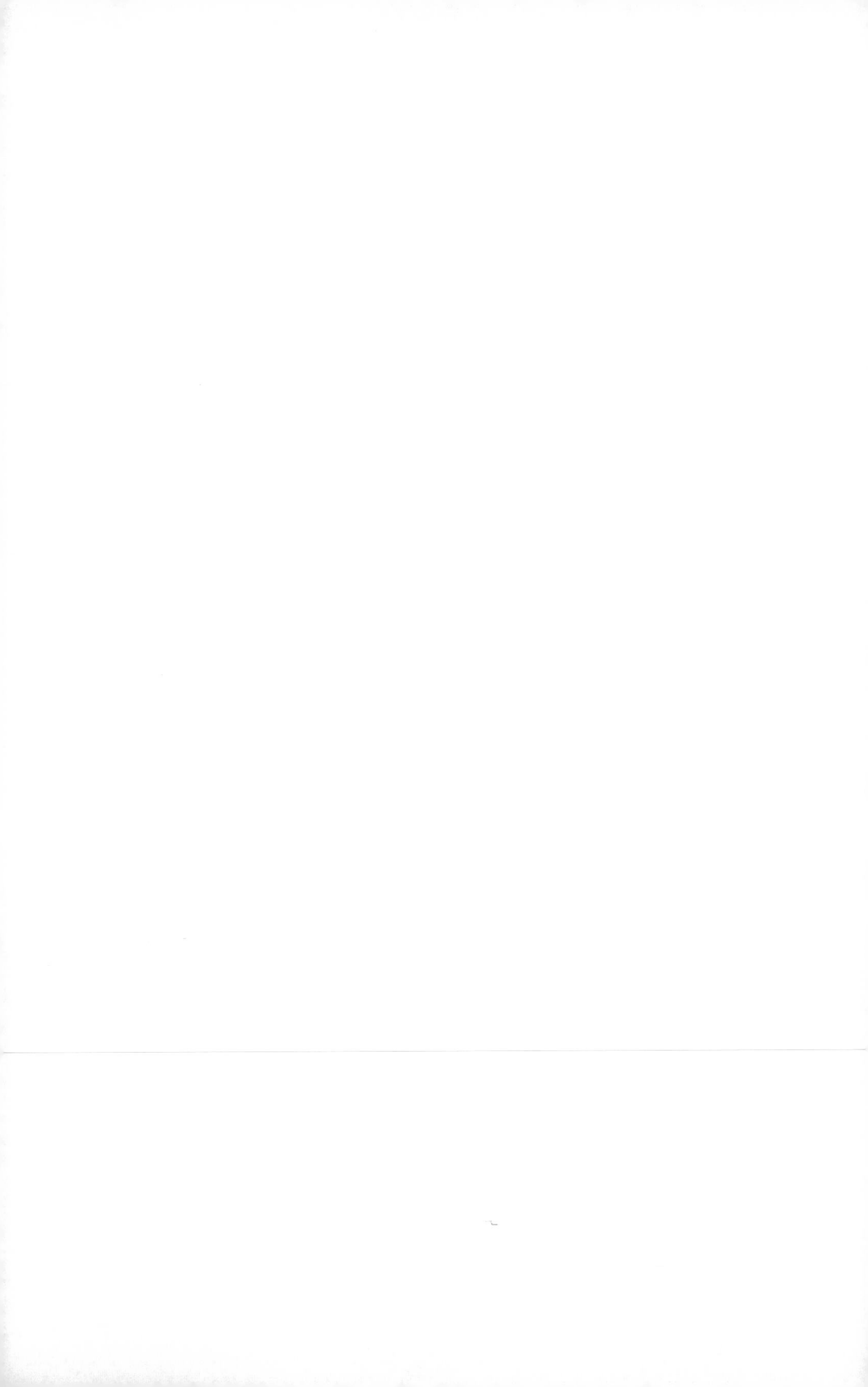

Family and Fertility in Puerto Rico

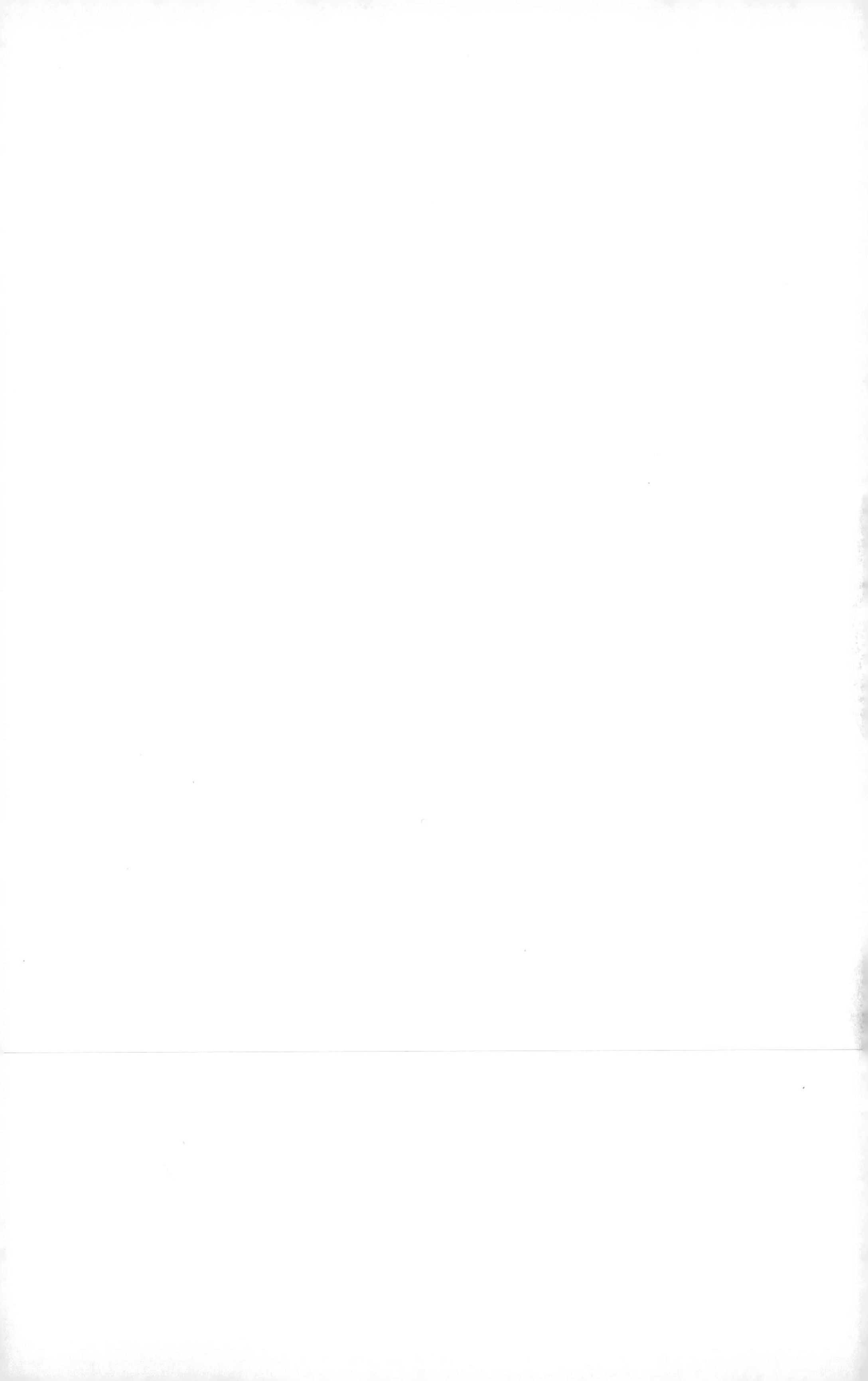

SOCIAL SCIENCE RESEARCH CENTER
COLLEGE OF SOCIAL SCIENCES
UNIVERSITY OF PUERTO RICO

Family and Fertility in Puerto Rico

A STUDY OF THE LOWER INCOME GROUP

by J. Mayone Stycos

1955

COLUMBIA UNIVERSITY PRESS, NEW YORK

COPYRIGHT © 1955 COLUMBIA UNIVERSITY PRESS, NEW YORK

PUBLISHED IN GREAT BRITAIN, CANADA, INDIA, AND PAKISTAN
BY GEOFFREY CUMBERLEGE: OXFORD UNIVERSITY PRESS
LONDON, TORONTO, BOMBAY, AND KARACHI

Library of Congress Catalog Card Number: 55-6620

MANUFACTURED IN THE UNITED STATES OF AMERICA

To My Parents

Family and Fertility in Puerto Rico is the first volume of the final report of the Family Life Research Project undertaken by the Social Science Research Center of the University of Puerto Rico with the purpose of trying to explain the dynamics of child spacing in Puerto Rican families of low income and low education.

The primary purpose of the Social Science Research Center is scientific inquiry concerning the basic problems and characteristics of the society of Puerto Rico. Since its creation in 1945, the Center has initiated 39 projects; 28 are completed and the rest are in progress. The research has been published in 14 books, with two more to be published later this year; 7 pamphlets; and 9 mimeographed reports. Also, more than 20 articles have been written reporting different phases of the Center's survey work.

The research so far undertaken has not only contributed to the knowledge of the social sciences but has also assisted the people, the Government, schools, and the University of Puerto Rico to understand, maintain, and improve the society of Puerto Rico. *Family and Fertility in Puerto Rico* will, no doubt, contribute to the theories of population dynamics by adding knowledge about the behavior and beliefs of low-income families—the high-fertility group producing the swift increments to the population of the world—in a culture of rapid development.

Other publications of research done in the Social Science Research Center are: Samuel Ewer Eastman and Daniel Marx, Jr., *Ships and Sugar: An Evaluation of Puerto Rican Offshore Shipping* (University of Puerto Rico Press, 1953, 230 pages); Paul K. Hatt, *Backgrounds of Human Fertility in Puerto Rico, A Sociological Survey* (Princeton University Press, 1952, 512 pages; in cooperation with the Office of Population Research, Princeton University); Clarence F. Jones and Rafael Pico, *Symposium on the Geography of Puerto Rico* (University of Puerto Rico Press, 1955, 486 pages); Eleanor E. Maccoby and Frances Fielder, *Saving Among Upper-Income Families* (University of Puerto Rico Press, 1953, 159 pages); Northwestern University, Department of Geography, *The Rural Land Classification Program of Puerto Rico* (Northwestern University, 1952, 261 pages; in cooperation with the Puerto Rico Department of Agriculture and Commerce, the Puerto Rican Planning Board, and Northwestern University); Harvey S. Perloff, *Puerto Rico's Economic Future, A Study in Planned Development* (University of Chicago Press and the University of Puerto Rico, 1950, 435 pages); Rafael Pico, *The Geographic Regions of Puerto Rico* (University of Puerto Rico Press, 1950, 256 pages); Lydia J. Roberts and Rosa Luisa Stefani, *Patterns of Living in Puerto Rican Families* (University of Puerto Rico Press, 1949, 411 pages; in cooperation with the Department of Home Economics, University of Puerto Rico); Caroline F. Ware, *Estudio de la comunidad* (Pan American Union, Washington, D. C., revised, 1952, 162 pages); Eric Williams (Editor), *Documents on British West Indian History, 1807-1835 . . .* (Trinidad Publishing Company, 1952, 466 pages; in cooperation with the Historical Society of Trinidad and Tobago). In addition to the present volume by Mr. Stycos two other research works are now in preparation.

Acknowledgments

THE GREATEST SHARE of my indebtedness goes to my interviewers: Armando Arroyo Gerena, Brigida González de Lladó, Angelina Saavedra de Roca, América Boneta de Saavedra, Emilio Santiago Velázquez, and Magdalena Escudero de Santiago. This group went well beyond the "call of duty" in the performance of tasks of considerable intellectual, physical, and interpersonal difficulty. Whatever success the project has had is in a large measure due to them.

Reuben Hill of the University of North Carolina also claims a large share of thanks. Both in the planning of the project and in the reading of the manuscript, his services as a critical sounding board were invaluable. Few Assistant Directors have had the fortune of working with a Director who could be of great assistance without intruding. Millard Hansen, the Director of the Social Science Research Center, deserves a good share of credit in this regard. His helpful criticism on a large portion of the manuscript and his cooperativeness in various aspects of the project made work a pleasure at the Social Science Research Center. My dissertation board at Columbia University was of great assistance in the revision of the manuscript. Professors Kingsley Davis and Herbert Hyman were especially helpful in this regard.

My wife Mary, who served as my assistant in the analysis and writing stage of the project, deserves the chief credit for the "detail work" which has gone into the report. Her patience and zeal for accuracy is responsible for whatever degree of precision has been created from highly qualitative materials. Three other part-time assistants, Angelina Saavedra de Roca, Rosa Pérez, and María Socorro Martínez were of great assistance in the tedious task of coding the material. Conchita Torruellas receives the major share of credit for typing the manuscript, assisted by Carmen Benítez de Guadalupe and Carmen López de Serrano.

I would also like to express my thanks to David Landy of the Social Science Research Center for his helpful suggestions stemming from his anthropological work in Puerto Rico; to Dr. Fernández Marina, who discussed with me some of the psychiatric aspects of the analysis; to the Department of Health for their contribution of time and personnel; to Raul Serrano, of the School of Public Administration, for information on family law; to the members of the Bureau of Scientific Taxation, who assisted in the sampling, and to other members of the Research Center staff who contributed in producing the final report.

I am indebted to the *Public Opinion Quarterly* and to the *Annals of the American Academy of Political and Social Science* for permission to reprint material originally printed in these journals.

Chapel Hill, N. C.
June, 1955

J. MAYONE STYCOS

Contents

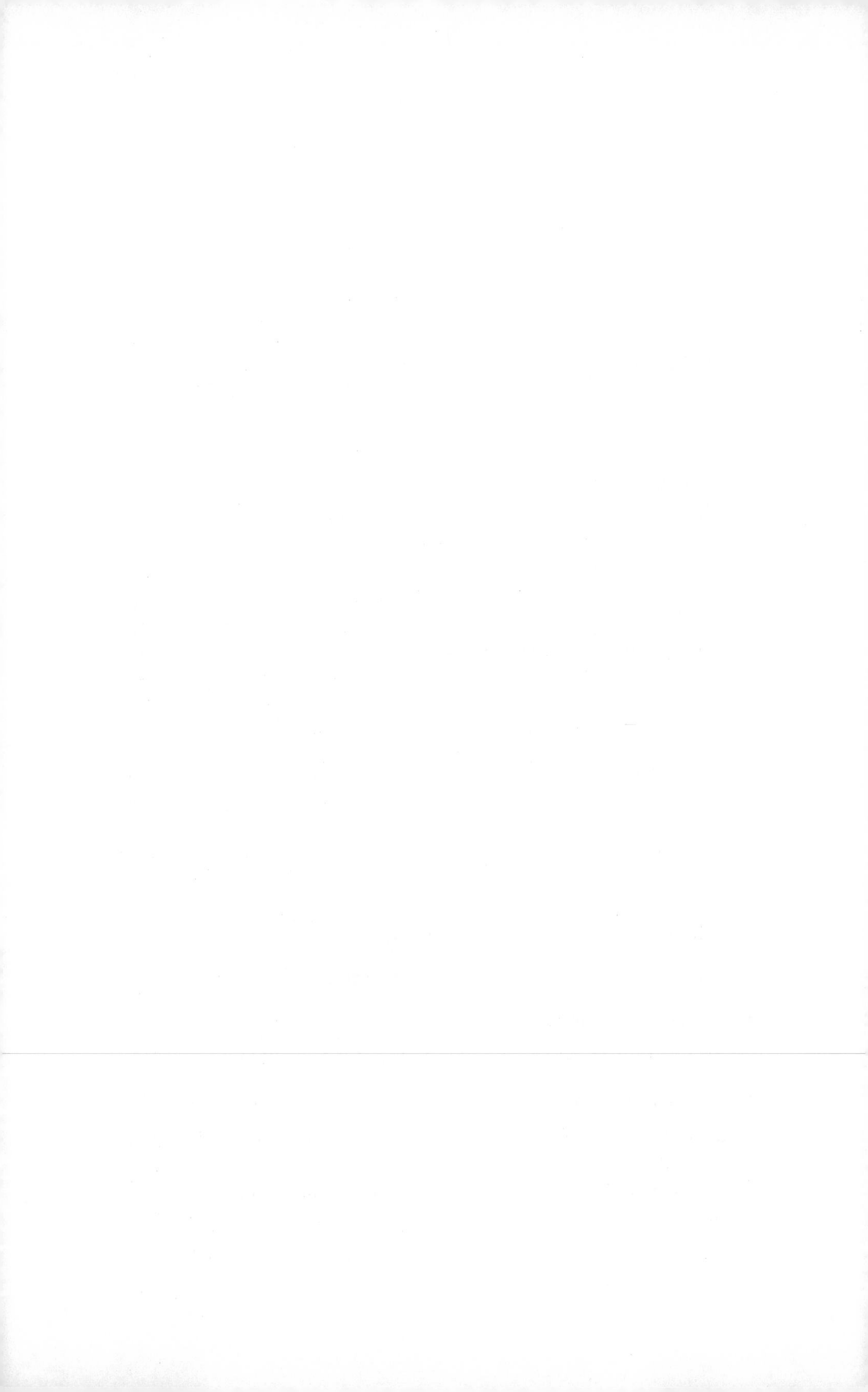

Tables

Figures

Family and Fertility in Puerto Rico

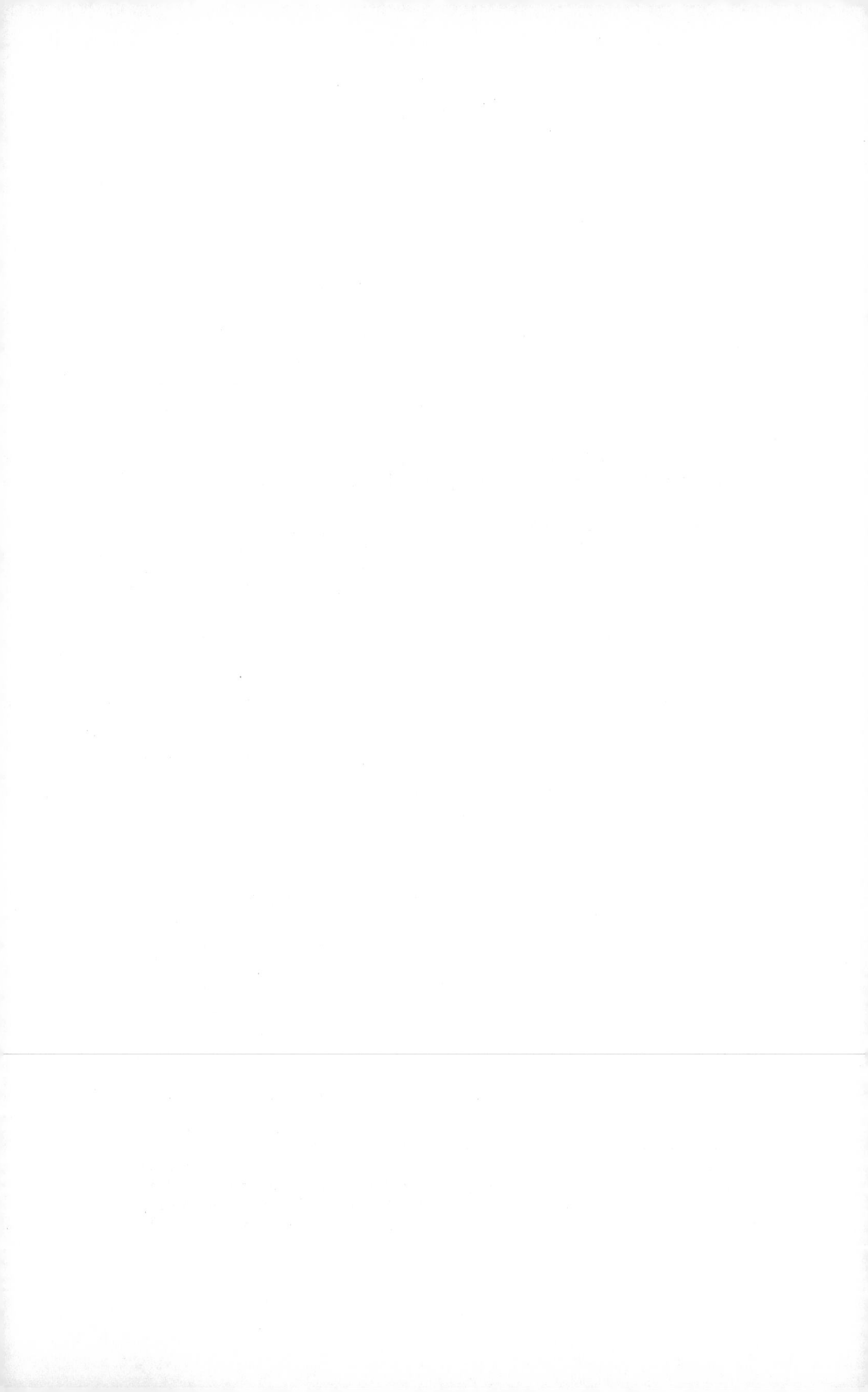

I

Introduction

> An Industrial Revolution in underdeveloped areas today will not offer the slack for demographic growth that it did in the West of an earlier period. . . . The cultural and religious tradition in which fertility is imbedded in one half the world is such that regardless of the speed of modernization the rate of decline will be much less than in the West.
>
> RUPERT VANCE

> Latin America is the fastest growing region in the world. Puerto Rico is the fastest growing political unit.
>
> CLARENCE SENIOR

> . . . South America is the dark continent, sociologically speaking. Its social organization is more obscure to us than that of African natives.
>
> KINGSLEY DAVIS

WHY THIS STUDY WAS UNDERTAKEN

The three quotations by demographers cited above summarize the major reasons for this book. The fear that the pessimistic Malthusian thesis may be borne out has alarmed the Western World and alerted it to the actual and potential population growth of the underdeveloped areas. The alarm of the West may be fed by a growing sense of guilt, for its own introduction of modern techniques for the reduction of deaths in underdeveloped areas has never been accompanied by equally efficient methods for the reduction of births.

The sources of the quotations at the head of this chapter are: Rupert Vance, "The Demographic Gap: Dilemma of Modernization Programs," in *Approaches to Problems of High Fertility in Agrarian Societies* (New York: Milbank Memorial Fund, 1952), p. 16; Clarence Senior, "Disequilibrium between Population and Resources: The Case of Puerto Rico," *Proceedings of the Inter-American Conference on the Conservation of Renewable Natural Resources* (1948), p. 145; Kingsley Davis, "Changing Modes of Marriage," in Becker and Hill, eds., *Marriage and the Family* (Boston: Heath, 1942), p. 100.

The blame, of course, lies not entirely on our own shoulders. Educating for the prolongation of life is a much simpler problem than educating for the control of its conception. But now that the prolongation of life has created even greater problems, responsible social scientists have been turning to the intricacies of population control, raising a number of challenging questions.

What factors underlie the great immediate and potential population growth of underdeveloped areas? What factors sustain a high birth rate when such actually imperils the existence of a society? What customs, mores, and attitudes of a people contribute to high fertility, and how susceptible are they of change? What complexes of thought and behavior prevent fertility from reaching its biological maximum in a society, and how can these further be emphasized? These are questions of interest not only to the sociologist and demographer but to the leaders of nations with accelerating population growth.

In Puerto Rico, where the economy must struggle to keep up with gains in population, there has been great concern over high fertility for the past two decades. It was such concern which prompted the current and other projects on human fertility in Puerto Rico; and it is to provide some of the answers to these questions that the present work has been undertaken.

While our chief purpose is to answer questions specific to Puerto Rico, we should hope at the same time to provide a good deal of information that might be applicable to other nations or cultures. What characteristics does Puerto Rico possess that might commend it as a crude laboratory for the study of the social dynamics of population growth?

1. Puerto Rico is in many ways typical of other underdeveloped areas of the world. Geographically located between North and South America, it is culturally more Latin than American, and much of what can be learned in Puerto Rico can be considered applicable at least to the southern nations of the Western hemisphere. For example, it is a Roman Catholic culture, and for that reason it is good ground for testing the obstacles to population reduction that are inherent in such cultures. Moreover, while changing rapidly, the society still has enough evidences of folk culture to make

it in many ways comparable to other areas dominated by the folk mentality.

2. While having many of the earmarks of the old world, Puerto Rico is definitely a society "in transition." Fifty years ago, only one fifth of the population over ten years of age was literate. At the present time, three fourths of the population can read and write. While still a poor country by United States standards, Puerto Rico through its recent economic gains has reached a per-capita income rivaled in the Caribbean only by Cuba. While the population is still strongly rural, the proportion of inhabitants living in cities has grown from 15 to 40 percent within the half century. Finally, while it has an economy primarily geared to agriculture, Puerto Rico's "Operation Bootstrap" has steadily accelerated the process of industrialization within the past decade. As a culture, then, with a foot both in the old world and the new, it provides a good testing ground for new world fertility ideals and practice.

3. Puerto Rico is a small island, making it a manageable unit of study for the social scientist. With an area the size of the state of Delaware, and with a predominantly Spanish culture that was insulated for centuries from foreign influence, Puerto Rico's two and a quarter million people are more easily studied as a culture than would be larger, less isolated, and less homogeneous societies.

4. Puerto Rico proves an excellent example of the mechanics of the demographic gap—the lag between the reduction of mortality and fertility characteristic of currently developing economies. In many ways Puerto Rico is too mild a case, for it has an advantageous position politically, geographically, and economically in regard to the United States. But if we can understand what is happening in Puerto Rico despite its unusual advantages, we shall have an idea of what even greater problems can easily occur in other underdeveloped areas of the world and, possibly, which directions for policy are most likely to be fruitful.

What, briefly, is Puerto Rico's history and present position with respect to population and resources?

When the United States took possession of Puerto Rico at the turn of the century, there were less than a million inhabitants; at the present time, with scant natural resources, the island's population has grown to nearly two and a half million despite heavy emigration. Only about half of the island's land is arable, and the present number of people per square mile is roughly fifteen times that of the United States.

Only three factors can bring about population change—changes in birth rates, changes in death rates, or migration. In Puerto Rico, as in such areas as Mexico, Jamaica, Formosa, and Ceylon, population increase has been brought about by spectacular declines in mortality. At the turn of the century, births were occurring annually at the rate of 40 per thousand of population, and deaths at the rate of about 25 per thousand, creating a relatively modest rate of increase. Only within the past few years has the crude birth rate shown any decline, dropping to 35.9 in 1952, but the crude death rate has dropped to 9.2, roughly that of the continental United States. At the rate of increase for the decade 1942-1951, assuming no migration, the island would have about nine million inhabitants by the end of the century. The sharp drop in mortality has been largely accomplished in the short span of the past two decades and is not hard to explain. As a result of improved transportation, sanitation, and public health, deaths due to diarrhea, enteritis, pneumonia, tuberculosis, malaria, nephritis, etc., have been greatly and quickly reduced.[1]

But population increase is not inherently bad and must be judged only in relation to a nation's resources. If the economy can expand as rapidly as the population, the nation will at least be no worse off than before. How has Puerto Rico fared? Puerto Rico has been favored by United States federal benefits, by American military installations, by American citizenship facilitating emigration, and by American capital and technology. It is also blessed by a stable government and by farsighted leadership. The government has invested its revenues in a broad program of industrialization aimed at providing more nonagricultural jobs for the population. Its efforts have added roughly 200 new industrial firms and 12,000 employees

[1] These data have been drawn from Kingsley Davis, "Puerto Rico: A Crowded Island," *Annals of the American Academy of Political and Social Science*, CCLXXXV (Jan. 1953), 116-22.

to the island's economy within the past decade. But the impact of this formidable accomplishment is largely vitiated by the fact that *every year* there are 16,000 new entrants into the labor force. Thus the gains of industrialization tend to be consumed by the rapidly growing population.

This brief example of the dangerous dilemma of one-sided public health programs should make it clear that the successful program in underdeveloped regions is one which aims at both a reduction in deaths and a reduction in births. Only in this way can we avoid "keeping more people alive so that they may live badly."[3] But how can this be done?

One obvious way is to provide the population with birth-control information and materials. This is precisely what Puerto Rico has done. Since 1939 a network of government-sponsored birth-control clinics has provided information and free materials to all those who desire and need them. Despite this fact, there has been little appreciable change in the crude birth rate. Apparently then, materials are not enough, and the neo-Malthusian assumption, that given information, people will act rationally and apply it, would not seem to hold in Puerto Rico. We must, then, look more carefully at the attitudes and social institutions which maintain high fertility despite available means for its reduction. Before moving specifically to a consideration of Puerto Rico, let us consider very briefly the general relation between culture and fertility levels.

CULTURE AND FERTILITY

Societies, and even classes within societies, often demonstrate surprisingly consistent levels of fertility over time. If not purely the result of biological differences (and presumably all nations and classes are more or less similarly endowed in this respect), fertility rates must be influenced by other factors. Actually, fertility is directly affected by only three variables: (1) the physiological capacity to reproduce; (2) the degree of exposure to pregnancy through sexual intercourse; and (3) the extent to which birth controls, including contraception, abortion, and infanticide, are

[3] *Ibid.*, p. 119.

employed. We will not consider the first of these, since it is probably least crucial in explaining differential fertility[3] and is least affected by culture. Assuming a more or less constant fecundity, fertility is determined by the extent to which checks on coitus and on birth are present in a given society. Both these variables are to a large degree determined by the common culture shared by a class or society, and it is for this reason that, by and large, families within a given class or society reproduce at a rate similar to their neighbors and different from those of other classes or societies.[4] It will be one task of this report to show how these two variables are affected by cultural elements in a *particular* society. Let us first indicate in a very tentative and summary fashion how culture can affect the degree of coitus and birth controls.

CULTURAL DETERMINANTS OF COITUS

Broadly and simply stated, culture in part determines the circumstances under which, and the extent to which, coitus occurs. It might be said that culture influences how, how often, among whom, and when sexual intercourse will occur.

Modes of Intercourse. The permissible forms of sexual relations are culturally defined. Of interest to our present concern with fertility would be the extent to which deviations from normal coitus occur in a given society—deviations which obviate or reduce the risk of conception. Himes notes, for example, the apparently frequent and permissible practice[5] of homosexuality and oral eroticism

[3] As one recent evidence, a comprehensive study of the causes for the reduction of fertility in England concluded that it is very unlikely that declines in reproductive capacity have had any significance in the reduction of the birth rate in that nation. *Royal Commission on Population Report* (London: H.M. Stationery Office, 1949), pp. 31-34.

[4] Actually there is also a great degree of similarity in fertility rates among certain *types* of society despite differences in many aspects of their culture. Logically it would follow that there are strategic cultural elements common to such societies. What these crucial aspects are must await further comparative studies.

[5] While evidence is lacking on this point, it is likely that there is a relation between the prescribed, permissible, and forbidden forms of sexual behavior in any society and what is actually practiced. While there are always discrepancies, it is probable that the norms operate as a check on the maximum expressions of any given sexual pattern. Kinsey showed a wide discrepancy between American sexual norms and conduct, but while the number of individuals who

in ancient Peru and Greece, and the custom of prepubertal coitus among some preliterate societies.[6] In summarizing the anthropological data on this subject, Ford and Beach conclude that "there are some peoples who do not strictly forbid homosexual relations, autoerotic practices or animal intercourse; and under such conditions one or the other of these alternative sexual patterns often constitutes an important secondary form of sexual expression for part of the population."[7] Whether such "secondary forms" are of sufficient incidence to reduce heterosexual coitus to the point of affecting fertility is, of course, open to question.[8]

Frequency. There is some anthropological evidence suggesting that more or less explicit customary coital frequency exists in some primitive societies; that is, a standard frequency which mated couples are expected to follow.[9] In more indirect and less explicit ways culture may have a great deal to do with coital frequency. If the general attitude toward sex is permissive, for example, women are more likely to enjoy sexual relations than may be the case in

have engaged in illicit behavior is remarkably high, the frequency of their deviation falls far short of "normal" sex behavior, and, presumably, short of what might be if such norms were nonexistent. However, research in this area should always attempt to assess the degree to which sexual norms are carried out in practice in a given society.

[6] Norman E. Himes, *Medical History of Contraception* (London: George Allen and Unwin, 1936), pp. 51-52.

[7] C. Ford and F. Beach, *Patterns of Sexual Behavior* (New York: Harper, 1951), p. 19.

[8] It is possible, too, that different positions during sexual intercourse and different patterns of sexual foreplay can increase or lessen the risks of pregnancy. For a general discussion of the effects of varying positions on fertility, see H. Van de Velde, *Ideal Marriage: Its Physiology and Technique* (London: William Heineman, 1926), p. 186. For a description of cultural variation in coital positions, see Ford and Beach, *op. cit.*, pp. 13-25. Also see p. 59 for an account of how some lower animal forms cannot conceive without certain forms of precoital stimulation. For the human female, the presumably beneficial effects of sexual foreplay have been widely discussed. Vaginismus and other milder obstructions to complete penetration have obvious implications for fertility and may be class-linked. Kinsey has demonstrated that upper-level males practice more sex play prior to coitus than do lower-level males but reaches the tentative conclusion that ". . . preliminary calculations indicate that the frequency of orgasm is higher among lower level females . . . even though the lower level coitus involves a minimum of specific physical stimulation" (A. Kinsey, W. Pomeroy, and C. Martin, *Sexual Behavior in the Human Male,* Philadelphia: Saunders, 1948, p. 367).

[9] Ford and Beach, *op. cit.*, pp. 75-82.

puritannical or double-standard cultures; sexual frequency might accordingly be higher. Or in some groups sex may be regarded as symbolic of power, virility, or divine possession. It is also conceivable that in groups with little opportunity for social mobility or with relatively meagre recreational outlets, more time and energy are channeled into sexual activity. For whatever reason, subgroups in our own society show strikingly different frequencies,[10] despite the fact that norms of sexual frequency have not been explicit, at least before Kinsey. How and why the particular standards for sexual frequency are set, circulated, and inculcated is still problematical, but the fact that group patterns exist suggests that culture (in this case subcultures) in some measure affects sexual frequency.

Coital Participants. Culture reduces maximum fertility by limiting the number of people among whom sexual relations are permissible. All societies have rules, but in only three of 115 observed societies is there a general tabu on all sexual relations outside marriage.[11] In such groups, intercourse is theoretically restricted to married couples, a fact which removes all the unmarried from the risk of pregnancy.[12] But in all societies, coitus is expected at least within marriage; therefore the rules of marriage are of considerable significance with respect to fertility. Tabus on divorce or remarriage of widows will lower the fertility of a society. In India, for example, it has been estimated that Hindu fertility would be 16 percent higher were it not for the tabu on widow remarriage.[13]

[10] While total frequencies do not vary greatly among occupational and educational groups, the sources of orgasm (masturbation, nocturnal emissions, homosexuality, marital intercourse, etc.) are markedly dissimilar, a fact which has clear implications for fertility. Those who go to high school but not beyond show highest frequencies, and even when in school ". . . their outlets average ten to twenty percent higher than the outlets of the boys who will stop by the eighth grade and twenty to thirty percent higher than the boys who will ultimately go to college" (Kinsey, Pomeroy, and Martin, *op. cit.*, p. 335).

[11] G. Murdock, *Social Structure* (New York: Macmillan, 1949), Table 75, p. 263.

[12] In countries such as India and Ceylon, where 99 percent and 97 percent respectively of the female population have been married by age 64, the confining of coitus to the married has less impact on fertility than in Ireland and Sweden, where only 76 percent and 79 percent have been married by the same age. See K. Davis, "Statistical Perspective on Marriage and Divorce," *Annals of the American Academy of Political and Social Science*, CCLXXII (Nov. 1950), pp. 9-21.

[13] K. Davis, "Human Fertility in India," *American Journal of Sociology*, LII, No. 3 (Nov. 1946), 243-54.

Also, the degree of tabus against the intermarriage of certain groups (kin,[14] clans, castes, classes) and the extent of celibacy practiced may be important in determining the rate of birth.

Not only the tabus themselves but the cultural mechanisms for enforcing them must be considered. In Latin American society, the chaperonage system helps guarantee against premarital intercourse for females by preventing the association of a boy and girl except in the company of a guardian of the mores. The purdah system of India makes sure that a man's wives will be inaccessible to other men. The monastery is more likely to insure celibacy than the free mixing of clergy with the rest of society. In combination with the tabus, then, these cultural forms are powerful depressants on intercourse.[15]

Occasion. Culture is also influential in determining the age at which sexual relations will be initiated, and, broadly, the occasions when they will occur subsequently. In certain societies, a boy will be expected to commence premarital sexual relations around a particular age, and in most societies a person is expected to be married by a certain age. In Ireland only 12.4 percent of the females are married by age 24, in contrast with 52.8 percent in the United States and 95 percent in India.[16]

Special periods when intercourse may, should, or should not occur are likewise set by culture. "A number of societies sanction either general sexual license or a substantial slackening of ordinary restrictions on the occasion of weddings, funerals, festivals, or religious ceremonies."[17] Special restrictions on intercourse are at least as widely spread. During or preceding war is a favorite period for such tabus, and "hunting, fishing, and farming may be accompanied, preceded, or followed by temporary abstinence from sexual activities."[18] In parts of India, religious days, days of sowing the

[14] For detailed analysis of tabus and privileged sexual relations among kin, see Murdock, *op. cit.*, Chapter XI.

[15] Murdock believes that societies can be divided into two classes: those which internalize sexual tabus and which presumably require little or no external controls, and those which rely chiefly on social safeguards and rules of avoidance (*op. cit.*, p. 273). Which of these methods is most effective in preserving the norms is a question that begs research.

[16] Davis, "Statistical Perspective on Marriage and Divorce," Table 3, p. 14.

[17] Murdock, *op. cit.*, p. 267.

[18] Ford and Beach, *op. cit.*, p. 76.

fields, and days of shaving or bathing are considered by many as periods for abstinence;[19] and in many other areas the periods of menstruation and lactation[20] call for abstinence.

CULTURAL DETERMINANTS OF BIRTH CONTROL

Whether or not differences in rates of coitus mean anything in terms of fertility depends on whether there are checks upon conception, live parturition, and continued existence of the newly born. Whether or not any such checks will be used to any extent by a society, and which specific checks will be used, depends on the state of technology with respect to birth controls, on the degree of diffusion of knowledge of birth-control technology, and on the degree of motivation present among the members of the society.

Technology. Every society has at its disposal some method of birth control. Abortion and infanticide are age-old techniques of population limitation and are still practiced to varying degrees in most societies. Twins, females, sickly infants, and illegitimate children are frequent victims of culturally permissible infanticide, but even more drastic procedures occur. For example, of a Madagascar tribe Linton writes, ". . . all children born on three days in each week were killed . . . immediately after birth, being dropped into a jar of boiling water head down, or buried in an ant hill."[21] Japan, which before the nineteenth century reputedly kept its population stationary by means of infanticide, is now the most outstanding example of a contemporary culture employing abortion. In 1952, 794,793 induced abortions were recorded, roughly 40 percent of the number of live births recorded for the same year.[22]

Contraception, while less widely known or practiced, is probably as old as recorded history. While the more effective chemical and

[19] C. Chandrasekharan, "Cultural Patterns in Relation to Family Planning in India," in *Third International Conference on Planned Parenthood, Report of Proceedings* (Bombay: Family Planning Association of India, 1952), pp. 73-79.

[20] Lactation periods may extend from two to three years, and "In nearly every instance, the justification for this abstinence is the prevention of conception" (Clellan S. Ford, "Control of Conception in Cross-Cultural Perspective," *World Population Problems and Birth Control, Annals of the New York Academy of Sciences,* LIV, May, 1952, p. 766).

[21] Letter from Ralph Linton to Lloyd Warner, Cited in Himes, *op. cit.,* p. 8.

[22] Private report from Ministry of Welfare, Japan.

mechanical methods have been developed relatively recently, contraceptives such as the dung pessary have been traced back 3,000 years in Egypt, and *coitus interruptus* has probably always been known even to peasant populations. Thus, some technology has probably always existed everywhere. The extent to which it is employed depends upon other factors described below.

Knowledge. The awareness of modern methods of birth control has not yet permeated a large share of the world. What one author describes as true in present day Korea probably holds for most underdeveloped countries of the world: "Knowledge of contraception is practically non-existent in Korea. It is the sort of thing that men talk about occasionally when they sit in one of the little rooms and drink their rice wine. It is practically unknown as a general practise."[23] But even in contemporary England, which has one of the oldest histories of widespread birth-control publicity, a great deal of ignorance apparently still exists. In a recent study conducted mainly in London, the degree of ignorance of modern birth-control methods was extensive enough to lead the authors to conclude that ". . . the gap in elementary knowledge is so large, after more than half a century of propaganda, that twenty years seems a short time in which to bridge it."[24]

What determines the extent to which a population will be aware of birth control? Obviously the degree to which devices are available and the length of time they have been available in a society are important considerations. But several other questions are also pertinent: (1) What form does the system or systems of communications take in the society? (2) What content is culturally permissible over these communication channels? (3) What audiences receive the content of the varying channels? (4) With what predispositions do the audiences greet the content?

(1) Form: It obviously makes a great difference whether the communications to which varying segments of the populations are exposed are of the mass media or word-of-mouth variety. The latter

[23] A. Bunce, "Economic and Cultural Bases of Family Size in Korea," in *Approaches to Problems of High Fertility in Agrarian Societies* (New York: Milbank Memorial Fund, 1952), p. 23.

[24] Mass Observation, *Britain and Her Birth Rate* (London: John Murray, 1945), p. 61.

theoretically restricts the amount, diffusion, and accuracy of communications content but is ordinarily a more persuasive form.

(2) Content: In cultures whose orientation toward sex tends toward the prudish, the communications network, however efficient, will be hampered by its inability to be explicit concerning conception controls. Religion, superstition, or general ideology may make such subject matter tabu even for word of mouth. Often such topics are communications currency for certain groups in the population only.

(3) Audience: In other than the highly industrialized nations of the West, poverty and illiteracy remove the great masses of population from exposure to the mass media. Word of mouth becomes the principal mode of imparting information, and whether the spoken word will carry birth-control information to all groups in the population depends not only on the prevailing attitude toward sex but upon the system of social stratification as well. In an open class system, information has a much better opportunity to trickle down to the lower classes than is true in societies with more rigidly fixed social classes.[25] Moreover, the latter type of society usually emphasizes age and sex differences, so that, depending upon the prevailing attitude toward sex, information on birth control may be considered as an adult male monopoly, to the extent that husbands may not even impart such information to their wives or sons. In such cases, even where women or young boys are interested in securing information they may be too fearful or modest to do so.

(4) Predispositions: Even where methods are known and available and some interest in contraception exists, what will be considered an acceptable method in one group may not be so considered in another. Many of the criteria for acceptability are based on acceptance by groups rather than individuals and consequently fall within our sphere of interest. For example, in a society or class

[25] Since most peasant societies are characterized by strong class lines, it is important, especially for policy makers, to know who, if any, are the connecting links between the literate and illiterate classes. In a study of communications flow in a rural Greek village, for example, it was discovered that the village priest, teacher, and bartender were strategic figures in determining the flow of information from the outside world. See J. M. Stycos, "Patterns of Communication in a Rural Greek Village," *Public Opinion Quarterly*, Vol. XVI, No. 1 (Spring 1952).

where sex is considered a fine art, such contraceptive methods as condoms or withdrawal may be regarded with special antipathy because they reduce sensation, interfere with the aesthetics of the sexual act, or deprive the male of a full sense of his virility. In male-dominated societies female methods may be objected to by males who feel that they should have control over conception. There may be superstitious fears concerning chemical and mechanical methods, on the ground that they produce ill-health; or modesty may prevent their use in overcrowded dwellings. Such resistances and their social and psychological origins should be understood prior to introducing birth control into another culture,[26] but they should not be overestimated. Many such resistances may be rationalizations for a lack of motivation and might disappear if motivation were to rise sufficiently. On the other hand, technological advances in contraception may make it so simple to avoid children that a minimum of motivation may be necessary. At any rate, it can be seen that motivation is a factor of major importance that remains to be considered.

Motivation. Experience in the United States has indicated that information campaigns impart the most information to those who need it least—the most interested and the already better informed. Even if birth-control information is carried to all by an efficient communications system, if there is no interest in contraception the content may fall on deaf ears. One writer maintains, for example, that in nineteenth-century England, ". . . very intensive propaganda for family limitation was carried on apparently without effect for fifty years, while in France at the same time, the size of families was being reduced while there was relatively little public discussion of the subject."[27]

A basic problem, then, is to determine what cultural factors impel one group to desire large families and other groups to desire small ones. We may begin to answer this question by first establishing what are the needs of various societies in this respect.

[26] One good example is the attempt to instruct Indians in the use of the rhythm method, where the culture already endorses numerous periods of abstinence. See Chandrasekharan, *op. cit.*

[27] A. Myrdal, "Population Trends in Densely Populated Areas," *Proceedings of the American Philosophical Society,* XCV, No. 1 (Feb. 1951), 5.

THREE DEMOGRAPHIC TYPES

Societies may be classified into three basic types according to their fertility and mortality performances—populations of high growth potential (usually underdeveloped economies), of rapid growth (with developing economies), and of incipient decline (with well-developed economies).[28] This is illustrated by Figure I.

Areas of High Growth Potential. Let us here raise some broad speculations concerning the social and ideological supports of high fertility and suggest a number of possible explanations of the absense of penalties on the large family. In areas of high mortality, if husbands and wives wanted small families enough to limit their fertility, the society would soon die out. With reference to the pre-modern period, in Asia, Irene Taeuber writes that ". . . the balance of births and deaths was probably precarious, so that the basic problem was not the curbing of a super-abundant fertility but the maintenance of the fertility that would insure survival under the hazardous conditions of life that once existed."[29] Thus, in high-mortality societies we would expect the presence of social mechanisms which insure that the mass of the population desire large families. However, it is not the case that people realize they must reproduce to save the society, although there may be some awareness that a large family is required in order to insure a few survivors.[30] Broadly expressed, it is that the social institutions, ideologies, and character structure of these societies are such that large families bring greater gratifications than small ones—or, at the very least, that there are no particular penalties attached to having large families.

Societies with high fertilities usually possess agrarian economies

[28] See F. Notestein, "The Facts of Life," in R. Anshen, ed., *The Family: Its Function and Destiny* (New York: Harper, 1949), pp. 258-76. Notestein's categories are actually somewhat different from these.

[29] I. Taeuber, "The Reproductive Mores of the Asian Peasant," in *Proceedings of the Annual Meeting of the Population Association of America,* (Princeton: 1949), p. 96.

[30] When an island-wide sample of Puerto Ricans were asked why they did not want fewer children than the ideal number they expressed, over 30 percent said that this was in order that if some die, others remain. Paul K. Hatt, *Backgrounds of Human Fertility in Puerto Rico* (Princeton: Princeton University Press, 1952), Table 41, p. 58.

or are in the process of changing from agrarian to industrial. They are usually characterized by tightly stratified social classes with little opportunity for social mobility and by a tradition of being content with one's lot in life. The decline of fertility in the West was facilitated by the presence of ideological pressure for social mobility and by mechanisms that make this mobility possible. The social structures in underdeveloped areas are not such as to generate great concern in this direction.

The interlocking nature of the economic and familial institutions in agrarian societies can be such as to make it especially profitable to have a large number of progeny. Since the family operates as an economic unit, children serve as a kind of capital. Even when married, they often are integrated into an extended family group which works as a team. At the same time, with standards of living extremely low and family tradition such as it is, most entertainment must be provided for within the family. Thus, to a certain degree, children are both a man's wealth and his recreation.

The structure of the family is quite important in other ways. In families strongly dominated by males, it will be the husband's motivations which count rather than the wife's. This can be a major block to fertility controls, since the male is ordinarily less concerned than the female with excessive fertility. Especially in societies with

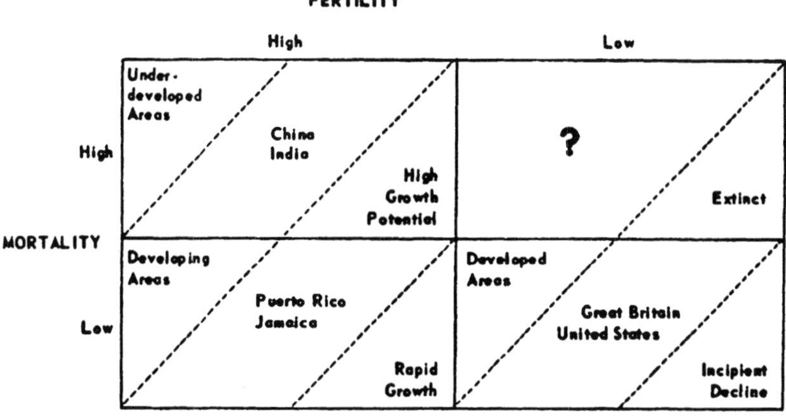

FIGURE I

DEMOGRAPHIC TYPES

unstable marital institutions, the male may feel no particular motivation to reduce fertility since he can always "leave the scene" if fertility pressures become too great.[31] Moreover, in structures of the extended-family type, the pressure of fertility on any one family could be relieved by the practice of dispersing the excess children among less fertile or less burdened relatives—a fact which might vitiate motivation for controls.

In all types of societies there probably is a culturally approved number of children, or at least a maximum or minimum number. In modern Western societies modal tendencies appear to cluster around three or four.[32] But in agrarian economies of the potential-growth variety the ideal number may be open—the more the better—and supporting ideologies give some of the reasons why this is desirable.

Religious ideologies provide some of the strongest props to prolificity. In India, religious belief has it that in order to go to heaven a man must marry and produce a son.[33] In Buddhist Ceylon, numerous progeny denotes merit in previous existences; for some, "if a dead soul wishes to be born into your family it would be a terrible sin to prevent its birth."[34] In China, the individual is encouraged to reproduce in order to have many worshipers after his death, and Mencius warned that of the three things which were unfilial, "to have no posterity is the greatest."[35] Fundamentalist Protestantism

[31] In the "keeper union" common in the British West Indies, for example, "the presence of several children tends to drive the man away, as it makes greater demands on his income" (F. Henriques, "West Indian Family Organization," *American Journal of Sociology,* LV, No. 1 (July 1949), 35.

[32] The average ideal number of children for the United States, England, France, and the Netherlands is about three; for Canada and Australia about four—according to public-opinion polls taken in these countries. "The Quarter's Polls," *Public Opinion Quarterly,* XI, No. 3 (Fall, 1947), 477. For an excellent compilation and analysis of international data in this regard, see Jean Stoetzel, "Les Attitudes et la conjoncture démographique: la dimension idéale de la famille," *Proceedings of the 1954 World Population Conference* (forthcoming).

[33] N. Sovani, "The Problem of Fertility Control in India: Cultural Factors and Development of Policy," in *Approaches to Problems of High Fertility in Agrarian Societies* (New York: Milbank Memorial Fund, 1952), p. 64.

[34] B. Ryan, "Institutional Factors in Sinhalese Fertility," *Milbank Memorial Fund Quarterly,* XXX, No. 4 (Oct. 1952), 371.

[35] O. Lang, *Chinese Family and Society* (New Haven: Yale University Press, 1946), p. 19.

enjoins its members to "increase and multiply," and Roman Catholicism sees procreation as the only real purpose for sexual relations.

Health ideologies with reference to fertility may also play a role. While public opinion in the Western world tends toward the belief that a multitude of children is injurious to health, opposite beliefs are prevalent among women in less developed areas. Among Jamaican lower-class women, for example, the release of the afterbirth is considered a healthful purge of products that otherwise might go to the brain and endanger health.[36]

Children may have symbolic value if it is believed that they are signs of a man's strength, power, or general ability. Even within tightly stratified social structures, there are ways in which one man can stand out from another. In agrarian societies, with little differentiation among families by wealth, some degree of status may be achieved by the ability to produce children. Thus both women and men may pride themselves on the number of children they have produced—for females a sign of fecundity, for males a sign of virility. Moreover, it may be believed to be a sign of good management or of relative prosperity if a man has many children whom he can feed and clothe; or they may be a symbol of power in a community where power may be reckoned by the number or relatives whom one can marshal to his aid. In this way, children may serve as symbols of status, especially where alternative status symbols are scarce.

Such ideologies explicitly enjoin or rationalize large families. Other ideologies may have similar consequences without a manifest fertility ideology. As far as religious ideology is concerned, it might be important to ascertain whether the religion fosters concepts of progress and manipulation of the material world, or whether it fosters a passive acceptance of what comes, living from day to day and avoidance of tinkering with "the nature of things."[37] Is the accent on the individual soul equal before God, or is the individual

[36] M. Kerr, *Personality and Conflict in Jamaica* (Liverpool: University Press, 1952), p. 25.

[37] In Trinidad, for example, one writer has noted a "lack of desire to plan or control one's life," an attitude that may be characteristic of descendants of slave cultures. L. Braithwaite, unpublished manuscript on a Trinidadian village. The consequences of such an ideology might be that action, if taken at all, is taken after the event—as with abortion and infanticide.

only an insignificant speck in the divine scheme? This ties in closely with other general ideologies concerning the value of the individual personality. Thus both democracy and Protestantism accept the importance of developing the individual personality to its fullest. As a consequence, the addition of each new life to a family may require a greater economic and emotional investment than in Far Eastern societies, where the individual is deemphasized.

Areas of Incipient Decline. There is no need to detail the presumed causes for the low fertility in the economically developed areas. Briefly, they are generally considered to be the converse of the picture presented for the underdeveloped societies. The Industrial Revolution, especially, created a less rigid class system and broke up the family as a productive unit, with the result that children soon became burdens rather than capital. At the same time sanitation and medication developed to the point where mortality was greatly reduced, obviating the need for producing many to salvage an adequate number. Ideologies began to lose many of their religious, superstitious, and traditional elements. Birth-control propaganda came to be widely disseminated, and the status of women improved. Such revolutionary changes are considered to be among the chief causes of the decline of fertility in the West.

Areas of Rapid Growth. The two broad classes of societies described above have fertility rates appropriate to their needs. It is the third type of society, where fertility is much in excess of mortality, which currently is posing world problems. Puerto Rico, Jamaica, Ceylon, and Mexico are examples of populations whose mortality rates have dropped swiftly and whose rates of natural increase have sky-rocketed, thus vitiating or slowing down whatever economic progress is underway. In one sense the explanation is simple: it is much easier to effect measures to reduce death than to reduce birth, and the former can be done much more quickly than ever before.[38] The changes which led to fertility reduction in the West did not

[38] One striking example should suffice: "In Ceylon, an effective island-wide malaria control program, based on DDT spraying, has apparently reduced the general mortality by one third within a few years" (M. Balfour, "Problems in Health Promotion in the Far East," in *Modernization Programs in Relation to Human Resources and Population Problems,* New York: Milbank Memorial Fund, 1950, p. 85).

cause a drop in birth rates overnight,[39] and we cannot anticipate such successful and extensive economic revolutions in underdeveloped areas as occurred in the West, where colonial expansion and virgin markets facilitated rapid economic progress.[40]

Our present study will deal with a society of rapid growth. Part of our task will be to give some indication of the extent to which the fertility-relevant aspects of the culture resemble those aspects which we have suggested may be typical for areas of potential growth, and the extent to which they resemble the patterns in areas of incipient decline.

CONCLUSION

The fertility rate is directly affected by the frequency of coitus and the degree to which birth controls are employed. These may be considered essentially in the biological and technological spheres, but their differential rates are to a large degree determined by social and psychological forces. Under the former we have discussed the influence of the prevailing sexual norms, family structure, knowledge and communication system, ideologies, and certain aspects of the social structure. Such factors vary in the degree to which their consequences for fertility are latent or manifest. What we will call the "fertility belief system," however, represents the sum total of *consciously* held beliefs and attitudes common to a group which have *explicit* reference to fertility behavior—for example, a belief that children bring good fortune.

"Character structure," like "fertility belief system," will be used as an omnibus term to denote those persistent psychological traits (anxieties, drives, motives, attitudes) common to the members of a culture or subculture which affect fertility in ways *not consciously intended* by the actor. For example, attitudes of resignation toward

[39] Europe required three centuries to bring its fertility and mortality into equilibrium, and ". . . there is no past transition that involved less than a century, and less than a threefold multiplication of population" (F. Notestein, "Summary of the Demographic Background of Problems of Underdeveloped Areas," *Milbank Memorial Fund Quarterly*, XXVI, No. 3, July, 1948, 251).

[40] This is not to say that an industrial revolution is a necessary antecedent to lower fertility. Any changes, such as increased education and opportunities for women, which make a large family seem burdensome might have the same effect; but such changes also usually require a good deal of time.

fate characteristic of some societies might not consciously deter individuals from planning conceptions but might in practice have that very effect. Or various anxieties characteristic of a group might lead it to emphasize or deemphasize sexual relations; certain types of dependency relationships could have consequences for age at marriage and for the frequency and kind of sexual relationship. Both character structure and the fertility belief system are interdependent, but the influence of the former on the latter is probably greater than vice-versa. Both, of course, are dependent upon the sexual norms, family structure, communications system, and ideologies prevalent in the society.

THE PLAN OF THIS BOOK

The present study is of an exploratory nature and represents only the first stage in a three-stage project on human fertility in Puerto Rico. Subsequent stages will aim at increasing specificity in an attempt to isolate the more crucial factors bearing on fertility performance. Moreover, subsequent studies will be directed at verification, whereas the present study is aimed at covering a fairly wide range of variables hypothetically bearing on fertility. Consequently, the present work is relatively broad in focus, although the chapters move toward increasing specificity with regard to fertility.

On the other hand, no attempt has been made systematically to cover all the aspects described above. Certain parts receive special emphasis and others (general ideologies and social structure) practically no attention at all. A decision was made at an early stage to emphasize sexual norms, character structure, the fertility belief system, and birth control practices, *as they are involved in and influenced by the family.*[41]

[41] The focusing of the project on the family has been made possible by the number of trail-blazing studies in demography, fertility, and general Puerto Rican culture which preceded our study. The most outstanding of these was Paul K. Hatt's attitude study of 13,000 Puerto Ricans, *Backgrounds of Human Fertility in Puerto Rico: A Sociological Survey* (Princeton: Princeton University Press, 1952). Moreover, four anthropological studies (soon to be published) have recently been conducted in rural areas under the general direction of Julian Steward of Columbia University. In addition to these works, L. J. Roberts' and R. L. Stefani's *Patterns of Living in Puerto Rican Families* (Rio Piedras: University of Puerto Rico, 1949), Emilio Cofresí's *Realidad pobla-*

Since the family was chosen as a major area for focus, the order of topics treated in this volume follows the life history of the family. The question of fertility itself will not be explicitly treated until the latter portion of the book, after a fairly comprehensive picture of the Puerto Rican lower-class family has been provided. A considerable amount of space is devoted to child rearing, since it was felt that this was crucial to an understanding of character structure. Courtship and marriage forms are also treated in some detail, since their bearing on coital and birth-control rates has been suggested to be of some importance. Since an understanding of marital relations would seem helpful in the analysis of the fertility belief system, this area has also been considered. Finally, the knowledge and communications system with respect to birth control, the fertility belief system, and the dynamics of birth-control behavior are examined. In a final chapter the various presumably strategic elements are synthesized into a hypothetical model of lower-class fertility determinants.

Since the task was seen as one of providing a background against which fertility beliefs and practices might be understood, factors specifically bearing on fertility are often pushed back through several antecedent stages. It is felt that what has been lost here in terms of direct relevance has been gained in terms of a more comprehensive understanding of that side of the family-fertility equation which has had least systematic attention.

While there has been an attempt to deal more exhaustively with those patterns which have the most direct significance for fertility, in no sense does the study aim at providing a definitive or all-encompassing study of the family in Puerto Rico. We hope, however, that we have given the reader enough of a picture so that structures relevant to fertility are seen in context.

DATA AND DATA COLLECTION

The raw material for this book comes from lengthy interviews with 72 husbands of the lower-income class and their wives: 24 from

cional de Puerto Rico (San Juan: Imprenta Venezuela, 1951), Charles Rogler's *Comerio—A Study of a Puerto Rican Town* (University of Kansas, 1940), and various articles on Puerto Rican fertility by Kingsley Davis and others have provided excellent background.

three rural areas, 24 from an urban area, and 24 from three small towns.[42] Because of budgetary limitations and technical considerations, the total area was restricted to northeastern Puerto Rico, a relatively industrialized sector of the island. However, every effort was made to insure that within this general area the rural areas would be among those least exposed to urban-industrial influence.

Once the rural and village areas were chosen, lists of all household heads living in houses valued at less than 250 dollars were drawn from the files of the Tax Assessment Bureau. This list was then further reduced to those homes with husband, wife, and at least one child, and in which husband and wife had been living together for a minimum of three and a maximum of twenty years. From this final list the appropriate number of names was chosen randomly. For the urban sample, a slum area was chosen, prelisted, and the same procedure for respondent selection was followed.

Tables 1 and 2 below describe the characteristics of the sample in greater detail. Interviewing was begun in December, 1951, and completed in March, 1952. Wherever available, comparable data from Hatt's study, conducted in 1947-48, are given.

Several general points may be indicated. Education is very low, averaging three years for women and four for males. Age at first union is low for women. Fertility is high, judging from the fact that women have averaged four pregnancies before reaching their thirtieth birthday. Roughly speaking, there are some signs of differential fertility by residence, for the country group has had the largest median number of pregnancies, despite oldest median age at marriage.

Despite the fact that the sample was chosen to give equal representation to three residence areas, Table 2 shows that most of the respondents were born in the country, a strong minority in small towns, and very few in large towns or cities. About half of the couples are living together without legal sanction, and while a single union appears to be the rule, a large minority of the sample has had two or more unions while still relatively young. As might be ex-

[42] See Appendix A for a detailed description of interviewing methodology and procedures for analysis of the data.

TABLE 1

SAMPLE CHARACTERISTICS: RESIDENCE BY MEDIAN AGE, AGE AT FIRST UNION, YEARS OF EDUCATION, AND NUMBER OF PREGNANCIES

	AGE		AGE AT FIRST UNION		YEARS OF EDUCATION		PREGNANCIES	NUMBER OF RESPONDENTS	
	Males	*Females*	*Males*	*Females*	*Males*	*Females*		*Males*	*Females*
Country	36.5	28.0	23.5	17.5	4.0	3.0	5.5	(24)	(24)
Village	36.5	32.0	24.0	18.5	6.0	3.5	4.5	(23)	(24)
City	33.0	28.0	19.0	16.0	4.0	4.0	4.0	(24)	(24)
Total	34.5	29.5	22.0	17.0	4.0	3.0	4.0	(71)	(72)
Hatt[a]	—	—	23.8	19.1	4.7	4.2	—	(6,187)	(7,085)

[a] Paul K. Hatt, *Backgrounds of Human Fertility in Puerto Rico: A Sociological Survey* (Princeton: Princeton University Press, 1952), Tables 32 and 21, pp. 48 and 37.

TABLE 2

SAMPLE CHARACTERISTICS: PLACE OF BIRTH, MARITAL STATUS, NUMBER OF MARITAL UNIONS, AND RELIGION, BY SEX

	MALES		FEMALES	
	Sample (percent)	*Hatt*[a] *(percent)*	*Sample (percent)*	*Hatt*[a] *(percent)*
Place of birth				
Country	65	71	62	68
Village	27	5	25	6
Towns and cities	8	24	13	26
	100	100	100	100
Marital status				
Legal marriage	54	79	54	79
Consensual marriage	46	21	46	21
	100	100	100	100
Number of marital unions				
One	68	–	72	–
Two	21	–	22	–
Three or more	11	–	6	–
	100	–	100	–
Religion				
Catholic	77	81	72	83
Protestant	20	8	21	8
Other	3	6	4	7
None	–	5	3	2
	100	100	100	100
Number of respondents	(71)	(6,187)	(72)	(7,085)

[a] Paul K. Hatt, *Backgrounds of Human Fertility in Puerto Rico: A Sociological Survey* (Princeton: Princeton University Press, 1952), Tables 20, 31, and 22, pp. 36, 47, and 38.

pected, most of the respondents are Catholics, but a substantial minority are adherents of other faiths.

In comparison with Hatt's data it is clear that the small sample is more characteristic of the lower class than of the population as a whole. Less education, earlier age at marriage, and a higher proportion of consensual unions all point in this direction. As seen in Table 3, occupations, too, are strongly skewed in the lower-class direction.

TABLE 3

OCCUPATIONAL BREAKDOWN, MALES[a]

Unskilled laborers	36
Entrepreneurs and farmers[b]	12
Skilled and semiskilled	8
Service	7
Store clerks	3
Foremen	2
Unemployed or students	4
Number of respondents	(72)

[a] Only 7 women work outside the home. A few others take in laundry.
[b] The terminology of this category is deceptive. Seven of the eight "entrepreneurs" are peddlers, and the four farmers represented here own only small subsistence plots. The service individuals and foremen are also in a very low income category in the present sample.

Unskilled laborers compose just half of the sample and are over represented in terms of their distribution in the total population. Hatt's representative sample, for example, showed only 30 percent in the laboring group. The sample then, meets general criteria for the lower class.

A word should be said concerning the generalizations based on such a small sample. It is obvious that no pretentions can be made about the representativeness of the sample; consequently, the generalizations made in the report must be taken as suggestive and hypothetical rather than as scientifically established. That every generalization is not couched in the qualifying language it deserves is not due to an effort to appear categorical but to avoid the awkwardness and repetitiousness attendant upon scrupulous qualifications. For purposes of style and facility, the analysis of the 143 cases will be presented as if they reliably represented the lower-class population, with full awareness that this may or may not be the case.

THREE MAJOR BIASES

Three major biases in the sample should be pointed out:

1. The husbands and wives chosen have been living together for a median of nine years. This means that, on the whole, the study is dealing with relatively well-adjusted couples, at least to the extent that divorce or separation has not taken place.

2. The sample deals with members of the lower class who are probably more subject to urban influences than is true for the island as a whole. Despite the fact that many of the rural families are located in dwellings an hour or two from a highway, the sample as a whole is located in or near the northern coastal plain and is reasonably close to San Juan or Río Piedras.

3. While the sample is equally divided in terms of urban, rural, and village residence, most of the individuals in the sample were born and reared in the country. Although this is typical for Puerto Rico's lower class as a whole, the reader should be aware that the respondents might be expected to be more traditionally oriented than groups that have always resided in cities and towns. This factor may to some extent counterbalance the bias present in the geographical area selected for study.

II

Differential Status Ideologies of the Sexes

> Men have seven senses. Women are weaker because they have only five.
>
> A FEMALE RESPONDENT
>
> We men know what is good and what is bad.—Don't women know?—*We* do, but they don't.
>
> A MALE RESPONDENT

Every society uses sex as a means of status ascription. Along with differing sex statuses go ideologies concerning the general character and differential capacities of the sexes. Almost universally the woman is seen as inferior to the man, and a system of rationalization is typically constructed by the society to justify the belief and the accompanying dearth of privileges for the female. The beliefs and rationalizations of this type current in Puerto Rico also provide the ideological backdrops for the prevalent types of child-rearing practices, courtship, and marriage relations. These latter can better be understood if preceded by a description of the sex ideologies.

STABILITY AND STRENGTH OF THE MALE

An important part of the sex ideology holds that male and female thought processes are different. Table 4 classifies the responses to the question, "What are the most important differences between men and women in their way of thinking?"

Only one in seven feels that men and women think the same, and only one in ten that women think better than men. A good majority of the males feel that the thought processes of men are superior to

TABLE 4

DIFFERENTIAL THOUGHT PROCESSES OF MALES AND FEMALES

Distribution of responses to Q.23A,M,[a] and Q.43A,F[a]

	Males	*Females*
Women think better than men	4	3
Men think better than women	21	9
Men's interests lie outside the home	3	21
Both think the same	6	4
Number of respondents	34	37

[a] "Q.23A,M" refers to question 23A, Male Interview. "Q.43A,F" refers to the same question in the Female Interview. English translations of the Interview Forms can be found in Appendix D.

those of women.[1] Women, however, do not in general say that men think better than women. Rather, the majority describe the male thought processes in more neutral terms, perhaps suggesting that the man's thinking is so different that they cannot make an invidious comparison; or, on the other hand, that they do not subscribe to male superiority. If we rule out such neutral or ambiguous statements, most of the remainder tend toward the belief that male thinking is superior. This is probably not very different from most lower-class cultures,[2] but the reasons or rationalizations for the belief seem particularly well developed.

First, the man's thinking is seen as more stable, sober, and rational than the woman's. The man is seen as clear-thinking and

[1] Similar beliefs are current in our own culture, but not to the same degree. Cross-sectional opinion polls have indicated that men are believed to be more even-tempered than women and superior in creativeness, decisiveness, and interpersonal relations. However, a higher proportion believes men and women are equal in these characteristics, and differences of opinion between the sexes do not appear as marked. See H. Cantril, and M. Strunk, *Public Opinion 1935-1946* (Princeton: Princeton University Press, 1951), pp. 792-93.

[2] To take two examples from American, rural, lower-class studies: (a) "Such [child-rearing] patterns breed in boys feelings of their own superiority, and contempt for the work, interests and intelligence of girls and women. . . . Most girls subscribe with the boys to the superiority of being a boy" (J. West, *Plainville, USA,* New York: Columbia University Press, 1945, p. 176). (b) "There is theoretical acceptance of the rightness of male dominance by both sexes. This has as a corollary belief in innate sexual differences in ability, which prescribe divinely decreed different realms of participation" (M. J. Hagood, *Mothers of the South,* Chapel Hill, University of North Carolina Press, 1939, p. 163).

steady, the woman as scatter-brained and flighty. Asked for the differences in the thinking and behavior of men and women, both sexes reflected the belief in the weakness and inconstancy of female thought.

Men have better thoughts. They are more constant and responsible. Women's thoughts are variable; they think one thing today and another thing tomorrow. (C7F)[3]

Women are weaker because they have two senses less for thinking. Men are more serene in what they say and have more responsible ideas. Women are more variable in their sentiment, feeling one thing now and suddenly changing their feelings. Men always tend to sustain firmly their own feelings through time. (TRA)

The idea that women's thinking is poor is buttressed by the folk belief that there is an organic basis for her inferiority—an interesting reversal of the American folk conception that women possess an extra or "sixth sense."

Men have seven senses while women have only five. I have heard that women are weaker because they have two senses less for thinking. (H24F)

It is, of course, strongly supported by a Spanish-Catholic tradition[4] which sees woman as inherently inferior to man.[5] Several respond-

[3] Quotations are followed by a respondent identification code. Except in cases of training interviews, the first letter represents the *barrio* of residence, the number represents the respondent number, and the second letter the sex of the respondent. Training interviews are designated by "TR" followed by an identification letter. Detailed characteristics of each respondent can be found in Appendix B.

[4] For a good summary analysis of the traditional Latin American family, see K. Davis, "Changing Modes of Marriage: Contemporary Family Types," in Becker and Hill, eds., *Marriage and the Family* (Boston: Heath, 1942), pp. 100-108. See also E. Willems, "Structure of the Brazilian Family," *Social Forces*, XXXI, No. 4 (May 1953), 339-45.

[5] An article in a monthly publication for Catholic University students in Puerto Rico had the following to say about female thought processes: "We shall concede that she does not see in the way a man does, but she foresees. She does not reason, she guesses. Her logic does not emanate from the brain, but from the heart" (*Verbo*, Vol. III, No. 2, Jan. 1952). Of course, not only Catholicism contains such creeds. Religion in general has embodied the myth of male superiority. "Religion generally appears to be a powerfully depressing influence on the position of woman, notwithstanding the appeal which it makes to woman. Westermark considers, indeed, that religion 'has probably been the most persistent cause of the wife's subjection to her husband's rule' " (Havelock Ellis, *Studies in the Psychology of Sex*, New York: Random House, 1942, II, 399).

ents quoted the Adam and Eve myth to support the belief in the inferiority of women.

Along with the idea of mental debility goes a conception of moral weakness. It is important to note that this does not have the connotation of moral perversity or inherent evil characteristic of medieval thought. It suggests, rather, that the combination of innocence, naivété, and a weak mind makes the female prone to "fall" morally. Conversely, the man is seen as shrewd as well as intelligent.

Any man can deceive a woman in love affairs because she is weak. *You cannot* fool the man. (B1M)

Anyone can convince a woman no matter how hard she is to convince. (TRB)

We men know what is good and what is bad. (Don't women know?) We do, but they don't. (H19M)

There is, finally, the belief that woman is weak sexually—that is, that her sex drives do not equal the potency of the male. Not only are the male sex drives stronger, but he is the true agent of procreation.[6] ("Los hombres los hacen y las mujeres los paren"—"The men make the children and the women bear them.") This point shall be discussed subsequently in more detail.

There are only two significant ways in which men see themselves "inferior" to women. One is in sentiment or feelings, the other in purity. The former refers to felt suffering, to demonstrations of emotion, and to emotional volatility. It is, of course, with condescension that this value is attributed to women, for such emotionality betrays an inability to meet problems rationally and firmly.

While men respect a pure woman, they do not greatly respect the same characteristic in themselves. When lauding the purity of women and decrying the rapacity of the male, it is easy to detect an underlying sense of pride in the male characteristics.

We men are more evil. If I have a chance I take it and have my little affairs outside. Don't you think a man needs to look for that once in a while? (H31M)

[6] In early Catholic teaching, the importance of the male role in procreation was heightened by attributing mystical qualities to semen. "Robert Briffault points out that the Christian fathers regarded the semen as constituting the actual substance of the Deity who used the male as his medium during the condition of sexual excitement" (H. Aptekar, *Infanticide, Abortion and Contraception in Savage Society,* New York, William Godwin, 1931, p. 104).

Women think about being housewives and we men think about running around. A woman thinks strictly about her husband. A man, even though he is a good husband, thinks about other women too. A man is never satisfied with just the wife he's got. (Y5M)

There are no bad women. We men are the bad ones. (B9M)

Women, of course, hold a similar conception of male rapacity. Only seven women and four men felt that man and woman are equally "good." The remainder saw men as highly sexed exploiters of the opposite sex. The belief is prevalent that, whereas there are some evil women, there is no truly good man.

Good women are pure. Man is never pure; he goes out with other women. . . . Man is perverse, mean in all senses. He just tries to have sexual joy from women, and then he may leave them. (B8F)

There is no real sense of rebellion against this state of affairs, however, for women see men as "built that way." Men are creatures who must have a great deal of sexual activity, and it is fairly well accepted that a wife is insufficient to satisfy his high sexual drives.

Men have more freedom than women. They need that because they can't be without having women. . . . Women can go without that. (B4F)

Nearly all men have had sexual relations before marriage. . . . I think that is correct, because men can't avoid that. (Why?) Well, they are that way. (Z4F)

While the women seem to take this situation somewhat philosophically, there is an underlying sense of martyrdom,[7] which is supplemented by the conception that the woman "feels more." "Every woman has her cross to bear" is the feeling of most women. The cross is frequently the extramarital relations of the male, which a wife is expected to bear sorrowfully, silently, and hopefully. Consequently, some women do not ask that their husbands be faithful

[7] Oscar Lewis found the same complex present among the wives in a Mexican village. "Husbands and Wives in a Mexican Village: A Study of Role Conflict," *American Anthropologist,* LI, No. 4 (Oct. 1949), 603. According to one writer, the Catholic Church in Latin America bolsters the conception of suffering for the lower class in general. "The Catholic Church has been adamant in its attitude of considering this world as a vale of tears, and that therefore people—especially poor people—must be patient and have hope in the hereafter" (A. Torres Rioseco, "The Family in Latin America," in Ruth Anshen, ed., *The Family: Its Function and Destiny,* New York: Harper, 1949, p. 129).

but that they spare them suffering by not informing them of their extramarital activities.

These ideologies concerning the differential virtues and capacities of the sexes have ramifications in many familial institutions of the lower class. They find their best expression in the patterns of belief and behavior which may be termed the complexes of *machismo* and virginity. After a brief description of the meaning of these patterns, we may proceed to investigate the manner in which they are transmitted to the younger generation and the effects which such transmission patterns have on general personality development.

MACHISMO AND VIRGINITY

Literally translated, *machismo* means "maleness." The expression "¡Qué macho!" is usually used in the same sense as the English expression "What a man!" and ordinarily bears the connotation of virility. Perhaps the best way of defining the term is to describe how the male respondents interpret it. Responses to the question, "Speak-

TABLE 5

EVIDENCES OF *Machismo*

Distribution of responses to Q.10A2,M[a]

	Percent
By conquering women sexually	16.8
By dominating women	8.4
By sexual potency	8.4
By begetting children	5.6
Through courage	11.2
Through honor and chivalry	14.0
Through honesty and reliability	18.2
By being a good neighbor	9.3
Through civic virtues (working hard, carrying out duties at work and at home, gaining community respect, etc.)	14.0
Through abusiveness (picking fights, boasting, gambling, drinking, etc.)	15.4
In other ways (charity work, acting like a male, etc.)	7.0
Number of respondents	(72)
Total responses	(92)

[a] Percentages are based on the number of respondents. Since most respondents cited more than one characteristic, percentages total more than 100.

ing of being a *macho completo,* how does a man show it? How does he prove it?" are classified in Table 5.

About four out of every ten respondents gave the term a sexual referent and about one out of ten cited courage. Of the remainder, no particular virtue stands out, but all are expressions of proper behavior in social relations. A not insignificant group interpret the term in an unfavorable light—as referring to a man who abuses women, brags about himself, and commits drunken acts of bravado.

The complex of virginity[8] also has both a specific sexual meaning and a broader significance. Specifically, it is the powerful tabu on premarital intercourse for women. This aspect will be given extensive consideration in the following chapter. More broadly interpreted, it is the system of beliefs which defines the woman as innocent and pure, and the system of practices which insures that she will so remain until marriage. One of its strongest ideological supports comes from the Catholic religion, which, as interpreted by the Spanish clergy[9] on the island, stresses not only premarital continence but every manifestation on the part of the woman which might occasion the male to sin.[10]

[8] The phrase, "virginity cult," was first used with reference to Puerto Rico by Morris Siegel to describe "a set of ideas and practices which dominates the relationships between the sexes and determines the role of males and females in pre-marital and post-marital life" ("*Lajas:* A Puerto Rican Town," unpublished manuscript, University of Puerto Rico, 1948, p. 148). In analyzing the Brazilian family, Willems has drawn the distinction between the complexes of virginity and virility, suggesting that the male and female roles are centered around clusters of values which can be so termed. Willems, *op cit.*, pp. 341-42.

[9] Puerto Ricans, and undoubtedly the clergy themselves, are highly cognizant of the differences between the American and the Spanish clergy on the island. The former are seen as more "liberal," "modern," "progressive," and "democratic," since they fraternize more with the people and do not require such rigorously puritanical behavior on the part of women. The latter often are seen as "old fashioned" and "fanatical" in their insistence on the relative isolation of the clergy from the people and in their denunciation of the "immodesty" and excessive freedom of contemporary women.

[10] A sample from the "Questions and Answers" section of a popular Catholic magazine published in Puerto Rico gives an indication of the prudery which often typifies the teaching of the Spanish priests (*La Milagrosa,* Oct. 25, 1950):

Q.: Is it right (*lícito*) to chat with boys on the beach, if dressed with a decent bathing suit? A.: No, *señora,* one should go swimming as God ordains, and not chatter with little clothing and less shame. Q.: Who can be considered a decent bather? A.: Only she who leaves uncovered only her hands, face and toes. Q.: And what is an indecent bather? A.: That I will not describe, for we are not living in a tribe of savage Africans.

The Virgin herself, of course, is an extremely popular figure of adulation. Young girls are urged to emulate the Virgin Mary, she is probably the most frequent recipient of prayer, and the language abounds with popular expressions such as "¡Ave María!" and "¡Virgen Santa!"

Before discussing the manner in which the younger generation is indoctrinated with the values of *machismo* and virginity, and the effects which such methods have on personality, a brief and more general description of lower-class child-rearing patterns is indicated. This will facilitate an understanding of the methods more specific to the indoctrination of the complex of virginity and *machismo*.

III

Child-Rearing Practices

When my wife gives birth to a daughter, it is a great suffering for me. I know how wicked I have been with women, and I fear she will go through the same thing. . . . They must be protected always.

A MALE RESPONDENT

All boys are born bandits. . . . It doesn't matter if they are dirty. The *macho es macho*. They have nothing to lose.

A MALE RESPONDENT

PARENTAL ROLES IN SOCIALIZATION

The lower-class Puerto Rican household in most respects fits the traditional picture of the patriarchal household. The father, whose authority is unquestioned on all matters, rules the household in the manner of the all-powerful patriarch. Seriousness (*un hombre serio*) and sobriety constitute the ideal demeanor for the father, and his greatest duty to his children is to teach them to respect primarily their father and secondarily their mother. That he should "love" his children in the sense of the American parent, and that they should love him, is of much less importance than that they respect and obey him and that he provide for their physical needs. Developmental concepts[1] of childhood and parenthood are rudimentary or absent. The tabulations below giving the distribution of responses to the questions, "What is the ideal son? What are some examples of what a good son does?" show clearly that the ideal role is one of obedience and a high degree of traditional propriety (Table 6).

[1] See E. M. Duval, "Conceptions of Parenthood," *American Journal of Sociology*, LII (Nov. 1946), 193-204.

TABLE 6

DEFINITION OF THE IDEAL SON

Distribution of responses to Q.24,F and Q.20,M

	Females (percent)	*Males (percent)*
Respectful and obedient	32.6	27.5
Has good habits (is clean, neat, does not swear or gamble, etc.)	26.3	18.7
Has good manners	10.0	10.6
Helps parents	4.7	18.1
Has good sentiments (amiable, kindly)	7.4	12.5
Studious	6.3	4.4
Loves parents	2.1	0.0
Other (unspoiled, understanding, industrious, religious)	10.5	8.1
	99.9	99.9
Total responses	(190)	(160)

Note that only 2 percent of the female responses and none of the male concern loving one's parents as a characteristic of the ideal son. The rest of the responses are nearly all along traditional family lines, the largest category being obedience and respect,[2] with good habits the second most frequently mentioned characteristic. It is interesting that the conceptions of the mothers and fathers parallel each other so closely, indicating cultural concensus on the important qualities in a child. Perhaps the most interesting sex difference appears in the "helps parents" category. The fathers are considerably more concerned over the economic help which they hope to receive from their children.

[2] "Respect" as it is used in common parlance by lower-class Puerto Ricans bears a different connotation from common American usage. It indicates honor and *fear* rather than esteem. Whereas the American middle-class parent tries to have his children "like him," the Puerto Rican lower-class parent is concerned that his children honor and obey him. The whole emphasis here is on transmitting to the child the sense of the vastly different statuses of childhood and parenthood. In more liberal urban families in the United States the accent is on deemphasizing the differential statuses. Thus respect is emphasized as the ideal relation in the Puerto Rican family, esteem in the urban American family.

The role concepts of the ideal mother and father, while showing slightly more developmental traits, largely echo the traditional conceptions of the ideal child (Table 7).

TABLE 7

DEFINITIONS OF THE GOOD MOTHER AND FATHER

Distribution of responses to Q.31,F, and Q.27,F (asked of Mothers)

	Ideal Mother (percent)	*Ideal Father (percent)*
Takes care of children	32.9	20.0
Provides for children	12.3	30.8
Teaches and disciplines children	14.7	17.6
Is gentle, kind, or good	10.0	15.0
Helps children	5.8	4.9
Defends and doesn't abandon children	13.5	6.8
Loves children	6.3	2.9
Other (teaches good example, is responsible, careful)	4.1	1.4
	99.6	99.4
Total responses	(170)	(204)

The chief task of the ideal father is to provide the material necessities for his children—food, clothing, medicine, and schooling. The chief task of the ideal mother is to care for her children in the home. To love children is of minor importance, but occurs ideally with the mother rather than the father. The latter, however, is expected to be kind to his children and not to beat them excessively. A mother must protect her children from danger, defend them against the outer world, and, above all, never abandon them.

The latter is an interesting concept. It is a primitive kind of "mother-and-cubs" feeling of devotion toward one's children and is expressed in heroic terms.[3]

[3] The necessity for expressing such an ideal may be due to more than "primitivism." It may be an expression of the society's fear of an excessive number of mother-child separations. The brittleness of consensual unions and the new tendencies for daughters to migrate alone to the cities both encourage the abandonment or giving away of children to relatives or friends.

A mother sacrifices up to the death for her children. She even prefers to die in a shipwreck so as to save her son. . . . A mother dies for a son if she has to. She sacrifices everything, she even goes begging for the sake of a son. (Z3F)

She would never abandon them, never, for anything in the world. Wherever I go, I would take them with me, and I would always be with them. (H1F)

With such ideal-typical roles in mind, we can better examine the techniques of child rearing. The first and most obvious factor is the dominant role of the mother in child rearing. Men consider this to be a woman's job, and to participate in many of the routine duties of child rearing would be a clear sign that one is *sentado en el baúl* ("Seated in the trunk"—that is, under the domination of the wife). Moreover, the father is physically absent from the home much of the time. Hours are long in the fields, and patterns of recreation are usually separate. Even when the father is at home, his primary contact with his children would seem to be for his own amusement rather than for their benefit.[4]

Also of importance in keeping the father from much direct contact with his children is the status difference. Both age and position as head of the family put the father almost beyond social reaching distance of his children. This is essential to the lower-class family in order to maintain the *respeto* which is a strategic value in the home. The father is seen as the lawmaker and is feared and respected as such. The mother is the executrix of the commands, and since this involves close contact with her children (plus the fact that the woman is supposed to be sentimental and kind), she cannot hold their *respeto* in the same way as the father. Mothers recognize their "weakness" in this respect.

. . . they have more respect for their father than for me. I am easily convinced. (B8F)

[4] See Landy's interesting conclusion that children tend to be treated as dolls or toys for the amusement of parents rather than as personalities in their own right. This is partly based on the assumption that a child does not really become a self-responsible personality until he achieves *capacidad,* occurring somewhere around the twelfth year. D. Landy, "Childrearing Patterns in a Puerto Rican Lower Class Community" (unpublished manuscript, University of Puerto Rico, 1952). This research report, based on observational methods and on interview forms developed under the direction of Sears and Whiting at Harvard, provides a wealth of detail on child rearing among the lower class.

It is his job to make them respectful. (H17F)

They obey their fathers better. . . . Fathers are stronger in character, and they don't care to disobey. (B6M)

In general, beating is an approved method of obtaining the respect of children. In some cases children are even beaten *de vez en cuando para que respeten* ("once in a while so that they will be respectful"). The remarks of the respondent below express the general belief in the efficacy of corporal punishment:

If he spanks the children, I do not interfere. If I spank them, he doesn't interfere either, *so that we don't lose our moral strength with them.* If he beats them, I don't ask why and he doesn't ask me either. (X2F)

Respondents in the present sample were beaten more frequently by their fathers than by their mothers. Landy, who dealt with current practices of a small sample, found that mothers administered corporal punishment more frequently. However, the child, who is frequently warned by his mother about punishment by the father, sees the latter as more severe and awesome, if only because it is less frequent and reserved for "special occasions."[5]

The father is also the key figure in major decisions concerning the children. On a question of any importance, the father must be consulted, not because the mother is incapable of making such decisions, but because for her to do so would be to impinge upon the status of the lawmaker. That his rights and privileges are seldom usurped is shown by the responses to the question, "When the children want to do something, whom do they ask for permission?" (Q.21B,F) Only 10, or 17 percent, of the mothers who answered this question replied that their children came directly to them. Thirty-five percent said that they asked both parents (usually ambiguously phrased and improperly probed), 29 percent said father if present, 7 percent said father for important matters, and 12 percent said the children ask the mother to ask the father. Thus, though a mother may intercede for the child, handle insignificant

[5] A similar pattern has been noted in the rural South, where ". . . the mother whips most, but . . . the children mind their father best" (M. J. Hagood, *Mothers of the South,* Chapel Hill, University of North Carolina Press, 1939, p. 141).

discussions, and serve as temporary decision maker, by and large she does not take decision making into her own hands. As one woman who always consults her husband before granting permission to her children put it, "In case something happens he can't blame me for not consulting him." Women do not want the freedom which would render them responsible for decisions that might be wrong.

We may now consider the more specific child-rearing practices which serve to inculcate the patterns of virility and virginity.

THE TRANSMISSION OF MALE VALUES—THE COMPLEX OF *MACHISMO*

Given the general lower-class value of *machismo*, what are the mechanics of socialization which insure that the *machito* (the little male) will become the *macho*?

The most striking manifestation of attempts to inculcate *machismo* occurs in the adult adulation of the infantile penis. By praising and calling a great deal of attention to the penis, the parent can communicate to the child the literal or symbolic value of the male organ. The following quotations from ethnographic reports show how, by praise and physical manipulation of the male genitals, the adult begins to build up a conception of *machismo* in the very young child.[6]

> A two-year-old boy will be asked, "What is that for?" while an adult pulls at his penis; and sometimes the child will answer, "For women." Such a child is called *malo* (bad) or even *malcria'o* (badly brought up), but actually the terms are used with some measure of approval.[7]

> Parents and their friends may play with the genitals of baby boys until the child is about seven years old. The size of the boys' genitals is talked about as an index of his potential masculinity.[8]

> It was very common to see mothers playing with the genitals of their little boys, kissing them and also making believe they were going to

[6] Since observational techniques were not part of the present project, the reports of other observers must be relied upon here.

[7] S. Mintz, "Cañamelar: The Contemporary Culture of a Rural Puerto Rican Proletariat" (unpublished Ph.D. dissertation, Columbia University, 1951), Chap. VI, p. 42. Mintz also notes the custom of fondling the genitals of infant children as a pacifying technique.

[8] E. Padilla, "Nocora: An Agrarian Reform Sugar Community in Puerto Rico" (unpublished Ph.D. dissertation, Columbia University, 1951), Chap. VIII, p. 3.

eat them up. As soon as they started to talk, they asked them questions about their penis, for whom it was and for what it was needed. They answered it was for the *chacha* or the girl friend, or to play a trick on the girl friend. . . . If they had an erection, they were praised and the parents would celebrate it by telling them they had joined the masculine race.[9]

A father will uncover a newly born male baby to show the sex organs to visitors, showing great pride while doing so. The larger the organs, the more *machote* the baby will be considered, and the prouder the father will be. (From an interviewer meeting)

Moreover, little boys are discouraged from playing with girls and are scornfully called *mujercitas* (little women) if they do so. A not infrequent punishment meted out to male children of the rural lower class is to dress them as little girls.[10]

Another direct means of inculcating *machismo* is to praise all those activities in the child which are typically male. Thus verbalizations and activities which are harmlessly aggressive or sexually tinted will be permitted and even praised. Mintz felt that the male child's temper tantrums were not only indulged, but encouraged.[11] Parents may also amuse themselves by teaching their male children obscene words.[12]

From the time they are six years old they start learning. Sometimes

[9] A. A. Casanova, "Estudio general de diez núcleos familiares del barrio 'Chicamba' de Ponce" (unpublished term paper, University of Puerto Rico School of Social Work, 1951).

[10] In a case study of forty-five lower-class problem children, it was found that in six families dressing like girls was a frequent form of punishment. A. Cruz Apellaniz, "Estudio de los problemas de conducta evidenciados en niños procedentes de hogares donde faltan los padres" (unpublished thesis, University of Puerto Rico School of Social Work, 1935). It is interesting that the expression *con la batona puesta* (with his nightgown on) is an expression used to poke fun at adult males who seem under the domination of their wives, a condition which indicates the husband is lacking in *machismo*.

[11] "From the age of perhaps two to five, boy's tantrums are not usually suppressed. A child may scream loudly at what he regards as some infringement on his dignity or freedom of action, and adults will laugh off the performance. . . . Boy children are admittedly teased and provoked into shows of anger, partly to establish this response as a part of their 'maleness.'" (Mintz, *op. cit.*, Chap. VI, p. 44).

[12] Landy feels that such use of profanity around children is rare. The conception of the child as a toy, however, would seem to release inhibitions about profanity when such would serve the amusement of the parent. The following illustration shows this clearly: "The one I love most is a seven-year-old who is like me. If I say to her, 'You are a bastard,' she answers, 'You are a bigger bastard yourself,' and I have a good time with her." (C10M)

the grown-up people ask them to repeat [dirty] words and the little boys amuse themselves because they do not know what they are saying. That is the start. The family itself goes on teaching them. (C10M)

Less crude but phallic-oriented articulations of the male offspring are usually met with pride by the parents. The following is from an interviewer's notes:

The boy is only three years old but seems very bright and talks clearly. When the interviewer commented to the mother on how well he speaks, the boy remarked, "Como un macho" (like a man). . . . Later he tells his father that he would be willing to marry the interviewer. This is reported with amusement and pride by the father.

There are other factors in the socialization process which, while they are not directly phallic, build up in the male child a sense of superiority toward the opposite sex. The first of these, to be discussed later, is the general cultural assumption that males are "better" than females. The male child learns by the treatment which is given him that the *machito* is self-reliant and tough and has many special privileges. In contrast, he sees his sister surrounded by a number of restrictions indicating that she is dependent, weak, and inferior.

The prevalent sibling relationships in the lower class are such that the girls defer to and wait on their brothers. As soon as they can, they will be preparing the boys' meals, washing their clothes, and obeying their commands. Moreover, the male must quickly pick up the realization that he is the guardian of his sister, since he is a repository of strength and stability. Parents who stated they wanted an equal sex distribution in their family, for example, gave as their second most frequent reason (the first being that this provided a good division of labor) the fact that the female children could each have a male as protector. With the ever-present fear of male rapacity, mothers and fathers are greatly concerned that their daughters be under constant surveillance.

Furthermore, the boy comes to realize that he may be called upon to act as father surrogate, at least in *loco parentis*. With a low average life expectancy (until recently), and with high rates of desertion, fatherless homes are not infrequent. In the absence of a father the *respeto* system would be threatened. Consequently, the male child must be trained to be ready to substitute, for the male sex is the true source of respect.

Every time we were going to have a child I wanted a boy because it is supposed that in a home there should be a son. If the father is missing, the son takes his place. (H4M)

. . . in case the father dies, the males could watch the females. (Why is that?) Because the man imposes respect everywhere. The girls would not be respected the same if they had no brothers. (H2M)

THE TRANSMISSION OF FEMININE VALUES—THE COMPLEX OF VIRGINITY

Since the boy is a "born bandit" and can "defend himself," there is no need to take care in dressing him.[13] No such permissiveness applies to the girl. Seven out of every ten mothers felt that the boy could be left without clothes for a few years, but no mother felt this way about the girl infant. One would suspect here a cultural push toward the development of penis envy, for the girl cannot help but notice that she must always be covered, while the boy may expose his genitals.[14] Mothers themselves admit that they consider the

[13] Boys are left completely nude or dressed only in a short shirt for several years in most lower-class families. Even on the streets of San Juan, boys up to the age of six or seven are occasionally seen nude.

[14] To the neo-Freudians, penis envy has come to have a much broader meaning than originally defined by Freud. Penis envy becomes a general envious attitude toward males who enjoy a higher status than women, the penis being only a dramatic symbol of the broader privileges enjoyed by men. See F. Fromm-Reichmann, "Notes on the Mother Role in the Family Group," *Bulletin of the Menninger Clinic, IV* (Sept. 1940), 132–48; C. Thompson, "Penis Envy in Women," *Psychiatry,* VI (May 1943), 123–25. In Puerto Rico, where more privileges are attendant on male status than in the continental United States, and where little girls have a greater opportunity to see both the penis and its value to parents, a higher degree of penis envy would logically follow *if* women were not content with their present status. While this is probably not the case for lower-class women, at least one small piece of research with 163 students has indicated considerable envy on the part of university women for male status. Asked what form of life they would choose if reborn, over nine out of every ten males chose to remain males, whereas only a third of the females chose to be reborn females. (In response to a similar question, two thirds of a national cross section of American women preferred to be reborn females. See Cantril and Strunk, *Public Opinion 1935–1946* [Princeton: Princeton University Press, 1951], p. 793.) Forty-six percent of the females would prefer to be males, and the remainder chose birds, flowers, and inanimate objects. The reasons given are revealing of the frustration over female status: "Birds are free"; "Birds can go anywhere without asking permission"; "A painting would be admired by everyone"; "The value of a painting would be appreciated"; "Water is needed by everyone"; "A building does not feel or suffer." E. Sánchez Hidalgo, "El sentimiento de inferioridad en la mujer puertorriqueña," *Revista de la Asociación de Maestros,* XI, No. 6 (Dec. 1952), 70–71.

female organs ugly and the male organs pretty. Thus, even female orientation is phallic.

I think the boys are pretty when naked, but the girls—it's something I can't look at. (H24F)

The boy is prettier. Everybody says, "Oh how ugly that naked girl looks." (H12F)

. . . the girls look very ugly when they are naked. Not the boys, because "that" is beautiful. But the girls—oh, they look ugly. (A11F)

Many such remarks were volunteered spontaneously in answer to the question as to why girls had to be dressed so much earlier than boys. In answer to a more leading probe,[15] six out of every ten women agreed with the statement that male children are prettier without clothes than are girls.[16] *No* woman felt the female genitals to be prettier than those of the male. Additionally, some mothers held the female genitals to be physically inferior and more susceptible to disease.

Thus the woman has become so phallic-oriented that even her own genitals seem ugly and inferior to those of the male. Needless to say, the male echoed the sentiments of their wives, and frequently added a touch of *machismo* pride. "Nothing looks ugly in boys," claimed one respondent, and another echoed Clement of Alexandria ("Every woman ought to be filled with shame at the thought that she is a woman") when he remarked, "The sexual parts look ugly in women. I find them awful. To be a woman is enough!" (H6M)

THE CLOISTER PATTERN

The freedom of general mobility which is customarily accorded the male child is denied the female. Not only must she be better groomed and dressed, but she should not stray from the *batey* (yard). This is the classic Spanish pattern[17] of the cloistered female,

[15] Q.23A1,F: "Some people say they do not clothe little boys because they are prettier than little girls. What do you think of that?"

[16] The remaining women felt both sexes were equally *ugly* without clothes.

[17] The classic pattern finds its expression in the adage, "La mujer honrada, las piernas quebradas, y en su casa" (the honorable woman has no need of legs, for she remains always at home). Cited in José Rosario, *The Development of the Puerto Rican Jíbaro and His Present Attitude toward Society* (San Juan, 1935), p. 67.

and it has permeated the lower classes to an extent that is surprising.[18] Boys are born for the streets (*de la calle*), but the woman's place is in the home.

Daughters should be kept at home without being permitted to go out like the boys; the boys can run around and go to town as long as they want to, even late at night. (A10M)

We were reared as I was telling you. The girls were not permitted to go out in the streets and stay out late, but the males were permitted to stay late and mama didn't punish them. They even went out and didn't ask permission. (A11F)

From the age of six or seven on, girls are strongly discouraged from playing with members of the opposite sex.[19] The rationale here is that they would be corrupted by the male child, who is born with evil instincts.

You have to keep the girls inside the house, forbid them to mix with the boys, so that they do not learn bad things and can be reared honestly. (A11F)

I am bringing them up as I was brought up, in the house and once in a while outside with other girls, because I don't want them to play with boys. . . . I am bringing them up in the home, the school, and the church. (H4F)

Of course, with an increasing number of children being enrolled in the schools, it is becoming increasingly difficult for parents to maintain this ideal. That it is still an operating ideal, however, is demonstrated by the replies of mothers to the question, "Are you rearing or do you plan to rear your children differently from the way in which you were brought up? In what way?" (Q.22,F) Only ten mothers of the sixty-nine who answered the question said that they were rearing or intended to rear their children less strictly than they had been brought up. The remainder stated that they would rear them in the same way. Two mothers stated that they planned to rear them even more strictly than their parents. Social change may in some ways thwart their plans, and many mothers complained of the increasing difficulty of keeping their girls in the

[18] For possible qualifications to this generalization, see Chap. IV, p. 83.

[19] See K. Wolf, "Growing up and Its Price in Three Puerto Rican Subcultures," *Psychiatry*, XV, No. 4 (Nov. 1952), 410, 420–21.

house,[20] but the fact that the ideal is still plainly in the traditional direction indicates that efforts will be bent toward that end.

As might be expected, the cloister pattern helps to insure that female children will be ignorant of sexual matters. Most of the women in our sample planned to do little to enlighten their daughters. This point will be given more consideration in the chapter on marital relations.

Rationale of the Cloister Pattern. There are three major reasons seen by parents for the special care and cloistering of the female child. The first is the logical consequence of the assumptions concerning female innocence and weakness. Since she is this way, she requires special protective measures. The second is the consequence of the virginity ideology. Since a woman must be delivered pure to the marital bed, every precaution must be taken to prevent her from being exposed to actions and information which might dispose her toward the loss of virginity. Finally, there are fears of incest and a general distrust of male intentions stemming from the assumptions that all males are rapacious. This leads to protective measures for the female child as well as to the inculcation of behavioral and attitudinal patterns which preclude giving males "occasion to sin." This latter point requires further exposition.

If it is true that "siempre la malicia vive en los hombres" (Evil is always present in men), then there is danger for the female infant just as there is for the grown girl. Not only is it assumed that young boys are dangerous for their young sisters, but grown men are also suspect. This is one of the principal reasons given for why young girls are dressed from birth or at a very early age.

There is much evil in men. When they see naked females, although they be small girls, their bad instinct is awakened, and there is the danger that they would dishonor them. (H1F)

We men like to see the flesh of the women, and though it be a girl, there is always the woman in her. (B5M)

Sure there is danger. Don't you know that if a man is visiting your house and you see your daughter sitting in a bad position, what do you have to do? Tell her to get up. (Why?) Because the man's instincts might be excited. (A13F)

[20] For example: "I am crazy about living in a place where there are no neighbors, where I can have my girls alone and shut up in the house."

The conception that men are evil also pertains to members of one's family. Among the lower class, incest fears are conscious, the tabus externalized and articulated, and practical measures are taken with the female child to insure their observance.

Even of their fathers women bear sons. No, no one can be trusted. . . . When I read of a case I say, "*Ay, Virgen Santísima!* I have to take care of my children!" (C10F)

Things have always been the same. Mother taught us to sleep in slip, sleeping gown, and panties. If she found us without panties she beat us. (Why was that?) As we all slept together, and you don't know the way you sleep, the father or some other person might wake up at night and see us showing our organs. (X7F)

The fears are not restricted to fathers but refer as well to brothers and members of the extended family.

We can't be careless even in the same house. (Why do you think so?) Men are half treacherous, deceitful, and one can't trust them. Who is going to trust a man? Nearby one niece gave birth to a child of her own uncle. . . . Men can't be trusted. Those are the things of life. (C10F)

There are so many malicious men one can't have confidence in them, not even in his own brothers. . . . The girls cannot be left naked. (C6F)

Today boys are born knowing . . . they may do these things with their sisters. (Y2F)

The whole situation in reference to the female child resembles a vicious circle. The dominant ideologies concerning her innocence and weakness lead to special care and cloistering; yet this very cloistering insures that the child will develop these same qualities.

EMOTIONAL CONSTELLATIONS

The fact that boys and girls are exposed to very different socialization contents has certain ramifications on their adult "character structure" intended by the socializers. Another important factor in childhood which influences personality development is the kind and intensity of emotional relationships typically maintained between the two parents and their male and female children. These relationships are to a large extent governed by family structure and by certain assumptions about the sexes, but their effects are probably neither intended nor realized by the family participants.

PREFERENCE FOR SEX OF OFFSPRING

To what degree are the two sexes *wanted* by mothers and fathers? In patriarchal cultures we would expect that males would be the more desirable offspring for both sexes. In the mildly patriarchal United States, a nation-wide cross-sectional poll of parents disclosed that there is a strong tendency (30 percent) for parents to maintain that sex of offspring makes no difference; but that for those who do

TABLE 8

PREFERENCE FOR SEX OF OFFSPRING

Opinions of Puerto Rican fathers and continental American fathers

Question 1: What kind of family would you like to have, one with more girls than boys, more boys than girls, or an equal number of each? (Q.19,M)

Question 2: When your wife is going to have a child, what do you hope for, a boy or a girl? (Q.19A,M)

Question 3: If you had another child, would you rather have a boy or a girl?

	PUERTO RICO		UNITED STATES[a]
	Question 1 (percent)	*Question 2 (percent)*	*Question 3 (percent)*
Boys	51	80	49
Girls	9	5	21
An equal number	40	—	—
Indifferent	—	15	30
	100	100	100
Number of respondents	65	63	—

[a] "The Quarter's Polls," *Public Opinion Quarterly*, XI, No. 4 (Winter, 1947), 641.

express a choice, boys are more frequently chosen than girls by parents of both sexes.[21] At least as judged by our small sample, the situation is somewhat different in Puerto Rico. In the first place, boys are more frequently the favorites of fathers than would appear true for the United States. The responses to three similar questions

[21] "The Quarter's Polls," *Public Opinion Quarterly*, II, No. 4 (Winter, 1947), 641.

show the relative preference for males present among our sample fathers.

The first-column question, asked first, evoked a high proportion of "equal number" responses, perhaps reflecting in part a tendency of some fathers to rationalize their having an excess number of girls.[22] The second column item, a probe following the first column question, is more likely to circumvent rationalizations; it effected a heavy shift from the "equal number" category to a preference for boys. Men who produce females are teased and called *chancleteros* (makers of *chancletas*—cheap slippers, a revealing slang term for

TABLE 9

PREFERENCE FOR SEX OF OFFSPRING

Opinions of Puerto Rican mothers and continental American mothers

Question 1: What kind of family would you like to have, one with more girls than boys, more boys than girls, or an equal number of each? (Q.56,F)

Question 2: If you had another child, would you rather have a boy or girl?[a]

	PUERTO RICO	UNITED STATES[a]
	Question 1 (*percent*)	*Question 2* (*percent*)
Boys	18	37
Girls	34	34
An equal number	48	—
Indifferent	—	29
	100	100
Number of respondents	71	—

[a] "The Quarter's Polls," *Public Opinion Quarterly*, XI, No. 4 (Winter, 1947), 641.

little girls), and occasionally such a fate is seen as punishment.

When a baby girl is born the male friends will say, "That is to pay for your sins." (*Esa es pa' pagar las que hizo.*) (A11F)

As seen in Table 9, the situation is not so clear-cut with mothers.

[22] Since sex of children was not recorded, this hypothesis cannot be tested. Other studies, however, have found it valid. See J. E. Clare and C. V. Kiser, "Social and Psychological Factors Affecting Fertility: Preference for Children of Given Sex in Relation to Fertility," *Milbank Memorial Fund Quarterly*, XXIX (Oct. 1951), 440–92.

In contrast with American mothers, who have a slight preference for males, the mothers in our sample say either that it makes no difference or that they would prefer girls. Relatively few chose boys, though in a somewhat higher proportion than their husbands chose girls. The reasons for choice of either sex are similar. Some see boys as labor saving and others (a higher proportion) see girls as labor saving. Those who chose boys felt that since they are born clever (*listos*) and always capable of defending themselves (*defenderse*) against the world at large, they do not need the care and protection which must be lavished on the weak and naive daughter.[23] In practice, this means that boys can be left to roam where they will, dressed poorly or left naked for several years. Note, in the following quotations, how ease of rearing for the boys is realized in both the economic and labor saving senses.

It is much better to have boys because we don't have to care for them so much. (C4F)

Boys you can have any way. You must have the girls better dressed, and they are more expensive. My husband says boys are better, too, because they run fewer risks, they take care of themselves. You must take better care of the girls because they are weaker and anyone could take advantage of them and deceive them. (X3F)

The girl should be better dressed and combed. . . . The son doesn't matter. It doesn't matter that he is dirty. (Why is that?) Because the *macho* is *macho*. He has nothing to lose. The girls must be taken better care of. (A5M)

These mothers who prefer girls feel that girls are less trouble than boys. In the first place, they can help the mother with housework. Three out of every ten mothers who chose girls gave this reason. Six out of ten felt they were easier to rear because of their comparative tractability. Once the boy is socialized, almost by definition he causes disciplinary problems for his parents because to some extent he becomes aggressive and independent.[24] Once the girl is effectively socialized, she becomes humble and submissive.

[23] The same cross section of continental American parents cited above were also asked whether they thought it was easier to raise a boy or girl. Forty percent said boys, 22 percent girls, 35 percent no difference, and three percent gave no answer.

[24] On the one hand, parents want their boys to be *humilde* and *respetuoso*, but on the other, they want to insure the development of *machismo* and inde-

The girls always ask permission when they are going out. The boys ask permission when they are small, but as soon as they are fifteen years old, they judge themselves to be complete *machos,* as the saying goes. They meet with other children, and if the parents do not agree with them, they leave the house. (C10M)

Girls . . . are more obedient. The boy wears pants and immediately he thinks he is a man and goes out to the street. They are stronger. (H14F)

I would rather have more girls . . . they are more obedient. They go to bed earlier and one doesn't worry as with the male; for he goes out and doesn't come back until ten o'clock at night. (H19F)

In sum, it would seem that on the whole boys are preferred by fathers, and that, to a somewhat lesser degree, girls are preferred by mothers. But to know preferences is only a beginning. More crucial to character formation would be the extent of affection and attention which each sex receives from its parents.

DIFFERENTIAL ATTENTION AND AFFECTION

When men were asked whether the father is more important for the daughters or for the sons (Q.18A,M), half said for the daughters; the other half was divided equally between "sons" and "equally important for both." Again, since the daughter is weak and naive, she must be protected and given extra care. Note, in the following illustrations, the sense of jealous pride which the father feels in protecting his "mentally and physically weaker" daughters.

I must look after her so that she doesn't do anything wrong. . . . There is the danger that a man may fool her. I know plenty of that, and I don't want my daughters to fall through ignorance. That is why I am here, to look after them. (Y8M)

Believing her weak, the man always tends to be more careful and is more jealous of his daughters than of his sons. (TRB)

Since the father always believes that the girls are weaker, he has to keep better watch over them because they are physically and mentally weaker. (B9M)

pendence. As one woman put it, "Parents spoil females more. They don't do it much with males because they want them to be more male, more independent." Independent behavior is also the by-product of greater freedom for males, giving them access to peer-group influences. With its accent on sexual exploration and self-manifesting activities, the peer group may foster an aggressiveness and independence which conflict with the parental values of obedience and respect.

Mothers noted that their husbands kept the daughters dressed and were more liberal in buying them luxuries. As one woman put it:

If the girls go out to church, he looks after them. If they don't come, he goes for them. I also notice that if they need notebooks, pencils, etc., he gives them money to buy some much sooner than to the boys. (Z8F)

Since the father is training his male sons to be hard, he can vent little affection on them. Girls, however, are meant to be soft and need more tenderness. There are relatively few barriers to a father's showing affection for his daughter.

The daughter deserves more consideration. She is a woman, and women have to be treated with more affection. . . . With the son we have to be stricter, to teach him to respect his father. . . . We have to make the daughter obey, too, but I think she should be treated with more kindness. . . . (Y8M)

He was always caressing me, but he beat the boys a lot. (Z5F)

When [my father] came home in the afternoon he used to take my sister and start kissing her, while he used to scold my brother and beat him. (H21F)

Some men hold their own sex responsible for woman's unhappy lot and fear that their daughters are likely to be exploited just as they exploited other women. Thus it is occasionally with a sense of guilt that males feel their daughters deserve extra devotion.

I feel so sorry for women because they sometimes meet with a bully. (A13M)

When my wife gives birth to a daughter it is a great suffering for me. I know how wicked I have been with women, and I fear they will go through the same thing. (H20M)

When asked, "For whom did your father have more affection when you were a child?" (Q.26A,F) only 23 percent of the women said their fathers felt closer to the boys, with 10 percent feeling the same about both. The remaining 67 percent felt closer to the girls. This relatively strong leaning on the part of fathers toward their daughters might, especially in view of the Oedipus theory, be expected to be reciprocated on the part of the girls. This is not the case: 77 percent of the women said that as a child they felt more affection for their mothers than for their fathers, and only 8 percent said the contrary.[25]

There appear to be several reasons for this. First, as we have seen, the father spends little of his time in the home; so that, despite the fact that the majority of this time may be allocated to the daughters, it still is not enough to compete with the time spent by the mother. Several respondents gave such reasons as the following for not feeling so close to their fathers:

As the fathers are always out in their work and the mothers are the ones who are always with us, one feels more love for them than for the fathers. (Y3F)

There is also the barrier of sex between the father and daughter. While in a psychodynamic sense it provides for greater attraction, the strength of such incest tabus as have already been described keep the father from having too much intimacy with the daughter.

The mother can bathe them and the father can't. The mother is more important because she can see their bodies, the father can't bathe them. (X6F)

To a certain extent, too, the father's role as the authoritarian is in conflict with his own desires to be affectionate to his daughters. The ideal of the stern disciplinarian, the protector and mentor of the family, may conflict with the derived need for loving the daughter out of pity and remorse. As the following cases show, it is the former social expectation which succeeds in being transmitted, despite attempts at the latter. Thus, the girl children fear and respect their father but cannot love him as they do their mother.

My father wasn't very much at home and had a bad temper. One feared him more than loved him. Mother was just the opposite; she was kind. (Z9F)

I felt more intimacy with my mother and I loved her more. I feel greater respect for my father and I didn't even dare to speak to him.

[25] In a sample of 501 college women in the United States, only 25 percent said they loved their mothers more than their fathers. When asked for the amount of attachment between them and their parents, only 12 percent were classified as "low to father and high to mother." R. Winch, "Further Data and Observations on the Oedipus Hypothesis," *American Sociological Review*, Vol. XVI, No. 6 (Dec. 1951), Table 2, p. 788.

. . . To the mother one tells everything, but to the father one doesn't dare. (Z7F)

Finally, although it is true that girls are not beaten as hard as boys and probably not as frequently, the father is more usually *associated* with punishment in the eyes of the daughters. In the instances below, the fathers succeeded in gaining the respect of their daughters by means of physical punishment, but again lost their affection.

I felt closer to my mother. She didn't beat us so much as father did and treated us with more kindness. . . . Whenever I saw him coming I started running home and hid myself. I felt too much respect for him. *Even now, old as I am, I don't dare to look him in the face.* (H10F)

We were more attached to my mother because my father was always out. . . . There is a saying that fathers there are many, but mother there is only one. (What do you mean?) *Sometimes you go out and someone slaps you in the face and you call this person "father" because the father is the one who beats you.* (Y4F)

Again the beating may only be the more tangible or spectacular expression of a whole tone of relative severity on the part of the male parent.

Although my mother beat us, she was more kind. My father didn't beat us but he was very strict with us. My mother let us go out more often. If he didn't let us, she talked to him and he then gave his permission. We could do it through her. (Z7F)

Again we see the mother's role as the appeaser, as the "soft" influence in the family, as the intermediary between her children and her husband—the factors which make stronger affectional bonds likely between her and her daughter. Thus it would seem that girls receive more affection than boys from both parents, but since the mother can give even more affection than the father, she is the principal love object for her daughters.

With this much information we can make some tentative inferences concerning boys.[26] The illustrations above have suggested that they receive *even less* affection and attention from their fathers than do their sisters, even though they are preferred by the fathers. In-

[26] Males were asked fewer questions concerning relations with their parents.

deed, the relationship seems such as to produce respect at best. Mothers, who preferred male offspring much less than fathers, also seem to give them less affection. When asked whether their mothers felt more affection for the girls or boys, only a third of the women said "boys," whereas slightly over half said "girls." While more affectionately oriented to sons than their husbands, the majority of the women appear to favor the daughters.

Again, a major reason appears to be that the daughters are given more affection out of pity for their unhappy lot in life. Throughout the statements by mothers one can perceive a feeling of sadness and fatalism over the suffering that will surely be a major part of the daughter's adult life. Throughout the quotations can be seen the martyr complex which has been previously mentioned. The mothers identify themselves strongly with their daughters, for whose future lives they feel as much pity as for their own.[27]

I love the girls more, because I love them with pity. (Why with pity?) Because as I am a woman I think they may get married to a bad husband and may suffer . . . and because of the toil and hardships that await them in life. (Don't you worry about the male children?) No, because they can defend themselves better and have the opportunity of selecting their wives, while the girls cannot. (A3F)

My mother used to say that she gave us more consideration because we were women, and women have to suffer very much in life. She herself suffered very much with my father. Women have more suffering in childbirth and with the husband if he is not good to her. . . . Women have to suffer for everything—if she is pregnant, she is waiting for the pains of delivery; if she is not pregnant, she is expecting her menstruation, scared that she *is* pregnant, because of the extra work and pains of childbirth. . . . Women are always on the losing end. They get the rougher deal. Men have to work for a living, but they don't have the sufferings of women. (B8F)

(Why are the girls loved with pity?) Because we women are weaker. Sometimes we don't know how to defend ourselves. (X6F)

Thus, while males bring more prestige to the family and receive more spectacular attention, they would appear to be on the losing end as far as affection and day-to-day attention are concerned.

[27] The feeling is reciprocated in many instances. Many women said that they felt closer to their mothers because of the sufferings the latter underwent.

When we combine these data with the fact that men seem inordinately attached to their mothers in adulthood (see Chapter IV), we may speculate as to whether some sort of causal nexus exists.

CONCLUSIONS

From the foregoing brief sketch of status ideologies and child-rearing patterns, a few speculative conclusions will be drawn, and some possible implications of these for fertility indicated.

The complexes of *machismo* and virginity are rough expressions of cultural expectations for the two sexes. Males should be masterful, sexually aggressive, and free; females should be submissive, chaste, and confined to the home. Men are conceived of as strong and shrewd, women as weak and naive. Such ideologies are reflected in child-rearing practices which help to insure that the "character structure" of the adult fits cultural expectations for the sexes. The male child learns superiority over the female and a positive attitude toward his sexuality. Moreover, he is given freedom of mobility by means of which he can develop a sense of mastery over a relatively broad environment. The female learns that she is inferior to the male, her sexuality is discouraged, and her mobility is heavily restricted by the cloister pattern. Thus the assumptions concerning the native capacities of the sexes become confirmed—males become self-reliant, tough, positively oriented toward sex, and knowledgeable about the world. Females become submissive, weak, negatively or non-oriented toward sex, and relatively ignorant about the world.

Besides bolstering the double standard of sexual activity, such patterns could have other tangential implications for coital and birth-control rates. For example, if the situation holds in adulthood, the *male* will determine the frequency, mode, and occasion for coitus as well as whether birth control will be used. Furthermore, he might be expected to exercise more initiative and scope in sexual matters than the female.

The relative insulation of the sexes in childhood as well as their broadly differing social statuses might serve as barriers to communication or form the basis for anxious or suspicious attitudes between the sexes in adulthood. Such factors might affect the frequency of exposure to coitus and birth control.

Despite a greater cultural value on males, in the actual family situation females appear to get the greater share of attention and affection. Moreover, their social roles would seem easier to fulfill and less likely to bring them into conflict with their parents. They must merely be docile and submissive and need prove their femininity by relatively few objective achievements. Moreover, all female socialization is consistently in this direction and is carried out with a considerable degree of affection and tenderness. Males, however, have to be toughened and are expected to become self-reliant, dominant and virile. The methods used to insure these are harsher than in the case of girls, the expectations more difficult to achieve, and their very achievement may bring the child into conflict with his parents. Thus one might speculate that the female would feel emotionally secure and contented in the parental household and that the male might feel insecure and discontented.

In combination with these factors, the differential valuation of the sexes might produce in the male a blend of superiority feelings and basic anxieties over maintaining this superiority, a complex we would not expect to be present in the case of the female. Such emotional complexes, in combination with other factors, could affect the age at which the sexes leave home, their choice of mates, the manner in which they mate, and the role which sex plays in serving their needs.

Whether the hypothesized consequences of child-rearing patterns receive any support from our findings in regard to adult attitudes, and whether in turn these appear to affect fertility patterns, will be examined in the following chapters.

IV

Courtship

What would you teach your son?—I would talk with a prostitute and send the young fellow to her house so he can get it off his chest.

A MALE RESPONDENT

What would you teach your daughters?—Nothing. It should come as a surprise.

A FEMALE RESPONDENT

THE FEMALE AND COURTSHIP

In summarizing the anthropological literature on the sexual norms of preliterate peoples, Ford and Beach write that "the methods used to prevent premarital sexual activity during adolescence include segregation of the sexes, strict chaperonage of girls, and threats of severe disgrace or physical punishment."[1] Lower-class Puerto Ricans combine all these techniques to insure that their girls will remain chaste. In contrast with the stereotypes concerning the Latin attitude toward sex, the lower-class Puerto Rican family shows striking parallels with the puritanically oriented Viennese family of the 1890's described by Freud.[2]

The restrictions placed on the female in infancy and childhood are magnified in adolescence, for it is at this time that violation of the virginity prescription becomes most likely and most dangerous.

[1] *Patterns of Sexual Behavior* (New York: Harper, 1951), p. 182.

[2] As paraphrased by Clara Thompson: "Young women of good family grew up apparently in sexual ignorance; they were allowed no legitimate opportunity to gratify their sexual curiosity in theory or in fact. At puberty they entered a life of severe restrictions by which an artificial form of behavior was fostered. Further general education was discouraged, and, while on the one hand they were to show no interest in sex in any form, they at the same time must devote their lives to getting husbands" ("The Role of Women in this Culture," *Psychiatry*, IV [Feb. 1941], 6).

Since the complex of virginity was only briefly described in the previous chapter, more space will now be devoted to a description of its structure and function.

THE COMPLEX OF VIRGINITY IN COURTSHIP

All the women in the sample believed firmly that a girl should be a virgin prior to marriage. Several respondents openly voiced their astonishment that such a question should even be raised.

She has to be *señorita.* It's clear that she should be. How could she get married if she wasn't? Ay, *Virgen Santa*! (C10F)

The woman after losing her honor is not worth anything any more. No, no, it isn't the same then! (A8F)

When asked the question, "Do you believe the majority of the girls around here are virgins before marriage?" (Q.34A2,F) the country and village women practically all answered in the affirmative, and all but a few of these said that *all* the girls were virgins. In the city sample, however, a quarter of the respondents answered in the negative, and another quarter implied that most of the girls were not. This suggests that, while the tabu is still effective in the more rural and the small-town areas, city living makes its enforcement difficult. Nevertheless, the universality of the tabu and the measures taken to insure compliance suggest the importance of this complex. What are its underpinnings?

The most obvious is the traditional Catholic tabu on premarital relations and the general Catholic stress on the Virgin and on the virtues of virginity.[3] While many of the respondents cited religious ideology to rationalize their beliefs, others saw the loss of virginity

[3] Saint Jerome, for example, "tolerated marriage because it provided the world with virgins." G. May, *Social Control of Sex Expression* (London: George Allen and Unwin, 1930), p. 39. The position has not become completely outmoded. As phrased in a recent Catholic text on the family, ". . . the Church . . . has ever taught that the state of virginity which is consecrated to God is higher than the marriage state as such" (Mihanovich, Schepp, and Thomas, *Marriage and the Family,* Milwaukee, Bruce Publishing Co., 1952, p. 418). Addressing a group of demographers in 1949, the Reverend William Gibbons remarked that "perfect chastity, or virginity, Christian tradition teaches, is in itself preferable to marriage, when chosen for supernatural reasons" (W. Gibbons, "The Catholic Value System in Relation to Human Fertility," in G. Mair, ed., *Studies in Population, Proceedings of the Population Association of America,* Princeton, Princeton University Press, 1949, p. 111).

as a *personal affront* to the Virgin Mary, particularly if the girl then marries in church wearing the symbols of virginity—the white crown and veil.

She [the participant in an illicit affair] got married in the church with the veil and crown. People talked a lot about her, and they said she was deceiving the Virgin. (H19F)

If a girl gets married not being virgin and wears the veil and crown, they are deceiving the Virgin and the public. (Y4F)

There are various folk stories about the consequences to those who "deceive the Virgin." In one case, a woman soon contracted cancer and died. In another, during the wedding ceremony, the crown would not stay on the head of the girl. Religion, however, does not seem to be the only factor in insuring the maintenance of the system. Social pressures and social sanctions appear to play at least as great a part.

An important social sanction lies in the attitude of the male. Not only does losing one's virginity illicitly bring disgrace upon the girl and her family, but the nonvirgin jeopardizes her chances for marriage. It is the predominant feeling among women, and many men echo the feeling, that once a woman has lost her virtue no man will want her because he cannot trust her.

Men imagine that the woman who gave it to a man would also give it to another. They don't trust her. (X3F)

I believe that if a virgin makes it easy for a man to have sexual intercourse with her, I would be afraid to marry her, because I would think that if she does it so easily with me she could fall for someone else if she has the opportunity. (C2M)

We have here not only the assumption that the woman is weak, but the very important implicit assumption that once she slips she is lost forever.[4] There are no degrees of virginity, and no degrees of goodness. One respondent likened the woman to a door: "She is like a shut door before, but once somebody opens it, everybody

[4] Spanish movies often convey this theme. A girl, basically good, is sexually exploited (through her innocence) by a depraved male. She then adopts a life of prostitution. It is always clear that she hates this life and that the man rather than she is responsible for it, but once virginity is lost, she almost automatically becomes a "bad girl."

comes inside." In another quotation, a woman describes how the young males hover almost vulture like around the girls, waiting for one to lose her virginity.

> The truth is that after a lady loses her virginity, nobody is going to marry her and everybody wants to have a good time with her. Do you know what the boys around here say? "*We have new flesh!*" (What do they mean?) That as soon as a girl loses her virginity, and it is known, all the boys know that it is easy to get her. If she lives with the man for a while and then they separate, the boys can have her as one more with whom to spend a good time. My son is one of those who say it. He wants to have a good time with them. You know, he is a shrewd boy. He isn't going to marry them. (C10F)

Additionally, if a woman is known not to have been a virgin at marriage, the man may use this fact as a cudgel for exploitation after marriage.

> [After marriage] the man has the right to go against her, and if she tries to stand up to him, he can throw in her face the fact that she was not a virgin when he took her and that he doesn't owe her anything. (X10F)

> It is important that she be a virgin. In this way she has more rights from the man. (In what way?) She can claim from him all she needs because he owes her this. If she is not a virgin she can't claim anything from him. (C6F)

Moreover, there is a tendency to consider that a marriage is not *real* unless the girl is a virgin; that is, that all the rights and privileges usually attendant upon marriage need not be observed. As one woman put it when asked about religious marriage, "That is a thing for virgins." This point will be given more consideration in the chapter on consensual unions.

The penalties described above, of course, apply only when the woman is known not to be a virgin before marriage. The most rigorous and humiliating sanctions are applied when the woman deceives the man into thinking she is a virgin. This is the unpardonable sin, because it goes beyond immorality and offends the male's ego. It threatens the status of the man, since any woman who has done that has shown herself to be shrewder than he. Equally status-threatening is the very fact that she *dared* withhold such an important piece of information from him. Practically every man who was asked which was the more important, the lack of virginity or the deception, replied that the latter was by far the more important thing. Many men went so far as to say they would marry a nonvirgin so long as she made this fact known ahead of time. The following quotations show that the disgrace of the male in being deceived is equal or greater than the disgrace of the fallen girl, and that, whereas immorality may be tolerated, deception of the male may never be.

(Would you marry a girl whom you had outraged?) If she is a good girl I would marry willingly. (And if she is not?) If a court forced me I would marry her. (And if another had outraged her?) I would marry provided she shows me that she is a good wife; that she is honest, humble, and a good worker. (And if she deceived you?) *That could not be pardoned.* If she is not a virgin, she should let you know before marriage. (B6M)

(Would you marry a girl some other man has dishonored?) No, because I would expose myself to public criticism. I would not plug the hole someone else has made. (What is more important, the deceit or the fact that she is not virgin?) The deceit is more important. *The other is not too important.* (X3M)

The deception is more important because she is making me unhappy because all the public would pick me up on it. In cases like that the man degrades himself. The people make fun of him. (C6M)

Indeed, the males are so fearful that this might happen to them that one of the more frequent answers to, "What should a young man know about women before getting married?" (Q.26A,M) was the ability to tell a virgin from one who is not, in order "to prevent being deceived" or "made a fool of." A total of eighteen men gave this response to the question. The cultural valuation placed on virginity is so high that some prostitutes or *cobos* (literally, "snail"; that is, one who hides the fact that she is a loose woman)[5] apparently attempt to make believe that they have not been previ-

[5] Other Puerto Rican phrases indicate the anxiety about being deceived concerning virginity. "*Señorita tapada*" and "*Señorita Americana*" are expressions used to refer to a girl who tries to give the appearance of being a virgin but in reality is not. The latter phrase also indicates a prevailing opinion concerning continental American women.

ously penetrated. This knowledge (or perhaps phantasy)[6] makes men doubly careful to make sure that they can tell the virgin from the nonvirgin.

There are many wise ones who say they are señoritas. They put their legs together and the man could believe she is a virgin. They cry out as if in pain. But as I know of this, I never fall for those tricks of women. (C2M)

The classic sanction for a girl who has been "found out" on the wedding night is that she be returned to her parents on the following day.

At the time of marriage he would find out she is "broken" (*rota*). Then he will reject her and take her back to the house of her father and tell him that he has no obligations to his daughter since she was not a real señorita. . . . He goes back to his house ashamed. (TRA)

Occasionally mentioned were more severe sanctions—beatings and murder. Respondents cite these alleged murders without much reproof for the husband, for he has received one of the most serious types of insults.

If he knows she is not virgin and he accepts her that way, it is all right, but if he doesn't know, he may even kill her. A case I heard about had a boy friend and he disgraced her and she said nothing. Later she married a soldier and she refused to have contact with him for a week telling him she was sick. After a week she began to cry and told him what had happened to her, so he killed her. (What did you think of that?) *She did wrong. She should have told him before marrying.* (A10F)

Another somewhat lengthy illustration will be cited because of its richness of detail. It shows that while the acceptable way of handling such cases is to return the girl to her father, more extreme measures occur, even in the upper class.

There was a case in my home town. I know the case because I was working at her house. . . . She was a rich girl who had everything she wanted. She went to the States and met a man with whom she

[6] Three men mentioned such "tricks" by women as weeping and holding the legs together, but whether or not this came from the respondents' own experience cannot be ascertained. The fear and the defensive precautions sound almost paranoid, and may be another expression of the hostility and distrust which separates the sexes.

had some dealings and even lost her virginity. When she returned home she didn't tell anything to her boy friend.

At last they got married. It was a splendid wedding, with hundreds of guests. A car filled with guests took the couple to the hotel. After leaving them, the guests went to a nearby restaurant where they were having drinks. They hadn't been there for long when a person came to tell them that the new husband was beating his bride. Her brother ran to the hotel and had a fight with the brother-in-law. Then he took his sister to her god-mother's house, where she stayed for months until her father sent her to the States again.

The husband discredited her. Both families were angry with her but also criticized the way he behaved because they said that he could have returned her home, avoiding any kind of a scandal. (X2F)

Violent retributions are probably dying out, but they are still being pointed out to the female younger generation as examples of what happens to girls who stray from the proper path in life.

PREMARITAL TREATMENT OF SEX

If virginity is of such importance in lower-class Puerto Rican life, what measures are taken to protect it? The first is the withholding of information on sex and childbirth. As judged by their responses, few of the mothers in our present sample had a clear idea prior to marriage of the mechanics of sexual relations and childbirth.[7]

TABLE 10

PREMARITAL KNOWLEDGE OF SEX AND CHILDBIRTH (Q.42B,F)

	Knowledge of Sexual Relations (percent)	*Knowledge of Childbirth (percent)*
Nothing	32	26
Little	50	48
Considerable	18	26
	100	100
Number of respondents	(72)	(68)

[7] Crowded living conditions do not insure that children will learn about sex from observation. Strong tabus on sex help to insure that parents will take measures to mask their sexual activities. See p. 154.

By their own admission, less than a fifth of the women knew much about sexual relations and only a quarter knew much about childbirth.[8] It is possible that women were too ashamed to admit possession of such knowledge. If this is true, they are very adept at fabrication, for their statements seem quite convincing. Below are samples of the types of statement classified as "knew nothing." They would seem to indicate that the cloister system can effectively insulate the girl from tabued information.

Childbirth

I knew nothing of that. Once I remember I was about fourteen. I asked my mother where babies were born from. She slapped my face, that was her answer. . . . They wouldn't let me out. I had no opportunity to hear. Mother didn't talk about these things, and she used to say that when there were visitors at home the children should go under the bed. (TRC)

They told me it was bad to have a child because it was very painful, but that was two weeks after I was married. (B9F)

I married at twenty-four and scarcely knew what was going to happen to me. . . . I was like a nun. . . . I was even ignorant of how a woman gives birth to her children. My mother had told us it was through the ribs. (C4F)

I was reared with so much *respeto* that even when my mother had a child we were not permitted into her room until three days after. . . . So we knew nothing of that. (A11F)

Sexual Relations

I was so ignorant I thought it would be as brother and sister. I thought it was like the movies—kissing and like that. (H16F)

I thought marrying him meant living together and loving each other but nothing else. (C3F)

Lots of things are brought to the attention of girls but about men nothing is told to them. When a girl is virgin nothing is told her about men. (Z8F)

I thought when a man got married it was just to have a woman to cook, wash, and take care of him. I swear to you I couldn't imagine what marriage was. (H39F)

[8] Both the figures hold when controlled by age.

Over and over, respondents refer to being "shut in" so that they could learn nothing before marriage. Of course, we are speaking here of a previous generation,[9] and it is probable that the present mothers will be more liberal with their children. We have a possible test of this in the question, "What should a young girl know about sexual matters before marriage?" (Q.34B,F) The responses, while indicating a somewhat more liberal trend, do not, on the whole, show a great willingness to have daughters well informed. Of the 70 mothers who answered this question, 14 percent said, "Nothing"; 37 percent said, "Something but not everything"; and 49 percent said, "Everything."[10] Among those mothers who feel that their daughters should know nothing or very little, there is again the notion that such knowledge would corrupt the girl, for, being weak, it might lead her to evil habits.

I think she shouldn't know. I think she becomes too wicked. . . . It is supposed that she goes to the altar, in front of the Virgin, so she must be as ignorant as the Virgin herself. (H9F)

But an even more frequently cited reason is one which shows clearly the negative value which is put on sex. For some women, relations are seen as so unpleasant, and the idea of sexual relations so shocking to the uninformed, that a fair number of mothers felt it dangerous to tell their daughters about it prior to marriage. It was felt that the information might be so frightening to the girl that she might never marry. As one woman put it, "It should come as a surprise."

In a way I think it is better not to know, in order not to be scared.

[9] It must be recalled, however, that the average mother in the sample is only 29.5 years old and is discussing events which occurred only 15 years ago.

[10] Of those who said she should know something or everything, only four out of every ten felt that the *mother* should do the telling. When it came to the question of whether the mother actually *would* tell her daughters, however, virtually none felt that they could face such an embarrassing situation. Two women said they could not do so because the daughters would then realize what had happened to their mothers. They preferred to leave the impression of an immaculate conception. Landy writes that "all mothers and all fathers declared they would either punish their child (of either sex) or tell them a lie if the child asked about sex." (Personal communication.) By way of contrast, a Swedish poll in 1942 disclosed that half of the parents sampled from towns and 22 percent of those from the country admitted having spoken to their children about sex. Cantril and Strunk, *Public Opinion 1935–1946* (Princeton: Princeton University Press, 1951), p. 794.

If they know they might even refuse to do it with the husband, and this might cause trouble. (B4F)

It is better if she doesn't know. Otherwise she may change her mind. . . . I think some of them would even stop the marriage if they knew. (A10F)

It is better if they don't know anything. Knowing about it, they get frightened; and not knowing anything, they are not frightened and better able to face the situation. (X5F)

There is a certain amount of truth in such allegations. Those girls who knew anything at all about sex and childbirth prior to marriage knew only the worst aspects. Such information as was imparted seemed of the traumatic type which served to create anxiety about the sexual act and childbirth. Practically all the women who were told anything were warned about pain, the terrible shame of undressing, and the rapacity of the male. The social function[11] of such traumatic information as is illustrated below would again seem to be one of insuring that the girl will not be tempted into illicit relationships.

They told me it was very bad, and that if one didn't undress, the man would tear the dress to pieces. (H24F)

My married friends told me it was the worst thing in the world, that I should never get married. I tell the same thing to many now. If you only knew what marriage is, you would never get married. (H13F)

Before I got married my friends were always telling me, "Start trembling." They also said, "Have fun now, because later you will be carrying a big belly." (X9F)

My sister told me my husband would examine me with a lamp to see if I was a maiden. I was afraid. (A3F)

When asked whether they feared sexual relations or pregnancy before marriage, only 44 percent of the women replied in the

[11] Such tales may also serve a psychological function for the recounter. They may serve as an outlet for sadism or fill a need for revenge for the sexual hardships and traumas undergone by the teller, usually a married woman. Since so much has happened to her, she may take pleasure in frightening the novice. Wolf has noted the mixture of sadism and hysteria present in Puerto Rican middle-class "shower parties" for the bride-to-be. K. Wolf, "Growing up and Its Price in Three Puerto Rican Subcultures," *Psychiatry,* XV, No. 4 (Nov. 1952), 426.

negative to the former probe, and 54 percent to the latter. About a quarter of the cases in the "not afraid" category so classified themselves because they had no idea of what to expect.

Girls are given traumatic information not only about sex but also about other frightening qualities of men. We have previously mentioned the martyr complex characteristic of many mothers. The conception that marriage is a period of suffering, however, is also held by young women prior to marriage. This stems from the belief that men tend to be harsh exploiters of the opposite sex, and in contrast with directly sexual information, this type of knowledge seems to be freely passed on from the martyred mother to her to-be-martyred daughter.[12]

I knew nothing of men. (What had your mother told you about marriage?) She had told me that married life was one of work and suffering. (B5F)

I knew a little from stories I heard from other people or from my parents who told them in front of us, so we might acquire some experience. I knew there were men who treated their wives badly and made them suffer. (X7F)

The interviews are full of premarital fears as expressed by those females who knew anything about men. Beatings, desertion, infidelity, and nonsupport were the most frequently expressed fears.

I knew almost nothing. I had heard that after marrying the man is the one who gives orders and that the woman must obey. I had heard that men, some men, beat the women and after marrying them don't let them go any place. Oh, that men were bad, and that they harmed their wives! (A8F)

I knew that there were many bad men that left their wives; men that beat them and made them suffer of hunger. I knew that there were men that stayed out all night. (A3F)

THE INSULATION OF COURTSHIP

Once a girl is in her early teens, she becomes eligible for courtship. This period is one of stress and conflict for parents. Up to

[12] Eric Wolf notes that Puerto Rican country girls are exhorted to "be like María, who also suffered and was a good mother." "Culture Change and Culture Stability in a Puerto Rican Coffee Community" (unpublished Ph.D. dissertation, Columbia University, 1951), p. 90.

this time they have been careful to keep their daughter from the company of boys and men. Once she has reached puberty, the problem is intensified by the girl's own growing sexuality and her attractiveness to men. Consequently, parents must be doubly vigilant. At the same time, however, she must in some way be made available to men, for a single woman is a disgrace to the family.[13] The compromise which is made by lower-class Puerto Rican society is the insulated courtship system—or, more precisely, the *parentally regulated courtship*. With courtship as well as with patterns of cloistered rearing, the lower class has adopted the old and aristocratic Spanish system.

Up to this time, the girl has had little opportunity to acquaint herself with members of the opposite sex other than those relatives who visit her house. Several women in the sample complained that prior to their marriage they had known no men other than brothers and cousins.[14] Sometime after puberty, however, there are several culturally acceptable means for the girl to meet boys under the supervision of the parents. One way for town girls to get acquainted in a rudimentary fashion with boys is at the village *plaza*. Here, on certain evenings, she is customarily permitted to walk around the plaza accompanied by a brother, older sister, or relative. The boys, too, lounge around the plaza and ogle the girls. There is little communication between the sexes at this time. In its most classic form the custom is termed the *paseo* (promenade), and this form can still be seen in several of the more conservative towns of Puerto Rico. In this more stylized version the girls parade in one direction, the boys in another (or just stand on the sidelines). Ideally, if a boy sees a girl he likes, he may send her a note or speak to one of her friends to determine her feelings toward him. It probably is more customary at the present that he will find some opportunity to speak with her directly. At any rate, there is a minimum of communication at this time, and subsequently the couple must not be

[13] Symbolic of the disparagement both of the *jamona* (spinster) and of asceticism is the phrase humorously applied to unmarried women—"She is left to dress the saints" (*se queda para vestir santos*).

[14] The reportedly high rates of cousin marriage in lower-class society may be partly the result of cousin contact in adolescence, to the exclusion of non-family contacts.

seen together too frequently without some statement of intention on the part of the male.

The other chief means of mixing adolescents of the opposite sex is at folk-religious events. The most popular of these are *velorios* (wakes), *rosarios* (group recitations of the rosary), and dances coinciding with religious holidays. Again it must be emphasized that a minimum of communication takes place. In describing a lower-class dance, typical of a coffee region in Puerto Rico, Wolf shows how the sexes are carefully segregated by internalized norms and by the ever watchful father or brother.

> During this pre-marital period, the task of supervising the marriageable girls falls to their fathers. Married women no longer attend dances in other houses, and only the men accompany their daughters to such events. Since dancing is considered as "a thing of the devil" (*es del diablo*) because it carries with it strong connotations of sexuality, care is taken at a dance to ensure that a girl never dances twice with the same boy. Nor may a girl engage in any conversations with her partner. If this rule is broken, altercations are sure to follow. Even the boys prefer to go to dances at which the girls are "respected." This was a good dance, one boy commented after a Three Kings celebration, "there were no sweethearts." After each dance, the girls are supposed to retire to one room, which has been made the girls' quarters.
>
> Other occasions on which boys and girls may meet are devotions to the saints and during Sunday or feast-day visiting. On both occasions there is a complete lack of physical contact. At devotions, boys and girls sit in different parts of the house. During visits, the girls usually arrive first, and the boys follow them after they have discovered where their "jewel" has gone. The girls are usually offered a meal by the lady of the house, while the boys remain on the balcony outside and are served coffee and soda crackers.[15]

Practically all courting occurs in the house of the girl. If the couple wants to "go out," they must either go in a group or be accompanied by an elder relative. Thus parents, while exercising little influence over the initial choice of suitors, hold a definite *veto power* once the initial choice is made. In order to convey the sense of the very restricted contact with their fiancés which most of the lower-class women in the sample had, the courtship experi-

[15] Eric Wolf, *op. cit.*, p. 91.

ences of several of the more articulate respondents are presented below.

It was at a dance that we talked to each other and he proposed love to me. I didn't accept him at first; but he continued sending me letters; in that way I began to like him and I felt love for him, so I accepted him. We were sweethearts for about two years. We saw each other at home, he visited me three days in the week. There we talked, but together with all the family. They didn't leave us alone. We didn't have the opportunity to know each other. (But you went to dances before knowing him . . . ?) Yes, but it was with my father. When I fell in love, I scarcely went to dances; I have told you, they were too strict with me. (H20F)

He used to visit me three times weekly, the days my father told him. When he came home I sat on a bench, he on another and my father and brothers on another bench in front. They never left us alone; if my sister was out, father was there. (H45F)

We were neighbors since we were small. I met him by chance, after four years, when he went back to the town. It was at a dance. And he went to my home after the dance, and so we continued and were in love. He came to Santurce to continue work, but I stayed in my home; we wrote to each other. He visited me at home every fifteen days. We scarcely had the opportunity to be together because my mother was too strict. If we went out, it was with my two sisters; we felt much respect for my mother. (H5F)

Well, I met him shortly before we fell in love. He used to go to our home to teach my sister's husband how to play the guitar; so that's the way we met. Afterwards he went to work at my sister's store, and we continued the relations for eight years till we got married. We saw each other every day at home, but we didn't go to dances, or theaters, or *plazas.* If we went out, it was with my sister to *velorios,* and things like that, but to no other place. He used to go to my house; that was the only place where we talked, and this was in the presence of my mother and even with another woman present who lived in our home. (C4F)

We went together to the church accompanied by my mother or other relatives. They never let me go alone with him. Once I visited his home, but I went with my sister. (What do you think of that?) I thought it was a good thing, that it was done to avoid talking or to prevent any disgrace ahead of time. (How did he treat you, how intimate were you?) Well, we kissed each other; we never stayed alone;

if my mother was going out, we went with her or he stayed and I went with her. (Z1F)

I knew him, he was our neighbor. We courted for a year, but when he went home to ask to marry me my parents refused to see him. He came near my house, but we saw each other only at a distance. We communicated with each other by letters that he gave me when he passed by and that I sent him through his sisters. (B3F)

Thus, even with the relative amount of liberty permitted girls during courtship, girls have little real opportunity to learn much about men.

I knew very little, only that there are good men and men who like to deceive women. (Why so little?) Because I have never been close to men. I went out and had friends and boy friends, *but never had the opportunity to know them well.* (Z4F)

Before I got married I didn't know about men. . . . They visited me but *I didn't know how they really were.* (B1F)

The courtships illustrated above, and practically all of the remaining cases other than a small minority of clandestine courtships, were carried on mainly under the supervision of the parents and were characterized by a very low level of communication and intimacy. In the case of the clandestine courtships, although they were free of parental control, even less direct contact was typical. These flourished by means of secret letters, verbal communications through intermediaries, and occasional meetings in the homes of friends.

There appears to be no clear-cut modal length of courtship, although as Table 11 shows, fairly long courtships are more typical than others.

TABLE 11

LENGTH OF COURTSHIP (Q.37A,F)

	Percent
Four months or less	21
Five to eleven months	18
One year to three years	44
More than three years	17
	100
Number of respondents	(61)

Again we have been dealing with the mothers of the sample. It would seem likely that such traditional patterns are weakening. The evidence the study has for such a hypothesis would indicate that while there is a tendency toward more liberal attitudes toward courtship, the traditional pattern is still strong. Of the sixty-two mothers asked how strict they are or plan to be during their daughters' courtships, only four out of every ten said that they planned to be or were less strict. A few of those who said they intended to be less strict indicated that they would permit the girl to bring her boy friend into the home instead of objecting to all love affairs. What the average mother means when she says she will bring up her daughter as she was brought up with respect to courtship is illustrated below.

(How should she be with her sweethearts?) As I was brought up, not going alone with the sweethearts. He should always come to her house. They shouldn't talk outside the home. They must not be too close because they don't know if they are going to get married or not. They shouldn't kiss, or have necking or petting. The girl loses in the eyes of the same sweetheart when she does that, and also she loses in the eyes of those who see them, and she loses the opportunity to get married. (Y5F)

If I had a daughter, I wouldn't let her go out alone. Her sweetheart would have to come to her house to talk to her; she shouldn't talk with him in the streets. He'd have to come on those days I gave him permission. I wouldn't let him come to the house every day, or have his dinner with me. I wouldn't permit boy friends, either. I would be the same way as I was reared, as strict as before. (Z6F)

Mothers were asked how a girl should behave with young men in general before marriage, and how she should behave with her fiancé. To the former question, practically all the responses were identical: a girl should be respectful, serious, and not too friendly. To the latter question, the responses were surprisingly similar. "Avoiding intimacy" (kissing and petting), being respectful, modest, and serious were the most frequent responses, in that order. Only five women said that a girl may kiss or pet with her fiancé.

Since the tried and tested social mechanism to prevent intimacy is respect, respect and seriousness should characterize the relationship between the couple. Mild expressions of affection and caresses are an occasional and reluctant concession to changing times, but, in the main, physical contact should be scrupulously delayed until the wedding night, lest it excite the male and bring shame and disgrace upon the female.

THE MALE AND COURTSHIP

The boy's greater freedom of mobility allows him access to a great deal more sexual information than is possible for his sister. Young males are allowed to associate with boys of a somewhat more advanced age, and, through the latter as well as through the peer grapevine, learn the facts of life at a fairly early age. One pattern was well described by a respondent.

> At night the boys get together in groups and start telling off-color jokes, and the youngsters gather information about women. (B5M)

We have seen that some manifestations of sexuality are encouraged within the family during male infancy. Although sufficient information is lacking here, we have the impression that there is a social latency period in which greater sexual tabus are placed on the male child for fear that he will corrupt his sisters.[16] By adolescence, however, once he has well introjected the incest tabus, he is no longer a threat to his female siblings, and sexuality is not discouraged. Several years before his first permanent union, the boy has his first heterosexual experience. Nine out of every ten men in the sample admitted to premarital sexual intercourse,[17] the median age for first experience being seventeen in the country and village sample, and fifteen in the city.

Sexual activity in adolescence becomes one of the chief symbols of maturity and independence. Respondents' descriptions of their first experiences leave the definite impression of a *rite de passage.* As one man put it, "I felt proud in being *un hombre completo* (a

[16] This impression is shared by Mintz: "The sudden minimizing of sex play and the frank concern of the parents over the possibility (in fact, presumed likelihood) of incest, do not appear to coincide accidentally. From this time until the boy reaches puberty, he can joke sexually only with his own playmates." "Cañamelar: The Contemporary Culture of a Rural Puerto Rican Proletariat" (unpublished Ph.D. dissertation, Columbia University, 1951), Chap. VI, p. 44.

[17] Those without such experience were mainly from the country. This is understandable in the light of the fewer professionals and semiprofessionals operating in country areas.

complete man), because a man is not a real man unless he has sexual intercourse with a woman."[18] As the following illustrations show, men may receive congratulatory "ribbing" from their peers and elders after their initiation into the male world.

I had the first one when I was about twelve years old with a woman who had left her husband. . . . I was proud, one hundred percent. . . . One day we were caught in the sugar cane field. My cousin saw us and told it to my father. *My father told me, "You have done well. A man should not remain a fool."* (H1M)

I could hardly walk for three or four days after. I was proud because I had never touched a woman. I was also ashamed because my friends teased me at not being a *mozo* (virgin). . . . They even told the story to my mother. She scolded me because I had done it with a virgin. I told her I had done it because my friends told me I was not a complete man until I had that. . . . (A13M)

One respondent recounted how he had been encouraged to perform his first sexual act by older men who found his initiation amusing.

My first sexual experience was with a prostitute when I was twelve years old. . . . Now I remember that some older men were with me that day. Since I was a little boy, they were interested in seeing me doing that. They paid the prostitute for me, and it was like a festival. (C10M)

The elders, however, are interested in the adolescent's sexual experience for more than purposes of amusement, for it is a strategic part of the socialization process that the male adolescent have premarital experience. Of the sixty-five fathers who were asked the question, "What experience should a young man have before getting married?" (Q.26B,M), nine out of every ten felt that premarital experience was one of the important elements of the young man's education. Respondents speak of this as "training," so that the young man will be well experienced at marriage and "not be made a fool of."

He should know how to do that, so he will know what to do with his

[18] For the adolescent, sexual experience may also represent an effort to escape the strong emotional attachments to the mother. The event may symbolize his passage from mother love to heterosexual love. A large number of men, however, are unsuccessful. See pp. 81–83.

wife. Before marriage he should go to a cheap woman or a prostitute to be trained. (A13M)

He must try out his sexuality with prostitutes or with any other women. . . . I would talk to the woman and send the young fellow to her house so that the kid can get it off his chest (*limpie el pecho*). (TRA)

In addition to a thoroughgoing knowledge of the mechanics of sexual relations, the young man is expected to be knowledgeable concerning the tabued periods for intercourse. The principal tabu concerns menstruation. Twenty-five men spontaneously mentioned this as one of the things a young man should know about women before marriage. A less frequently mentioned tabu concerns the postpartum period. The country custom is to proscribe relations for forty days following delivery—*la cuarentena.*

The question now arises, if every young man is expected to have premarital intercourse, from whom can he receive his training? Table 12 below shows with whom the members of the sample had their premarital relations.

TABLE 12

CLASSIFICATION OF FEMALE PARTNERS FOR FIRST PREMARITAL SEXUAL EXPERIENCE (Q.28A,M)

Prostitutes and "cheap women"[a]	29
Married women (unattached)	10
Married women (attached)	2
Married women (unspecified)	7
Virgins	2
Number of respondents	50

[a] For convenience, "cheap women" and prostitutes are grouped together. The former are actually amateur prostitutes who usually accept "gifts" but are not strictly in business. They are termed variously as cheap women, *cobos,* loose women, and women of gay life. Nineteen males so designated their first sexual partners. All but three men used such derogatory terms in describing their first paramours, indicating that almost by definition a girl who allows such advances is a cheap woman.

As might have been anticipated from our previous discussion, virgins do not form the typical object of the male's sexual attentions, at least for the first experience. One respondent phrased the tabu quite clearly.

A man makes love to every woman that passes his way. But if the woman is *señorita,* then he should let that one pass by, because it is not good to fool with virgins. (C1M)

A mother, in speaking proudly of her son, showed how both she and he approved of exploitation of the nonvirgin, but for the fiancé a different code prevailed.

Ah! He has his fiancée in town. She is a good and honest girl. Now with the others he takes care of himself, and says that he is *macho,* and that the *macho* never loses. (C10F)

This raises the question as to why men, allegedly so rapacious, should leave the virgins untouched. First of all there are powerful social sanctions. Violation of the virgin would cause the male a great deal of trouble with her family. He might be beaten or killed by the disgraced male family members or pressured to marry the girl. But the fear of such sanctions is not the only deterrent. Attitudes toward girl friends in some respects resemble those toward sisters and mothers, and thus assist in preventing excessive intimacy.

In answer to the questions, "How should young men behave toward young girls before marriage? And with their girl friends? And with the fiancée?" (Q.26,M) the responses of the males were surprisingly indistinguishable from those given by the women. They are characterized by "respect", and "not too much intimacy."

The degree of respect appears to *increase* as one moves closer to one's potential wife. Thus, while most men felt that one should "get to know" one's fiancée better than other girls, one must at the same time render her more respect than the others. There is a kind of manifest ambivalence in most of the responses, for, while speaking of the greater "intimacy" one should have with the fiancée, the respondents simultaneously cite the necessity for what amounts to greater social distance.

One gets the feeling from reading the responses that the accent is on reserve; that the "intimacy" refers to increased opportunities for meeting, conversation, and greater affection—but not more intimacy in a sexual sense.

With the girl friends he should be like a good friend . . . *with the fiancée, he should be even more respectful.* (Y5M)

He should treat the girl friends with respect. . . . The fiancée should be treated with more consideration and *more respect because that one will be your wife.* (Z6M)

One must be correct and gentlemanly with young girls . . . the same with girl friends but with a greater grade of intimacy. . . . *With the fiancée one should have more respect* because she will be one's wife. (Z3M)

Thus it would appear that the closer one gets in terms of a potential mate, the stronger are the sexual tabus. Expressed another way, the more likely a woman is to be one's wife, the more likely is she to be surrounded with attitudes resembling those held toward the mother or sister. Perhaps the greater the *danger* of sexual relations, the stronger must be the attitudes which serve to tabu this relationship. Thus respect increases with courtship intimacy.

The formation and preservation of this attitude is probably affected by religious ideology and by the tendency on the part of the male to seek a mother substitute as a mate.

In the Puritanical tradition, Eve is the symbol of woman—Eve the inherently evil temptress who seduces essentially innocent man. Thus all women are more or less evil and vary only in degree. Catholic culture, in particular the Latin American variety, seems to have two symbols for womanhood—*Eve and the Virgin.* As might be expected, the two are seldom mixed in the same person; that is, a woman is either Eve or the Virgin, either good or bad. Degrees of evil do not exist in the same sense, since there is a qualitative difference between the two types.[19] Thus, some of those

[19] Both in behavior and attitude, the distinction has become blurred in the United States. Kinsey's data show that so many unmarried girls have had premarital intercourse that the distinction between the good and bad girl in terms of sex becomes difficult. For some girls, it becomes "technical virginity"; that is, the experience of the gamut of sexual foreplay without male genital penetration. In other instances, it must be based on a somewhat narrow monetary criterion—those who charge for sexual relations are bad. The narrow line between the good and bad girl is well expressed by Riesman's use of the concept of "marginal differentiation": ". . . the sharp discontinuity that once existed between respectability and sin . . . has now become a problematic gradient where one must look for marginal differentiation" (D. Riesman, *The Lonely Crowd,* New Haven, Yale University Press, 1950, p. 126). In Puerto Rico the behavior of "good" and "bad" girls is sharply defined, and a good girl is only she who goes undefiled to the marital chamber.

women symbolized by the Virgin will be better than others of their type, but none are "bad"; some of those symbolized by Eve will be worse than others, but none "good." In Puerto Rico, as in most of Latin America, the two types are easily identified. Prostitutes, *cobos,* and *mujeres baratas* (cheap women) are in the camp of Eve; virgins are in the camp of the Virgin.

While helping to account for the attitude of respect toward virgins in general, the impact of religious ideology does not account for the increased respect toward the fiancée. The latter would seem at least partly due to the male tendency to seek a mother substitute. We have seen that the male child is given relatively less attention and affection by his parents than are his sisters, and that his relationships with his father tend to be minimal and marked by status barriers. Conceivably, this situation impedes the formation and/or the resolution of the Oedipus conflict. Since he has never truly identified himself with his father, nor escaped the dependency feelings for his mother, he may be unable to desire her sexually—the integral part of the Oedipus constellation.[20] Thus, he surrounds her with a holy glow of virtue and immaculate love and seeks a mother figure in adulthood. Whether or not such rearing factors are the cause, we have abundant evidence that many lower-class males sought mother substitutes in marriage. The fact that a psychiatric interview was not necessary to elicit such articulations would indicate that the emotional attachment for the mother is on a conscious level, and that the sexual side of the attachment is either unformed or successfully repressed. To the family student who anticipates that such attachments will either be unrealized or go unexpressed, the free responses of the males in the sample are striking.

In answer to question 32A,M ("What were you looking for in

[20] "Although an undisturbed confidence in the mother is important for the normal development of infants of both sexes, the emotional security which results from it affects boys and girls differently. It gives the boy permission for self-assertion and a sense of courage. Thus he may free himself from his dependence on the mother in order to start a development in which identification with the father becomes a leading motive. . . . [At three to five years old] the child's identification with the parents of the same sex has evolved strongly enough to motivate his erotically colored demands toward the parent of the other sex" (T. Benedek, "The Emotional Structure of the Family," in Ruth Anshen, ed., *The Family: Its Function and Destiny,* New York: Harper, 1949, p. 205).

a wife?") and question 32A3,M ("Were your feelings toward your wife different from those toward the women you knew before you married?"), 14 men made explicit references to their mother. In answering the former question, another 14 cases gave mother-*substitute* responses, such as, "I was looking for a woman to take care of me, protect me, be kind to me," etc. Still another 8 cases gave mother references when asked why they married so early or late. Here, for example, they explained that they had been taking care of their mothers, that they were satisfied to live with their mothers, or that their mothers had died and they needed someone to take care of them. If so many (36, or half of the sample) spontaneously give direct and indirect mother responses, it can be assumed that the attitude is both prevalent and important. Better to illustrate how strongly mother-fixated these men are, most of the direct mother references are presented below.

I wanted a wife who would *love me as my mother* did. . . . I think this was the most important thing. (A8M)

Well, that she be *like a mother to me.* (Y8M)

I lived divinely happy with my mother. Besides God what one loves most is the mother, and then the children. (H24M)

I was searching for a good companion because I did not have a mother. (Did you want a wife with the same qualities as your mother?) Yes, of course; because in my opinion a *good wife is like a mother to one.* (H10M)

I was looking for an honest woman that could be faithful to me, that wouldn't use bad language, and *that would be like my mother.* (C1M)

One loves one's wife as if she were the mother. . . . She takes care of me and is a faithful woman like my mother. ((H15M)

My wife was like a mother. I adored her. She used to look after me. She used to protect me. (H18M)

My wife is a second mother. In the place of the mother there is a good wife to look after one. . . . [I was looking for] *a wife who would treat me like my mother.* She loved me very much. (Y5M)

. . . *I treat my wife as if she were my mother. She is the one who . . . takes care of me and protects me.* (Z7M)

You want your wife to be like your own mother because *she is the second mother one has.* (Y6M)

I was looking for *a wife who had the customs of my old mother.* I had to wait until I found one. . . . That's why I chose her for my wife. (Z1M)

A man tries to find a wife that resembles his mother, and he compares the women he thinks of marrying with her. (X6M)

Thus, in a high proportion of the sample, emotional independence from the mother seems never to have been completely achieved. It is noteworthy that, of the nine men who professed not to have had sexual relations prior to marriage, six give specific mother references, another gave a mother-substitute response, and another married a woman fifteen years older than himself. Thus there is the possibility of some relationship between sexuality (at least early sexuality) and mother-dependency.

A FEW CHECKS ON VALIDITY

Much of the foregoing may appear far-fetched to the reader. The cloister pattern, the seemingly inordinate pressures for premarital virginity for females, the ignorance of matters pertaining to sex may all appear to be the result of the particular methodology used rather than a true reflection of lower-class patterns. The present study concerns itself mainly with attitudes and relies upon these as well as on respondents' own behavioral descriptions for assumptions about behavior. Since observational techniques were not a part of the present project, there is always the question of whether the verbalizations represent behavioral reality.

A number of other studies employing observational methods have been conducted in Puerto Rico. Unfortunately, of those which are available, none concentrated especially on courtship and marriage, and all are limited to a particular town or rural area. With these limitations in mind we may examine their conclusions.

The earliest study, conducted by Rogler in 1936, in general concurs with our present findings. In describing the chaperonage system Rogler writes:

It is sometimes said that the girls of the lower class do about as they please in their courtship relations with boys, but the evidence proves the contrary. There is very little more transgression of courtship customs among these girls than among those of the better class.[21]

[21] C. Rogler, *Comerio—A Study of a Puerto Rican Town* (University of Kansas, 1940), p. 71.

And with reference to the importance of virginity he notes:

The foregoing description is more strictly applicable to the daughter . . . who belong[s] to the upper class than it is to the lower class. But since the upper class sets the moral and social standards for the community, the observations offered above are more or less applicable to the women of the lower class.[22]

Siegel's conclusions (1948) are of a somewhat different nature. First of all he writes that:

The impact of some fifty years of contact with North Americans and their culture is less visible in the sphere of sex relations than perhaps in any other aspect of ordinary life. [Except for small, urban, college educated groups] Puerto Rico's population still adheres to the Catholic morality which desexes "respectable" girls and women in its worship of the supreme virtue, virginity.[23]

But this generalization is subsequently qualified:

The middle classes believe in the validity and in the righteousness of the code, and their members, particularly the females, are expected to conform to it; the low income class also recognizes the validity of the code, but a great many of its members follow, in fact, quite different standards.[24]

The observations of Mintz (1951) for a sugar-cane region parallel our own conclusions more closely:

I am now quite convinced that young virgins, at least in the community where I worked, are quite cut off from casual sexual experiences; that there is a very considerable concern regarding a girl's virginity at the time of her first union, and that any claims about the lower-class rural proletarian female's wantonness or promiscuity are quite ridiculous. . . . I feel quite safe in saying that the likelihood of a casual sexual experience before the establishment of a consensual union or marriage is extremely slight, and that parents and community can exert considerable pressure in getting conformance.[25]

In the most recent study, Landy (1952) concludes that, if anything, the lower-class sexual code is more strict than that of the middle class:

[22] *Ibid.*, p. 74.

[23] M. Siegel, "Lajas: A Puerto Rican Town" (unpublished manuscript, University of Puerto Rico, 1948), pp. 149–50.

[24] *Ibid.*, p. 150.

[25] S. Mintz, personal communication, September, 1953.

They are extremely prudish in theory and practice, with regard to the insulation and protection of the female, apparently more so than the middle class. The latter often attend functions in Agua Lluvia where the sexes mix freely, an unheard-of occurrence for lower-class families, where sex separation lines cross every area of life. The puritanism of the rural lower-class family of our study seems as rigid as that practiced by the people who settled New England in the 17th and 18th Centuries.[26]

Thus, much of the observational evidence, while it leaves much to be desired, tends to support some of our general conclusions concerning the courtship period.

CONCLUSIONS

Courtship, an institution which usually serves to acquaint the sexes with one another prior to marriage, is unusually weak in this function in Puerto Rico. The cloister pattern continues to operate during this period, chaperonage and parental supervision insuring that the girl will have a minimum amount of contact with her fiancé. Moreover, the relationship between the courting couple is ideally one of considerable reserve; modesty and mutual respect being the appropriate demeanor to insure a minimum of intimacy.

Not only is the female denied the opportunity for a realistic testing out of sex and intimate interpersonal relationships with her future spouse, but the degree of general knowledge concerning marital relationships appears to be of a limited and distorted nature. The premarital conceptions of marriage appear to be characterized by fear and ignorance.

Males, on the other hand, indulge in heterosexual experiences with prostitutes at an early age, and regard sexual relations as a pleasureful activity required of the "complete man." However, social sanctions and attitudes of respect toward the fiancée discourage the initiation of premarital sexual relationships with the intended spouse. At the same time, males appear to want wives who resemble their mothers in the sense of protectiveness, tenderness, and modesty, another factor which might inhibit physical intimacy.

[26] D. Landy, "Childrearing Patterns in a Puerto Rican Lower Class Community" (unpublished manuscript, University of Puerto Rico, 1952).

Again drawing a few tentative implications:

(1) The gap between the sexes which began in childhood is not lessened to any degree in the premarital period, and may even become aggravated. This could have important consequences for the degree of successful marital communication as well as for general marital adjustment—two factors conceivably bearing on fertility.

(2) Similarly, the negative orientation or nonorientation toward sex on the part of women appears not to change greatly in this period, while the positive attitude of males is reinforced by sexual experiences. These differing attitudes, if unchanged in marriage, would presumably affect the couple's sexual patterns.

(3) The relative lack of affection given the male child may have found its expression in the search for a mother figure by adult males—a fact which could influence mature sexual behavior and marital adjustment.

(4) The cloister pattern and the insulated courtship could affect the time and form of marriage. It is to this question that we shall now turn, attempting to assess the impact of child rearing and courtship patterns upon marriage.

V

Early Marriage and Consensual Union

Why did you get married?—One gets blind with love and doesn't think. A FEMALE RESPONDENT

Why did you get married?—I was looking for a wife to do my laundry. A MALE RESPONDENT

EARLY MARRIAGE

One of the most strategic factors affecting a people's fertility rate is age at marriage. Ireland, of course, is the outstanding example of a nation which has successfully lowered its birth rate by means of late marriage for both sexes.[1] Puerto Rico shows no such pattern, its median age at marriage for males being about the same as that

TABLE 13

MEDIAN AGE AT FIRST MARRIAGE FOR UNITED STATES, PUERTO RICO, AND PRESENT SAMPLE

	U.S. (1947)[a]	*Puerto Rico (1947)*[b]	*Sample*[c]
Males	23.7	23.8	22
Females	20.5	19.1	17

[a] K. Davis, "Statistical Perspective on Marriage and Divorce," *Annals of the American Academy of Political and Social Science*, CCLXXII (Nov. 1950), 14.

[b] P. K. Hatt, *Backgrounds of Human Fertility in Puerto Rico: A Sociological Survey* (Princeton: Princeton University Press, 1952), Table 32, p. 48.

[c] The age at marriage for the present sample might be expected to be lower than Hatt's, because the present sample is confined to the lower class. Hatt's two lowest-rental-category women show their median age at marriage to be 18.6 and 17.9. *Ibid.*, Table 100, p. 129.

[1] In 1941, only 3.2 percent of Ireland's males and 12.4 percent of Ireland's females were ever married by age 24. K. Davis, "Statistical Perspective on Marriage and Divorce," *Annals of the American Academy of Political and Social Science*, CCLXXII (Nov. 1950), 14.

of the United States (a country of relatively early marriages), and the median age at marriage for females considerably lower than in the United States. Table 13 gives the median ages at marriage for the United States, for Puerto Rico, and for the present sample.

Note that while the discrepancy between male and female median ages at marriage is slightly more than three years on the continent, it is close to five years in Puerto Rico.

ATTITUDES TOWARD AGE AT MARRIAGE

Ideal age at marriage is of equal interest for our purposes. Table 14 shows that the ideal age at marriage is placed considerably beyond the actual age at marriage.

TABLE 14

MEDIAN IDEAL AGE AT MARRIAGE FOR MALES AND FEMALES

	Hatt[a]	*Sample*
Males	26.6	23.5
Females	20.9	20.0

[a] Tables 33 and 34, pp. 49 and 50.

Hatt found that 29 percent of the males and 63 percent of the females had married younger than their expressed ideal age,[2] and that 27 percent of the females and 12 percent of the males wished they had married at a later age.[3] In the present sample, discrepancies between ideal and actual age at marriage are even more striking. Table 15 shows the degree to which the members of the sample realized their ideal ages at marriage.

More than four out of every ten males and more than six out of every ten females marry three or more years earlier than their ideal. Only four out of ten males and two out of ten females marry at or later than their ideal age. This indicates not only that a high proportion marry considerably earlier than they would ideally desire but also that the *women* are particularly unlikely to realize their ideals. That this is regretted by the women is evidenced by the fact

[2] P. K. Hatt, *Backgrounds of Human Fertility in Puerto Rico: A Sociological Survey* (Princeton: Princeton University Press, 1952), Table 36, p. 52.

[3] *Ibid*, Table 35, p. 51.

that 48 of the 58 women who married earlier than their ideal said it would have been better had they married later.

TABLE 15

YEARS OF DISCREPANCY BETWEEN IDEAL AND ACTUAL AGE AT MARRIAGE FOR MALES AND FEMALES

	Males (*percent*)	*Females* (*percent*)
Married three or more years earlier than ideal	42	64
Married one or two years earlier than ideal	14	16
Married at ideal age	7	13
Married one or two years later than ideal	10	0
Married three or more years later than ideal	27	7
	100	100
Number of respondents	(71)	(70)

CAUSAL FACTORS IN EARLY MARRIAGE OF THE FEMALE

Of those 52 women who married two or more years earlier than their ideal, 18 said they did so to get away from home, 13 said they fell in love, 12 said they did so out of ignorance or because they "didn't think," and the remainder gave combinations of these reasons or other reasons.[4] Each of these reasons bears further analysis.

TABLE 16

LENGTH OF COURTSHIP BY AGE AT MARRIAGE

	Short Courtship[a] (*percent*)	*Long Courtship* (*percent*)
Early age at marriage	71	37
Average age at marriage	12	29
Late age at marriage	17	34
	100	100
Number of respondents	(24)	(38)

[a] Short courtships were classified as those which lasted for a year or less.

Chapter IV showed that, while women in the sample generally had long courtships, a wide range was present, running from a few months to more than half a decade. If it were assumed that all the women started courtships at roughly the same age, there would

[4] "I was orphaned," was the chief other reason.

theoretically be a marked relation between length of courtship and age at marriage. This is borne out in Table 16.

Twice as many of those with short courtships married early as did those with longer courtships. It would seem important, then, to determine the reasons why some girls have such short courtships. One of the major reasons appears to be the sudden precipitation of marriage which breaks off the courtship because of an intolerable home situation for the girl. We shall term this pattern rebellion.[5]

Rebellion. In Chapter III we advanced the hypothesis that the girl's more consistent and tender child rearing should dispose her toward being more contented in the parental household than her brothers, other things being equal. At the same time it was suggested that she may not develop such a compulsive dependence upon her parents as the boy, because of the greater attention and consideration she receives. Subsequently we pointed out that the cloister pattern is intensified during adolescence, and that courtship for the girl is hedged in by various sorts of restrictions. Our present data would suggest that these additional pressures on the girl are such as to counteract her feelings of satisfaction and contentment in the home, if such really existed, impelling the girl to rebel from parental authority.[6] Three basic questions are pertinent: To what extent does rebellion actually occur? What are the factors in family relationships which encourage rebellion? What is the connection between rebellion and early marriage? The tentative answers to these questions may be stated briefly and then substantiated: A high proportion of girls rebel against the restrictions placed on them during courtship. This rebellion leads them to desire escape by the only available means—marriage. Since early courtship and marriage are often disapproved by parents because so many male suitors do not meet with parental approval, and since the girl is predisposed

[5] Rebellion not in the sense of genuine deviant behavior but merely in the sense of conscious hostility toward the parents leading to a withdrawal from the home situation into marriage.

[6] It is conceivable, too, that feeling certain of parental affection, daughters are more capable of rebelling from parental authority in a conscious and overt fashion. In the case of the male there are two blocks to rebellion. Few restrictions are placed on his liberty, and early independence is encouraged, even though this creates problems of discipline. Thus, he has less cause for rebellion. Second, he may be emotionally indisposed to rebel because of the greater emotional dependency he develops on his mother.

toward escaping her parents' authority, courtship is abruptly cut off, and the couple elopes—a pattern in the lower class which is frequently associated with the consensual-union type of marriage. Two types of rebellion can profitably be distinguished—rebellion against the general restrictions of the cloister pattern and the drudgery of work in the parental home; rebellion against parental disapproval of the courtship and/or the suitor.

Cloister Rebellion. The first type of rebellion can be described as a reaction against the cloister pattern on the part of the girl in late adolescence. Thirty-four percent of the women gave the reason, "To get away from home," as the principle cause for marrying at the time they did. The illustrations below show how adolescence creates an emotional chafing at the bonds of the cloister pattern, so that marriage, with or without love, is seen as the only way out.[7]

At that moment I didn't think at all. I only wanted to be free from my family and my home where I was shut up. (C3F)

My parents didn't . . . allow us entertainment of any sort. We lived as nuns. . . . At home they didn't let us work or help anybody. We went to church and back home. . . . My parents didn't allow my first sweetheart to visit me and even had a wooden rod to beat him with. . . . If my home environment had been different, I would have liked to have stayed there longer or even not marry. . . . I didn't love him. . . . (H45F)

I did it because I was too tied down at home. My parents didn't let me go to dances or parties. . . . We weren't in love and he didn't visit me. . . . I wasn't interested in him. (H1F)

Girls rebel not only against the restrictions which are imposed on them but against the arduous duties as well. As the children grow into adolescence, the girl's value to the family increases,[8] since she

[7] Rebellion leads to marriage only because of the lack of other alternatives. As industrialization increases and factory work becomes a culturally acceptable prerogative of the female, we would expect a high proportion of females to turn to this rather than to marriage as an escape. This is particularly evident when it is realized that, in the case of rebellious girls, marriage occurs more as the result of a "push" from the parental home than as the result of the "pull" or attractiveness *per se* of marriage.

[8] Mintz feels that the value of the boy decreases at the same time. "From the age of 12 onward, the boy's role in the home dwindles steadily in importance, while the girl's value increases" ("Cañamelar: The Contemporary Culture of a Rural Puerto Rican Proletariat" (unpublished Ph.D. dissertation, Columbia University, 1951), Chap. VI, p. 49.

can share in the housework, child rearing, and so forth.[9] In many of the childhood homes of our respondents, the lives of the adolescent girls appear filled only with the drudgery of household work.

I wanted to leave my mother's home, to get away from all the suffering, because they left me with the burden [of the house], so I was dissatisfied and decided to get married. He became aware of this and proposed marriage in order to save me from being a slave, washing, ironing, and doing everything. (Z1F)

I was ignorant and I eloped with him. . . . My parents sometimes piled up the housework on me; that's why I didn't want to stay home any longer. (A13F)

In 39 out of the 72 cases, women expressed in varying degrees such sentiments of rebellion as are illustrated above. While the quotations suggest the correlation between such attitudes and early marriage, to what extent is this borne out in the total sample? Table 17 shows a fairly marked correlation.

TABLE 17

CLOISTER REBELLION BY AGE AT MARRIAGE

	No Evidence of Rebellion (percent)	*Rebellion (percent)*
Early marriage	36	69
Average	24	18
Late marriage	40	13
	100	100
Respondents	(33)	(39)

It has already been suggested that rebellion influences early marriage partly because it reduces the courtship period. This is borne out by the fact that only 53 percent of the rebellious females had long courtships, whereas 70 percent of the nonrebellious females did. Both brief courtship and rebelliousness appear to be related to early marriage, each exercising an influence in its own right.

9 Practically all of the mothers who wanted an equal number of boys and girls for a family cited as their reason the "help to the mother" which the girls could provide.

TABLE 18

AGE AT MARRIAGE BY CLOISTER REBELLION AND LENGTH OF COURTSHIP

Percent Who Married Early

	REBELLION		NO REBELLION	
	Percent	*Base*	*Percent*	*Base*
Short courtship	75	(16)	63	(8)
Long courtship	56	(18)	21	(19)

The highest proportion of early marriages occurs with those women who experienced both rebellion and short courtships, the lowest proportion with those who experienced neither.

Since elopements frequently result in consensual marriages,[10] another hypothesis would be that both consensual union and early marriage are products of similar causes.[11] Table 19 combines these factors to determine to what extent they are related to rebellion.

TABLE 19

CLOISTER REBELLION BY AGE AT MARRIAGE AND TYPE OF MARRIAGE

Percent who expressed cloister rebellion

	EARLY MARRIAGE[a]		LATE MARRIAGE	
	Percent	*Base*	*Percent*	*Base*
First union consensual	73	(22)	50	(6)
First union legal	64	(22)	26	(22)

[a] Marriage occurring at 18 years of age or younger.

Although the cases are few, they give credence to the hypothesis. More than seven of every ten of those women who married both

[10] For detailed discussion of consensual or nonlegal marriage, see pp. 105–19.

[11] There appears to be some relation between age at marriage and consensual union. In Hatt's higher-rental category, the median age at marriage was 20 for the "all unions legal" women and 18.6 for the "not all unions legal" women. In the lower-rental category, the median ages at marriage for these two groups were 19.5 and 18.6. Hatt, *op. cit.,* Table 308, p. 432.

young and consensually evidenced rebellious attitudes toward their parents, whereas less than three out of ten of those who married late and legally evidenced such attitudes. Those groups which experienced either consensual or early marriage, but not both, show a proportion of rebels between the two extremes. While bearing out the hypothesis, the table leads us to speculate as to the deviant cases. What of those cases of early marriage and consensual union which did not evidence rebellion, and those cases of late and legal marriage which did? Six such cases are in the former category, and six in the latter.

Those in the category of no rebellion but early, consensual marriage age are clearly special cases. In two instances the man was already married and consequently could not marry legally. In another two cases marriage was promised before elopement and was accomplished soon after. Of the remaining two women, one had been raped prior to marriage and, consequently, saw no point in legal marriage; in the last case, the parents apparently encouraged a consensual marriage—the only case of its kind in the sample. As far as the early age at marriage is concerned, one fact distinguished the group—all but one of them started their courtships at an exceptionally young age. Although all the women in this group were married at eighteen years of age or younger, five of the six courtships lasted four years or longer. Thus we may suppose that, since they started courtship considerably earlier than most of the others in the sample, they might be expected to marry earlier, despite the fact that they evidence no rebellion from their parents.

It was by an examination of the second deviant group (the rebellious but late, legal marriages) that another type of rebellion had to be distinguished from the cloister type. In examining these six cases in detail, it was discovered that, while all of the girls articulated rebellious feelings against their parents as a result of the cloister pattern, in all but one case the *courtship and the suitor* had been approved of by the parents. In these cases, despite general rebellion against the parents, the courtship period itself was sufficiently permissive, apparently, to preclude an early "bolting" of the girl into consensual marriage. The discovery of this fact suggested the need for an investigation of courtship approval and resulted in the delineation of a second type of rebellion.

Courtship Rebellion. This type of rebellion reacts against the almost customary opposition of parents to the suitor and the restrictions with which they surround the girl during the courtship. As we have seen, parents become particularly vigilant during this period and may even take away some of the small liberties which were considered innocuous prior to adolescence.[12]

Parental opposition to the suitor was mentioned in 24 of the 69 cases in which some information was obtained on this subject. In six other cases, in order to obviate parental opposition, the courtship was carried on clandestinely. These women were so afraid of punishment on the part of their parents that they felt compelled to conceal the suitor. As some of the following quotations show, their fears were not groundless.

> When I fell in love, I never told anything to my parents, because I feared them so much. I was very young, and they threatened me, saying if I got a boy friend they would beat me. My father had a very strong character. So I eloped with my boy friend. (B8F)

> They didn't like him, and they beat me when he came. . . . They didn't like him, so I eloped with him. (B6F)

> My father was too strict with me and obliged me to take that bad step. My father didn't like him, and instead of giving me good advice, he treated me badly. He made me kneel on *guayos* [a metal instrument for grating coconuts—one of the harshest of country punishments] and threatened me with a knife. . . . I was afraid of them, so I eloped with my sweetheart. (H12F)

The conception that "no one is good enough for my daughter" seems prevalent. Parents make such a considerable emotional and material investment in their daughter that their standards for a son-in-law are placed unduly high. Moreover, they may hope to gain

[12] "To keep her under control, all her former liberties, already very limited, are eliminated, and usually there is someone in the family keeping an eye on her" (S. Gregory de Torres, "Elopement in the Lower Classes of Puerto Rico" (unpublished term paper, University of Puerto Rico, 1950). The writer is indebted to Mrs. Torres for further documentation of several of the ideas expressed in this section. These were the product of a seminar on Puerto Rican Society conducted by the writer.

some surcease from poverty by a successful match.[13] Whatever the cause, the repression and punishment help to insure rebelliousnes on the part of the daughter. To escape the intolerable situation, they bolt prematurely from the household, in desperation or pure spite.[14]

I married at sixteen out of spite. My family didn't like him, so we decided to get married one day when I went to town. . . . My family beat me because of him. . . . Sometimes you are stubborn and don't think. (Y4F)

My father didn't like my sweetheart, and I *married out of spite.* (H21F)

I was an ignorant girl, under age, and as we were angry with my father, we did it as a rebellion. If my parents had permitted us to see each other often, *perhaps we would have married, and married a little later, when I was more mature.* (H18F)

Common to both types of rebellion is a volatile emotional state on the part of the girl, a state of mind in which she wishes fervently to escape from an intolerable home situation. This emotional state may cause a suspension of her more critical judgment, or at least a submersion of such values as a leisurely and legal marriage. Consequently, she leaves her home at a date earlier than she might wish ideally. But why consensually? In the first place, her eagerness to

[13] "It is known that in Puerto Rico the poor areas suffer from extremely poor living conditions. Sometimes the attitude of the parents may be explained in terms of their frustrated hopes of marrying their daughters to richer men, and thus benefiting by it" (Gregory de Torres, *op. cit.*). That the girls also marry early to escape from the poverty in the parental home is a possibility, supported by at least one such statement by a respondent. Such motivation appears common even among the lower class of England. Thirty-eight percent of a sample of mothers living in high-fertility areas said they married "for a home." ". . . Among the working class this often meant little more than an escape from difficult conditions to less difficult ones. Many gave as their reason for marriage that they wanted to get away from their parents' home" (Mass Observation, *Britain and Her Birth Rate,* London, John Murray, 1945, p. 62).

[14] Males are perhaps even more prone to marry consensually for this reason. Wounded by the fact that he is not approved of by the parents, the male's pride may lead him to spite them by stealing her away (*se la lleva*). This, particularly when it results in a consensual union, serves as an insult to the parents and acts as a kind of retaliation for wounding the male ego. Three males said they married in this fashion because the girls' parents were opposed to them. As one of them put it, "I wanted to marry her, but her family opposed me. . . . I fooled them. . . ." These cases were the only ones in which the males seemed "pushed" by emotional factors into consensual marriage.

leave home might make her susceptible to doing this *on the man's* terms, and, as we shall see, it is more frequently the man who decides the type of marital arrangement. Second, both the fact of sudden elopement and legal under-age at marriage make it difficult or impossible to secure a license in time. This is particularly true when parental opposition precludes the legal step of granting consent to an under-age marriage.[15] The combination of the two types of rebellion, then, should serve as a more accurate predictor of early and consensual marriage. Table 20 shows that this is true.

TABLE 20

EXTENT OF REBELLION, BY TYPE AND TIME OF MARRIAGE

	Both Types Rebellion (percent)	*One Type Rebellion (percent)*	*Neither Type Rebellion (percent)*	*Total Number of Cases*
Early and consensual first union	37	28	11	(17)
Early or legal first union	53	48	39	(33)
Late and legal first union	10	24	50	(22)
	100	100	100	
Number of respondents	(19)	(25)	(28)	(72)

For those women who experienced both types of rebellion against their parents, only one of ten married late and legally. Half of those who experienced neither type of rebellion so married.

We may now turn our attention to the final deviant group, those 14 cases of early and/or consensual marriage with *no* evidence of either type of rebellion. Five of the cases falling in this category have already been explained (p. 94) as special cases. Among the remainder, however, there is a pattern of responses which suggests that there are factors other than rebellion to be taken into considera-

[15] *With parental consent,* males may marry legally at eighteen and females at sixteen. Without consent, the legal age for marriage is twenty-one for both sexes. *Código Civil de Puerto Rico* (San Juan: Government Printing Office, 1930), Art. 70, Subsections 3 and 4.

tion. "I was blind and didn't think"; "I was ignorant"; "I was in love and he invited me and I eloped"; "I never gave a thought to it. I was very ignorant"; and "He offered me everything" represent the bulk of the reasons given for early marriages or consensual unions, and they lead us to a discussion of two other interrelated factors which serve to encourage such unions—romantic love and ignorance.

Romantic Love. Neo-local residence,[16] the relative freedom to choose one's mate, and the prolonged but insulated courtship characteristic of the premarital histories might lead one to expect that romantic love would characterize lower-class courtship. This hypothesis does not find substantiation in the case of the males but to a considerable degree would seem characteristic of females. Thirty percent of the women gave "I fell in love" as their principal reason for marrying at the time they did, but it is, of course, possible that the same expression has a different connotation in another culture. To get at the respondents' meaning of love and its importance to them, two questions were asked: "Tell me what you understand by love (Try to differentiate between affection and love.)" (Q.33C,F) and "Which is more important for a woman, that she be married to a good man, or to one she is very much in love with?" (Q.34D,F) In reply to the former question, 46 out of the 67 women who answered it gave such descriptions of romantic love as are exemplified below.

They want to be near each other, to have the loved person near you always. When the person is out working it seems as if he were never

[16] As contrasted with matri-local or patri-local residence, neo-local residence describes the pattern whereby newly-weds live neither with the parents of the bride nor with those of the groom. In Puerto Rico, the pattern of "living alone" is dominant in ideology and practice. It is voiced in such folk expressions as, "*El casado casa quiere*" (The married person wants his own home) and "*Quien se casa, pa' su casa*" (He who marries should have his own house). In our own sample a broad and somewhat leading question was asked: "It is said that in the United States in general, parents and children live alone without other relatives. What do you think of that?" Forty-nine of the women asked (69 percent) approved. In practice, too, the pattern in the lower class seems clear. In a 1948 census of 79,000 *agregado* (landless wage earner) families, only six tenths of one percent were living doubled up. *Plano regulador para el desarrollo de Puerto Rico,* Puerto Rico Planning Board, cited by Mintz, *op. cit.,* Chap. VI, p. 24.

coming back. When one loves a person one adores this person and has no peace. (B4F)

It is the best thing in the world to be in love. It happens when one is young. . . . One wishes that he would never leave one's side, and that other girls will not look at him. One would like him to come to the house and never leave it. It is that desire to have him, even to possess him. (C10F)

That is the most sublime thing in the world. When one is in love, there doesn't exist anything else in the world besides that man. (X10F)

If a majority of the women have a good notion of romantic love, a smaller proportion think it is the crucial factor in marriage. Of the 47 women who were asked question 34D just half felt that being in love with the man was more important than that he should be a good man. The general tone of these responses was that "Love conquers all." The other half felt that it was more important that a man should be good, for in this way a woman will suffer less, regardless of whether or not she loves him. We may conclude that at least a substantial majority of the female respondents know what romantic love is and consider it to be an integral aspect of courtship.

In the light of the fairly long and insulated courtship, the letters, intermediaries, chaperones, and guarded glances, this is understandable. Equally important, however, is the emotional state in which the girl is found prior to marriage. Rebellious against the tyranny of her parents and frustrated by the inability to associate with her boy friend, she is prone to the violent type of emotional attachment described by romantic love. Romantic love may be the *psychological mechanism intervening between parental rebellion and elopement,* providing the dynamism by which this radical move can be made.

One woman described her love as greatly intensified as a result of her parents' opposition, showing one way in which romantic love serves as the intermediary between rebellion and an impetuous action such as early marriage.

I married just because my parents were against him. I think *I loved him more because they were against him.* (A11F)

This is not to say that early marriage and rebelliousness are always accompanied by romantic love or vice versa. Indeed, the deviant-case analysis showed that there are several cases where early or consensual union was not accompanied by rebellion. In some of these cases romantic love by itself seemed to be the reason offered by women for the time and type of marriage; that is, they fell in love and just "didn't think." Romantic love, which seems to be another cause for a suspension of the critical faculties, is closely related to a third factor leading to early marriage—sheer ignorance on the part of the female.

Premarital Ignorance. We have already discussed in detail the manner in which the adolescent girl is carefully shielded from the masculine world, and Table 10 demonstrated the degree to which girls appear ignorant of the facts of sex and childbirth. This ignorance may breed fantastic and romantic notions about the prospective mate. Although girls are disposed to believe that men are inherently evil, their lack of actual experience with them, plus their volatile emotional state in the courtship period, may foster illusions about the courting male. In contrast to what she has been told, her boy friend is solicitous, respectful, and kindly. In contrast to her subjugation and poverty in the parental home, the lover may offer freedom and an improved economic status. Inexperienced with the honeyed words of the male courtship vocabulary, she accepts his enticing promises. Sixteen percent of the women said they married earlier than their ideal age "out of ignorance."

> Men win girls because the girls are less intelligent. . . . They have a weaker mind. . . . Men make girls promises, deceive them, and take them away. (A13F)

> One tells the girls a story, and they fall in love. (C8M)

> I expected [of marriage] a place to live in, to be well treated, and not to have too much work or troubles. (Why did you expect that?) Because that is what men promise when they make love. . . . The only thing I knew about men was what they promised me. (A9F)

The ignorance concerning men is intensified by romantic love. What little knowledge the girl may possess concerning the tabus on early marriage, elopement, and consensual union becomes immobilized by its presence. The lack of basic information and the presence of romantic love are important factors precipitating the girl into an impetuous decision.

(Why did you elope with him?) When one is young *one is blind,* one gets *blind with love* and doesn't have reasons. (X10F)

If my parents had not had me so shut up in the house, I would not have married so soon. I would have had a chance of knowing the man better and perhaps would not have eloped with him. *I knew nothing about life then, and the first one I saw I fell in love with.* One thinks that the world ends there, and it is the best thing to do. (TRE)

One male demonstrated an unusual awareness of the relationship between the cloister, ignorance, romantic love, and elopement.

(Why is it that girls are easily deceived?) There are two reasons. The girls go out of the house less than the boys. They do not have a chance to meet anybody. Then any John Doe comes to them, and they want to marry immediately. The other reason is that they are less educated. (C4M)

The complex of parental rebellion, romantic love, and ignorance, then, helps to explain the young age at marriage for females—an age considerably below that which they consider ideal. It also helps to explain many consensual unions, in the sense that the girl bolts suddenly and without much knowledge or premeditation. This means that there may not be sufficient time or possibility for a legal ceremony, and/or that she follows the inclinations of the male without thinking. What then is the situation of the males as far as early marriage is concerned?

CAUSAL FACTORS IN EARLY MARRIAGE OF THE MALE

In a consideration of the causes of early marriage among Irish farmers in the early nineteenth century, Connell[17] suggests several factors which seem applicable in the case of the lower class in contemporary Puerto Rico. In Ireland at that period, there was no necessity to delay marriage until the father relinquished his land. Matchmaking by parents was not much in evidence, cheap land was available for rent or purchase, and the development of skills and capital prior to marriage was largely unnecessary as well as difficult of attainment. Moreover, the wretchedness of living condi-

[17] K. Connell, *The Population of Ireland, 1750-1845* (Oxford: Clarendon Press, 1950).

tions gave a man a "companion in suffering" and a valuable helper on the farm. In the Puerto Rican group with which we are dealing, income is derived mainly from unskilled wage labor, and a home-made shack rather than agricultural land is practically the only marital prerequisite in the way of possessions. Particularly in the case of consensual unions, only a modest cash outlay is required upon marriage, and there is little or no parental regulation of marital choice. At the same time, there is little necessity or possibility of building up capital, and the wife can supply needed services in the way of laundering, housekeeping, and, possibly, tending a few chickens and a pig. Thus some of the checks on early marriage present in certain other societies are absent among our sample, while the usual positive motivations are present.

This helps to explain why males marry relatively young, but one might still ask why they marry an average of five years later than females, and why more males than females marry at or beyond their expressed ideal. The wishful motives and impulsiveness which seem to be characteristic of females prior to marriage are either absent or of a different nature in the case of the males. In order better to explain this, let us begin by considering the responses of those males who married *earlier* than their ideal age. The reasons for this occurrence fall into several categories. A half dozen men said that even though it was earlier than the general ideal they expressed, in their own case, they felt old enough to marry. In a strict sense, these men did not marry earlier than their ideal.

Another small group said they did so to get away from home, but their responses do not show the kind of rebellion evidenced by the girls. Rather, they show strong mother attachments which, in one way or another, were disturbed, usually by conflicts with the father. In two cases the mother died. In one of these cases, the man could not get along with a stepmother; in the other, he could not get along with his father. Another case had constant quarrels with his father and married to get away from this situation. Another did not get along with his stepfather. The final case in this group was a professional musician whose parents would not let him sleep late enough in the mornings.

A half dozen cases said they married young "out of ignorance," but, again, their responses do not have the same tone as do those of the women. Four out of six of the respondents in this group explained what they meant by ignorance. In all four cases they referred to the fact that they were not sufficiently aware of the *economic* difficulties which go with marriage. That is, if they had a chance to do it over again, they would save more money or secure a house or a piece of land.

A large group gave direct or implicit references to their mothers to explain their early marriages. Six said they married early to have some one look after or take care of them, and three cases explained that their mothers had died, leaving them without anyone to look after them. With respect to romantic love, we might expect that the insulated courtship, plus the projection of the mother ideal on the prospective mate, might involve a good deal of romanticizing. The latter hypothesis has been advanced by Sereno for the middle-class male[18] but would not seem to hold for the lower class.

In the first place, the sexual frustration which ordinarily fans the flames of romantic love is not so characteristic of the lower-class male. Sexual love for the fiancée is at once more repressed than in our culture and at the same time transferred to the Eves or impure women. Second, lower-class courtship is not characterized by the extreme competition so conducive to romantic love in American society. Once the male begins courting the female, other males do not in general compete for her affections. The competitive dating characteristic of American society is simply not a part of courtship in Puerto Rico.[19] Third, the wife-as-mother ideal leaves little room for romance. In addition to desiring a pure, kindly, and protective mother figure in a wife, men express such mundane and easily ob-

[18] R. Sereno, "Cryptomelanism: A Study of Color Relations and Personal Insecurity in Puerto Rico," *Psychiatry*, X, No. 3 (August 1947), 267.

[19] There is perhaps more "competition," or at least anxiety, on the part of *women* for men, for the latter are allowed much more freedom. This may be another factor contributing to the higher frequency of romantic love among women. For a discussion of the competitive aspect of romantic love in American society, see K. Davis, "Romantic Love and Courtship," in Davis, Bredemeier, and Levy, eds., *Modern American Society* (New York: Rinehart, 1949), p. 591.

tainable ideals as a woman who will be attentive to their elementary needs[20]—in short, a housekeeper.[21]

I was looking for someone who could fix my clothes. (Anything else?) One who could do housework. (H24M)

I had to marry. I had nobody to do my things. My earnings were not sufficient to pay the person who was doing my things. (H12M)

I was searching for a wife to do my laundry. (H15M)

Whereas 30 percent of the women gave "I fell in love" as the principal reason for marriage, only 7 percent of the men gave reasons even resembling romantic love. These were of the "I wanted a woman" or "I was anxious to get married" type rather than expressive of romantic love. The attachment to the mother and the absence of romantic love may be two of the factors which keep age at marriage higher for men and more in line with their ideals. Of the 19 men who married at an age three or more years later than their ideal, seven gave their mothers as reasons for the delay. The quotations below leave no doubt that romantic love would be difficult in the face of such strong mother-son bonds.

I married at the age of twenty-four because my mother died, and I felt the necessity of having a woman who could take care of me and who could love me. . . . As I had my mother alive before that, I saw no need in getting married. (C4M)

I married at twenty-seven because I had my mother who did every-

[20] Senior came to the same conclusion in dealing with lower-class Puerto Rican family heads in New York City. "The explanation for missing the families was never made in any except the following three terms: 'If my wife was here, she could fix my food'; 'If my wife was here, she could keep house for me'; 'If my wife and children were here, they could work in defense plants and earn money too.' If romantic love entered into the mind of any worker, it was not expressed on the questionnaire from which these data were gathered" C. Senior, "Puerto Rican Emigration" (University of Puerto Rico, mimeographed, 1947), p. 26.

[21] The housekeeper ideal does not appear to be restricted to the lower class, nor is there any seeming embarrassment about its admission. In a recent column of *El Imparcial's* Inquiring Photographer, the question was asked, "Why did you get married?" The respondent quoted is a well-dressed taxi owner. "When I was single, I was spending too much money on laundry, meals, and rooms; and I thought it would be better to get married in order to avoid so much expense. Despite the fact that I now have a wife and two children, I find married life much cheaper than when I was single, since I don't have to spend so much eating out, sending out laundry, and sleeping in hotels."

thing for me. For that reason I had no need for getting married. When my mother died, I decided to get married. (X7M)

I had sexual relations with women and I didn't need to have a steady woman at twenty-one. My mother gave me everything I needed. I had clean clothes and food and I didn't need a wife yet. (B5M)

This line of reasoning, pushed to its extreme, might raise the question as to why men ever marry. If their sexual needs are filled by prostitutes and "cheap women," and their emotional and physical requirements satisfied by their mothers, why should they marry? One reason which we have already observed in respondents' statements is the cultural prescription to marry. As most of the men who married at or around their ideal said, "It was time to get married." That is, even where the situation is desirable at home, a man is expected to get married. While he can postpone it and enjoy for a few extra years the maternal blessing, public opinion will eventually be pushing him toward marriage. Of some importance, too, is the need to prove one's virility and fecundity, and the only socially permissible fashion of having children is within marriage.

Thus, extremely few of the males have any of the impetuous and wishful predispositions which encourage early marriage for females. Frequently their age at marriage seems to a large degree dependent upon their relations with their mothers. If they feel satisfied with these relations, they take their time about marriage. If for some reason, however, they feel this relationship disturbed (by death, remarriage, or too much competition for the mother's affection), they seek a protective mother figure at an earlier age. In neither case does their decision seem accompanied by romantic love, by ignorance about women, or by the type of parental rebellion seen in the case of the girls. Despite, and perhaps because of, the search for a mother substitute and housekeeper, we would expect more reasoned and calculated choices concerning the time and type of marriage.

CONSENSUAL MARRIAGE

If a common-law marriage may be defined as "an unlicensed, unrecorded and nonceremonial marriage,"[22] the *unión consensual* so

[22] A. C. Jacobs, "Common Law Marriage," in *Encyclopedia of the Social Sciences.*

prevalent in Puerto Rico might be considered a synonym for common-law unions. It is distinct from concubinage in that among the lower class the woman has roughly the same *social* status as a legal wife, and in that usually neither partner is married to another. It is distinct from the casual sexual liason in that it is a relatively permanent union, though, as we shall see, it is somewhat more brittle than a legal union.

However, the consensual union differs from the common-law marriage in that it has never received the legal sanction throughout Latin America which common-law unions have received in Europe and the United States. Puerto Rican law does not distinguish the concubine (in common parlance, the *querida*) from the consensual wife or *concubina.* By law, both are *concubinas* and are denied support, inheritance, and name.

In previous decades, a distinction in status was made between children born from these unions. Legitimate children[23] were products of legal unions only; *natural* children, products of consensual unions; and illegitimate children, the product of *querida* or casual relationships. The latter children received no inheritance, support, or name by law, whereas the natural child had most, but not all, of the rights of legitimate children. Legislation within the past decade has removed the distinction between natural and illegitimate, granting both the status and rights of natural children.[24]

[23] Consensual unions are largely responsible for Puerto Rico's high rate of illegitimacy, another factor which makes the institution of interest to the sociologist. In 1950, one-third of the island's 85,455 births were classified as illegitimate (*Annual Book of Statistics of Puerto Rico,* 1950-1951, Table 17, p. 35), but consensual unions are largely accountable for this seemingly high number. A study conducted in 1936 demonstrated that, if births stemming from consensual unions were deducted from the number of total illegitimate births, the illegitimacy rate would only be 4.6 per hundred births, not greatly above the rate of 3.2 for the United States at that time. J. Rosario, *A Study of Illegitimacy and Dependent Children in Puerto Rico* (San Juan: Imprenta Venezuela, 1936), p. 31.

[24] Currently, half of a man's inheritance must go to his legal wife, The other half has three divisions. *La Parte legítima* is divided equally between the legitimate and natural offspring (if the latter were born after 1942); *la parte mejor* also must go to the children but can be distributed according to the preferences of the deceased; and the third, termed *libre disposición* (or free testament) can be distributed in any way the deceased wishes. Concubines and consensual wives have no rights to property.

Efforts to elevate consensual unions to the status of common-law marriages

There are two reasons for discussing consensual unions in some detail. First, we already have had some evidence that early age at marriage and consensual union are often the joint or separate product of the same cause or causes. Second, consensual unions may bear some relation to fertility. For example, we have Hatt's data which suggest that the consensually married are less fertile. In the lower rental category, those women whose marital unions had all been legal had 533 pregnancies per 100 women, while those women whose unions had not all been legal had only 465 per 100 women. Women whose present or last union was legal showed 3.8 pregnancies in the first nine years of marriage, while those in consensual unions showed only 3.4.[25]

Hatt suggests that the difference in fertility may be due to the more temporary nature of the consensual union, a factor which reduces exposure to pregnancy. Our own qualitative data would suggest that there may be a tendency for consensual unions to be *more* fertile, if exposure is held constant, since individuals living in such unions tend to remarry and desire a new family with each new partner. This will be given some discussion in Chapter IX. For the present, we may examine the extent and possible causes of this type of marriage.

Approximately one quarter of Puerto Rico's married couples live

in Puerto Rico occurred as early as 1903 and as late as 1943. The law passed in the former instance was revoked after three years, and in the latter instance, the proposed law was defeated in the Senate. *Código Civil de Puerto Rico,* Ley de 12 de marzo de 1903, p. 119, and Ley de 7 de marzo de 1906, p. 103. See also L. Muñoz Morales, *Reseña histórica y anotaciones al Código Civil de Puerto Rico* (Santurce: Imprenta Soltero, 1947).

The most recent decision, however, while denying the legality of the consensual union, has operated to enhance inheritance opportunities for the consensual wife. "An agreement between a man and a woman to share property acquired by them while living together is valid. If there is no contract to share the property acquired while living consensually, the woman can recover her proportional share of the property for which she contributed her capital and labor" (Torres vs. Roldán, 67 DPR 367, May 23, 1947).

[25] Hatt, *op. cit.,* Tables 310 and 271, pp. 434 and 316. In a study of six hundred Mexican factory workers, a similar finding was made. Whereas the mean number of children was 3.84 for men living in unions contracted by religious ceremony, men living in "free" unions had an average of 2.86. W. Moore, "Attitudes of Mexican Factory Workers toward Fertility Control," in *Approaches to Problems of High Fertility in Agrarian Societies* (New York: Milbank Memorial Fund, 1952), p. 81.

without legal bonds.[26] Table 21 shows, as might be expected, that type of union is highly correlated with economic class and education.

TABLE 21

MARITAL STATUS OF EVER-MARRIED ADULTS BY ECONOMIC CLASS AND EDUCATION

Percentage of each class currently living in a consensual union[a]

	Percent
Lowest rental category	47.2
Highest rental category	21.0
No school	46.6
13 or more years in school	11.3

[a] Extracted from P. K. Hatt, *Backgrounds of Human Fertility in Puerto Rico: A Sociological Survey* (Princeton: Princeton University Press, 1952), Tables 98 and 99, pp. 127f. For facility of presentation only the polar categories are illustrated above. Hatt's figures show a steady progression of legal marriages from the lowest to the highest class and educational categories. Basing his conclusion on anthropological field studies, Steward makes a similar kind of generalization: "Where property or social status are involved, marriage is usually religious or civil; where neither counts, it tends to be consensual." J. Steward, "Cultural Patterns of Puerto Rico," *Annals of the American Academy of Political and Social Science*, CCLXXXV (Jan. 1952), 97.

Consensual unions do not seem to be declining at any significant rate. Hatt's data (based on the proportions of consensually married, according to age) show no decline,[27] and census materials for Puerto Rico show only a fairly small and slow decline.[28] Both the extent and persistence of consensual unions, then, are additional reasons for our interest in this institution.

Historical reasons may briefly be considered. The early Spanish settlers, almost completely male, quickly took Borinquen women to live with them. Even after the arrival of Spanish wives, concubines were kept in the country and wives in the city.[29] Additionally, when

[26] 1950 Census of Population, Preliminary Report, Table 1.

[27] Hatt, *op. cit.*, Table 232, p. 266.

[28] For the decades from 1910 to 1950, the percentage of consensually married females of all mated females was 30.7, 26.3, 27.0, 27.4, and 24.9 (computed from United States Census Reports).

[29] Rosario, *op. cit.*, pp. 8–10.

the Negro slaves arrived, there was little effort on the part of the *hacendados* either to give them religious instruction or to encourage religious marriage. Thus, both by personal example and as a matter of policy, the early settlers set the scene for widespread casual unions.[30]

The historical basis, however, does not explain the institutionalizing and long survival of the pattern. One popular explanation is that the cost of a wedding and/or a wedding license keeps the lower class from legal unions. Although the point has some validity, its importance has been greatly exaggerated. While a full-dress wedding can be expensive, a civil marriage is cheap.[31] Were social consensus unequivocally behind legal marriage, the money would be found, as it is for other more socially significant events. Among the women who married consensually in the present sample, only a few even mentioned cost as a factor.[32]

ATTITUDES TOWARD CONSENSUAL UNION

The sum of evidence on consensual unions would suggest that it is by and large socially disapproved, but that this social disapproval is not of the intense type which insures a high degree of conformity. Hatt found that 67 percent of the males and females think it is a bad or very bad way of life for a *man*; and that 82 percent of the males and 86 percent of the females think it is a bad or very bad way of life for a *woman*.[33] Over 90 percent oppose it as a way of life for their daughters.[34] The attitudes are, of course, correlated with class, but even in Hatt's lowest rental group, in which favorable

[30] Mintz, *op. cit.*, Chapter VI, p. 6. Davis summarizes three historical influences which set the pattern for concubines in Latin America in general: (1) priestly concubinage; (2) the influence of Moorish polygyny; (3) frontier conditions in Latin America. The absence of Spanish women and cultural restraints, plus the presence of caste distinctions between settlers and native women, encouraged illegal unions. K. Davis, "Changing Modes of Marriage: Contemporary Family Types," in Becker and Hill, eds., *Marriage and the Family* (Boston: Heath and Co., 1942), p. 101.

[31] Actually it is free, if conducted during the office hours of the Justice of the Peace. The only cost—and this is optional—is fifty cents for a copy of the wedding license. This is approximately one-third the price of a bottle of rum.

[32] See p. 111 for other reasons.

[33] Hatt, *op. cit.*, Tables 43 and 44, pp. 61 and 62.

[34] *Ibid*, Table 45, p. 64.

attitudes reach their peak, 60.9 percent of the sample disapprove of it for men, and 76.8 percent disapprove of it for women.[35]

Our own data back up Hatt's general findings, but add a qualitative note. While the large majority of respondents seem genuinely to oppose consensual unions for themselves and others, the intensity with which this opinion is held does not seem strong. In relating the history of their marriage, for example, some women told of the immediate fury of their parents over their elopements into consensual marriages. However, not only was the bulk of the anger directed at the idea of *elopement* (a breach of parental authority), but parents and children were soon reconciled, without further demands about legal marriage. The responses of several men suggested that the anger was ceremonial and the whole procedure a kind of ritual. When asked what they would do if their daughters married consensually, they replied that they would be furious. When asked how long that fury would last, however, they replied, "For a few days," or "A little while," or "Until I thought she was punished enough." The examples below provide an idea of the intensity of the value of legal marriage.

> I would let her suffer for a time. *I would hate her to remind her that I'm her father.* Not him, because she's the one who hasn't taken my advice. . . . If he had persuaded her to elope, both are guilty *and I would hate them both for a time.* (H24M)

> I would show her as long as I live that she acted badly, especially if she eloped with an unreliable man. (And if he is a good man?) I would try to get them married. I would never hold it against her, but against the man—*except if he is a good man.* (C3M)

> I would like them to marry at home, but if they elope with a good man, it would not be bad. Now, if the man is bad, I would not agree with that. (What would you do?) *I would be angry with them for two or three months* and then I would be pleased because she is part of my blood. (A13M)

One might conclude that consensual union is, in Linton's terms, a *cultural alternative.* Marriage is split into two culturally permissible alternatives. While the legal marriage is generally prefer-

[35] *Ibid,* Tables 120 and 122, pp. 151 and 153. The most frequent reason given for not favoring this type of union was that "society disapproves." Religious reasons were infrequently mentioned.

able,[36] it is not so much more preferable to the consensual as to induce all to choose it. The two patterns exist side by side, practically everyone paying lip service to the superiority of the one, but with about a quarter of the married population practicing the other.

But why is one alternative chosen rather than another? While a separate research project would be required to answer this question, we may venture a few hypotheses. One would be that, just as women enter blindly into early marriage, they enter equally blindly into consensual marriage, allowing the male to determine the mode of marriage. Another hypothesis would be that women see considerable advantage in the consensual union, the possibility for desertion operating as leverage for them in their marital relationships. An hypothesis to explain the choice by many *men* of this type of union would be that the child-rearing and courtship systems are such as to generate anxiety about the prospective marital partner. This anxiety might result in a variation of the trial marriage, from which the person has easy recourse to desertion if the marriage does not work out. Unfortunately, men were not systematically queried in the area of consensual union, and we must rely on the testimony of their wives. With this limitation in mind, we may proceed to examine the above-stated hypotheses.

MOTIVATIONS IN CHOOSING CONSENSUAL MARRIAGE

A detailed examination of the female responses with regard to the question of consensual union disclosed three basic types on a "calculated" to "nonreasoned" continuum. A little over half of the cases married consensually simply because their husbands wanted it that

[36] The existence of alternatives, while it weakens the strength of both norms, does not, of course, preclude the general desirability of one of the alternatives. The data seem to indicate that a good proportion of consensual unions are subsequently legalized. Hatt found considerably more consensual unions among the young than among the old. Thirty-five percent of all present or last marriages were consensual or concubinal for those nineteen years of age and younger, while less than 19 percent of those fifty years of age and older were so united. Hatt, *op. cit.*, Table 232, p. 266. One explanation for this would be a tendency for consensually married couples to legalize their unions later in life. Sporadic drives by the Catholic Church to marry the spiritually unmarried in Puerto Rico undoubtedly contribute to this trend. However, the fact that so many older individuals remain nonlegally married, despite special drives, justifies the hypothesis that the institution is functional to the individuals and/or society.

way. These cases did not think about the advantages or disadvantages of such a union but blindly followed the husband's lead. Roughly another third of the cases saw advantages in this type of union, but feel (at least now) that these are outweighed by disadvantages. Nevertheless, this group also followed the lead of the husband. In some of these cases, we get a blend of romantic blindness and of reasoning. Love, in these cases, was not so blind that certain advantages to this type of marriage were not realized. The type is well expressed in the quotation below.

I loved him. I was blind as I had never been before. . . . I was so blind that I didn't think about a legal marriage, and he didn't suggest it. I have never mentioned it. The truth is that I was married to the first one and suffered so much that I thought it would be better not to be so tied down again. (Z6F)

There is, finally, a small core of women who were completely rational about consensual union. Most of this group seem to have prompted their suitors into this type of union and to have resisted their subsequent suggestions to marry.

If we take the latter two groups and examine their reasons for seeing advantages in consensual unions, we can learn a great deal more about the advantages and disadvantages of such unions.

Differential Authority Allocation. At the outset of the study, one of the hypotheses advanced was that consensual union was of greater advantage to the woman. This was based on the notion that the tensions conceivably engendered by differential authority allocation in marriage might be assuaged for the woman by consensual marriage. That is, in a legal union, by nature of the subordination pattern, an incompatible husband could be more trying to his wife than could an incompatible wife be to her husband—*Es la mujer la que paga* (It's the woman who pays). In the consensual union, on the other hand, it is easier to hold out the threat of desertion, thereby bringing differential authority allocation into greater equilibrium. This would seem to produce a more satisfactory, if less stable, relationship for the woman.[37] On the basis of a community

[37] Similar conclusions have been reached for the lower-class family of the British West Indies. According to Henriques, women fear domination by the male in legal marriages. "In practice unmarried union leads to equality between the sexes" (F. Henriques, "West Indian Family Organization," *American Journal of Sociology,* LV No. 1 (July 1949), p. 33.

study, Mintz, in writing that "the lower-class women are as opposed to formal Church marriages as their men,"[38] tended to support the general hypothesis. Petrullo stated more flatly that attempts to put an end to the custom of consensual marriage failed because of resistance from the women, who felt that the husband would wield too much authority in a legal union.[39] Our own data give only scant support for this hypothesis.

Only 4 women thought there was more advantage for women than for men in consensual union, and only 8 others felt there were equal advantages for both sexes. Twenty-two women felt there was some advantage, but less than for the men, and the remainder could see no advantage for the woman at all. Significantly, consensually married women saw no more advantages to this type of union than did legally married women.

TABLE 22

ADVANTAGES FOR THE WOMAN IN CONSENSUAL UNION, BY MARITAL STATUS

	Legally Married (percent)	*Consensually Married (percent)*
No advantage for the female	53	50
Some advantage, but less than for the male	28	35
Same or greater advantage for the female	19	15
	100	100
Number of respondents	(36)	(34)

Of those who saw advantages, only a few cited those which were hypothesized concerning differential authority allocation. However, the fact that *any* woman gave this reason is of interest. Such women suggested that the wife has more rights in legal marriage but that she also has more duties. They felt that the formal bond makes greater demands on the woman than the informal type. Moreover,

[38] Mintz, *op. cit.*, Chapter VI, p. 13.

[39] V. Petrullo, *Puerto Rican Paradox* (Philadelphia: University of Pennsylvania, 1947), p. 129.

the woman always feels free to threaten the husband with desertion if he disapproves excessively of her behavior—something which would be more difficult were the marriage legalized.

Being married, one must be more respectful, one cannot go out too much. . . . My husband doesn't want me to go out, but I go on my own. If I were married, I wouldn't do it. (Why?) I wouldn't dare. Being married you must be more respectful. (X6F)

If married, there is more obligation on the part of the woman. Not married, [the husband] has no right to claim anything. (Y8F)

If he is not married to her and she wants to go some place and he doesn't approve of it, she could tell him, "As I'm not married to you, I'll go, for the only thing you can do to me is to leave me." (C1F)

In contrast to those women who see fewer obligations in consensual marriage, however, there are considerably more women who accent the fewer *rights* which a woman has. When married, moreover, one has the greater blessing of the community, and some women desire this added prestige.

[Married], she has more prestige; and her husband will treat her better. The girl who elopes with a man, even if they marry later, can always be treated badly by the man. He may throw it at her. (H6F)

Now I wish I were married. If I had married my first husband, I would have had more rights. . . . I have wished a million times I had married. One has more rights. Other women respect the married woman more. (H9F)

A second hypothesis originally advanced to explain the extent and durability of consensual union proved more fruitful.[40] This hypothesis can be summarized as follows: The women, and perhaps the men, of Puerto Rico's lower class enter marriage with a certain sense of anxiety.[41] The insulated courtship system means that it is difficult to judge the compatibility of a prospective mate, and the

[40] It is interesting that both hypotheses were based on the assumption of rational action. As the preceding section demonstrated, however, nonrational factors are no less, and possibly even more, important than the rational ones outlined in this section. The unraveling of such unanticipated nonrational motivations is a striking illustration of the advantage of the flexible interview form.

[41] See Chapter IV.

difficulty and expense of divorce make it nearly impossible to rectify a poor choice. These factors make the cultural alternative of consensual union highly attractive, for it can be used as a kind of trial marriage.[42]

We have already seen that women are very ignorant about men prior to marriage. What knowledge they have may be productive of anxiety, for it suggests that males are exploiters of the female. On the other hand, we have suggested that romantic love often causes a temporary suspension of these fears to the extent that the woman trusts the man who takes her away into a consensual union. But in many cases love was not so blind as to exclude all practical considerations. Such considerations serve as additional stimuli for entering consensual unions and are of particular importance in explaining their duration.

The Trial Marriage. Given the premarital anxieties about the opposite sex and the inability for the reality testing due to the insulated courtship system, some kind of trial marriage would seem functional. In the United States, where a double standard is less in evidence, where young males need rely less on prostitutes for premarital experience and more on women whom they may subsequently marry, and where long periods of sexual and other interpersonal relationships precede marriage, there is less risk involved in a permanent commitment. Moreover, in the United States, if the courtship experience proves deceptive, divorce is a relatively simple expedient, and serial marriage may compensate for the inadequacy of premarital experimentation.

In Puerto Rico, however, the situation is blocked at both ends. On the one hand, premarital experiences with one's future mate are minimal, and, on the other, the poor or religious cannot resort to

[42] A trial marriage, not in the technical sense of the "companionate marriage" but rather in the sense that the marriage is seen as providing a way out if not successful. Havelock Ellis has observed precisely the same phenomenon in Europe: "The more or less permanent free unions formed among us in Europe are usually to be regarded merely as trial-marriages. That is to say, they are a precaution rendered desirable, both by uncertainty as to either the harmony or the fruitfulness of union until actual experiment has been made, and by the practical impossibility of otherwise rectifying any mistake in consequence of the antiquated rigidity of most European divorce laws" (*Studies in the Psychology of Sex*, New York, Random House, 1942 II, 379).

divorce.[43] To what extent is such reasoning articulated by the respondents in the sample?

The advantage of consensual union most frequently stated by Hatt's respondents was that it provides greater freedom.[44] The qualitative interviews of the present study have refined this concept of freedom and shown that the attitude stems from the constrictive nature of the courtship and marriage institution.

In this context, it seems that "freedom" means "*freedom to correct a mistake.*" Men and women know so little about each other that a mistake is quite easy to make, and it is little wonder that the trial marriage is a frequent expedient. A number of women suggested that, previous to marriage, they had had doubts about the worth of the prospective husband and had conceived of consensual marriage as the safest way of finding out.

I used to say that if he turned out too dominant, I could leave him. (Z5F)

I didn't expect to live long with him, and I used to say, "Well, if he doesn't suit me, I will leave." (X3F)

. . . one can't marry a man without living with him a while and knowing how he behaves. (H23F)

Many of the respondents who discussed the advantages mentioned the difficulty of divorce. At the time of marriage, they felt that to make an irreversible decision would be taking too great a risk and preferred to leave the door open just in case.[45]

I said to myself that I'd never get married, for I thought that, if I

[43] Over the past decade, the highest peak in divorce reached by Puerto Rico was in 1946, when the rate was 1.9 divorces per 1,000 population. At the same time the rate in the United States was 4.4. "Post-war Divorce Rates Here and Abroad," *Statistical Bulletin,* June 1952. Per hundred marriages, Puerto Rico's rate in 1949 was only 0.16 as compared with 2.8 in the United States. *Annual Book of Statistics of Puerto Rico, 1949–1950,* Table 8, p. 9. While no evidence is at hand, it is probable that the rate for the lower class is much lower.

[44] Sixty percent of the respondents who favored consensual union for females gave "more freedom" as their reason, and about 90 percent gave this reason for favoring this type of union for males. Hatt, *op. cit.,* Tables 46 and 47, pp. 64 and 65.

[45] Petrullo, without stating evidence, contended that, since breaking a consensual union is moving *from* a state of sin, the person need never fear the wrath of the priest, and that this was a major factor in explaining consensual unions. While plausible, this explanation finds no confirmation in the present study. See Petrullo, *op. cit.,* p. 129.

took a man who was bad, I could leave him without having to go to court for a divorce. (X5F)

I thought that, if it came out bad, I could leave him without having to go to any court to get a divorce. (X9F)

. . . if something happens between them, there would be no problems of rights. They don't have to get divorced. They just separate. (Z3F)

Other respondents suggest that the consensual marriage, if successful, is followed by legal marriage.

If the woman turns out bad, one leaves her. . . . If she is good, one marries her. (H13M)

If the wife does not turn out well, one separates easily from her. If she turns out to be a fine worker and faithful, one may marry her later. (H7M)

The advantage is the trial. If it works, one gets married, and if not, one doesn't. (C3F)

To a certain extent we know this is true. Hatt's data, showing the much higher percentage of consensual unions among the young, might indicate a tendency for consensual unions to be legalized. However, in *most* instances the marriages are not legalized. There seem to be several reasons for this. First of all, we have seen that the attitudes concerning legal marriage are not intense, so that a person who has married consensually faces some disapproval, but no disgrace, in the eyes of the community. As a lower-class saying goes, "A good consensual union is worth more than a bad marriage" (*Vale más un buen amancebado que un matrimonio mal llevado*). Second, the great importance placed on virginity and the Virgin makes the ceremony of marriage intimately associated with female virginity. The marriage ceremony is a *rite de passage* signaling imminent penetration. Once the latter has occurred without a ceremony, however, a subsequent ceremony loses some of its point. One woman expressed this eloquently.

He wanted me to marry after we had lived together for some time, but I refused. . . . I believe it makes no difference married or unmarried. . . . I told him to forget it, that that was for virgins. . . . After one has been opened (*destapona'o*), what are you going to be married for? After all, one behaves correctly and is modest. One is as much a lady as being married. (Y7F)

A male respondent expresses the same sentiment when he states that he married legally *because* his wife-to-be was a virgin.

She was a virgin. That was why I married her. (If she had not been a virgin, would you have married her?) I don't believe so . . . then there wouldn't have been the need for marriage. Then we would live together without being married. (Y2M)

Additionally, there may be the feeling, after the *fait accompli,* that a church wedding would be "deceiving the virgin." One woman, while able to face the Virgin, could not face the priest.

A week after eloping he suggested that I call the priest to marry us, but I was ashamed and didn't want to. (C3F)

A third reason for continuing consensual union is the suspicion and hostility between the sexes which continue even after marriage. Neither partner is completely sure that his mate is faithful or will remain that way forever. One can never be completely sure when to give a permanent commitment. In such a context, a perpetual test is required.

As she has had another husband, I must test her first. (But you have lived together for seven years now.) Yes, but I want to test her better. (H13M)

I heard a man saying that he had lived nine years with a woman without being married, waiting to see how she was before marrying her. (C3F)

Finally, there is the fact that the lower-class male tends to be interested in more than one woman, consensual unions being one version of serial marriage. Thus we might guess that many men want their freedom in the sense of freedom for other women. There is no evidence for any such motivation in the woman, but in two cases consensual marriage was seen as a stepping stone to other opportunities. In one case, the woman told of a detailed plot in which she planned to elope consensually with a man so that she would escape from her parents and be taken to the city. There she would find work, desert the man, and have her independence. The union was conceived of as a means to escape parental and male domination and to enter the labor force. This case represents the extreme type of rational motivation for the woman.[46]

[46] This case is a unique example of the transitional effects of industrialization and urbanization on the family. The rebellious girl in the traditional society must marry to escape her parents. In the modern society she can

If the analysis concerning the trial-marriage aspects of consensual unions is correct, it would suggest a higher rate of separation for such couples than would be expected in legal marriages. The opposite is a frequently held opinion. Some observers have suggested that consensual unions are as permanent as legal unions. There is considerable truth in this, but in their effort to extol the moral virtues of the lower class such observers have greatly exaggerated their point. The fact is that consensual marriages are considerably more brittle than are legal marriages, although not so brittle as the moralist might expect. In the present sample for example, despite a median age of only 29.5 for women and 34.5 for men, there has been a considerable number of separations. Sixteen of the women and 15 of the men have had three or four unions, and 4 men have had five or six. Hatt's more reliable data show a similar tendency. In his lower rental group, 5 percent of all the married women whose unions had all been legal were divorced or separated, while 15 percent of the women whose unions had not all been legal were separated or divorced.[47] Table 23, computed from Hatt's data, shows that this holds true when residence and class are controlled.

TABLE 23

PERCENTAGE OF EVER-MARRIED WOMEN AT PRESENT DIVORCED OR SEPARATED, BY MONTHLY RENTAL VALUE OF HOME, TYPE OF MARITAL EXPERIENCE, AND RURAL-URBAN RESIDENCE[a]

	All Unions Legal	*Not All Unions Legal*
Higher rental		
Urban	7.9	19.2
Rural	4.2	9.6
Lower rental		
Urban	10.2	16.7
Rural	4.0	10.3

[a] From Hatt, Table 307, p. 431

migrate and work. In the transitional society, ideally, she may have to do both, using marriage as a stepping stone to migration and work opportunities.

[47] Hatt, *op. cit.*, Table 306, p. 616.

CONCLUSIONS

Early age at marriage, particularly for women, is a pattern fairly typical of the lower class in Puerto Rico. Chief among the motivations for women are such nonrational factors as parental rebellion, romantic love, and erroneous conceptions of marriage. Singly or in combination, these lead the girl into the impetuous kind of action which results in an early rupture with the family and in a sudden elopement in which there may be little opportunity for legal marriage. Moreover, they leave her prey to the type of marriage desired by the male.

By and large, these nonrational elements are not present in the case of the male. He has had a good deal of premarital experience with women, he cannot or need not rebel from his family and is not so prone to romantic love. Consequently, he feels no great need to marry as early or as impetuously. In many cases, whether or not the male marries early or late appears to depend upon how satisfactorily his emotional and physical needs are being satisfied at home.

With regard to consensual marriage, most males would appear to choose this type of union in a more or less rational fashion. As a result of the insulated courtship custom, many males do not feel secure about their prospective partners and resort to a more satisfactory cultural alternative, which provides an easy outlet for a poor choice. A small minority of women also appear to see such advantages and prefer the consensual union for this reason. Men, moreover, tend to use this type of marriage as a kind of serial polygyny, perhaps thereby better satisfying their *machismo* drives. In many cases the male stirs up the girl's desire for liberty and security by promises of freedom, love, and economic sustenance, and convinces her that elopement into consensual marriage is the advisable method. Partly blinded by rebellion, romance, or ignorance, partly seeing advantages in the union, she will follow his lead.

The reasons why many unions are not subsequently legalized would seem to be based not only on the realization of their advantage (indeed, most women see these as less important than the disadvantages) but also on the fact that, once the union has been accomplished, the community sees it as a *fait accompli,* and the wives may be embarrassed to "deceive the Virgin" or to undergo a ceremony that "is a thing for virgins." The husbands, of course, keep other pastures in mind.

The foregoing analysis has drawn on elements of child rearing and courtship to show how they affect age at, and form of, marriage. The following chapters will show how such early patterns affect relationships within marriage, and how these in turn relate to fertility.

VI

Marital Relations

El matrimonio es como el flamboyán. Al principio todas son flores y después todas son vainas.
Marriage is like the flamboyant tree. First it's all flowers and then it goes to seed. A PUERTO RICAN SAYING

They fall in love as I did and think heaven is coming, without knowing that what really comes is hell.
A FEMALE RESPONDENT

DOMINANCE RELATIONSHIPS

That so many women marry with the idea of escaping the domination of their parents appears somewhat ironic when we consider the dominance relations between husband and wife. Subsequent to marriage some women are shocked to discover that they are still cloistered to a considerable extent.[1] One woman, who reported she married in order to escape *el gremio de los padres* (the lap of the parents), sees in retrospect that at least *they* were disciplining her for her own good.

I believed there was more freedom in marriage because parents discipline and inhibit (*cohibían*) us, but it's for our own sake. The husband, however, imprisons us. . . . *You think you can gain your freedom by getting married, but you only get more tied down.* (TRD)

Another woman, in contrasting the father with the husband, showed that the husband's authority is greater and more awesome than the father's.

[1] When asked what things their husbands forbid them to do, 38 women mentioned going out alone, 24 dancing with other men, and 8 gossiping with the neighbors. It is quite likely that many of the other women were taking such matters for granted and felt no necessity to mention them. This is made more likely by the fact that the most traditional women (see following pages) cited no more restrictions than did the least traditional women. Only 11 women in the sample claimed that their husbands forbade them nothing.

His authority over you is stronger than your father's. You can wheedle things out of your father but not from your husband. When he says no, it's *no*. (B8F)

In general, however, our evidence suggests that women adapt themselves to the new pattern of authority, assuaging their feelings either through the martyr complex or through the consolation that all women are in the same boat. As one woman put it, "Mal de muchos, consuelo de todos" (The misfortune of many is the consolation of all). Women have lived so long under the domination of their fathers that the new domination of the husband, while it may be a bitter disillusionment, is really nothing new.

One comes out of the home of one's parents to live with the husband. He acts like a father . . . he is like a father. (C7F)

Evidence of acceptance of their roles, for example, is seen when women are asked who has more freedom, males or females. Only three women feel that the sexes have equal freedom, yet all but two in the sample approve of greater freedom for males.[2]

MARITAL-STATUS IDEOLOGIES

The ideologies which rationalize the superiority of the male find their greatest behavioral expression in the relationship between husband and wife. The general ideology is clearly expressed in a Catholic publication for university students.

Woman . . . owes her gratitude to man for two reasons: for the gift of her existence and for the gift of her supernatural resemblance to God. . . . But resemblance is not equality. Every man owes protection to woman. Every woman should help her man. . . . Man is not for her, but she is for man.[3]

[2] This may, of course, be misleading, since we are dealing only with relatively well adjusted families, at least by the criterion of intactness. The high rates of desertion among the lower class may indicate that many women are not willing to accept their new masters. When we consider that it is precisely the rebellious women who tend to enter consensual marriages, and that consensual marriages are more easily broken, it is quite possible that many of these women rebelled again. Other studies should direct more careful inquiry at the causes for separation.

[3] *Verbo*, III, No. 2 (Jan. 1952), 48. Several men opined that "Women are for the use of men," directly parellelling the quotation from *Verbo*. A few mentioned the Bible as sanctioning female subservience, and one used the Adam's rib myth to rationalize the dominance of males.

The respondents in our sample echo this ideology. Table 24 classifies the responses to the question, "What is your idea of a good wife?"

TABLE 24

DEFINITION OF THE GOOD WIFE

Distribution of responses to Q.22,M, and Q.30,F[a]

	Males (percent)	*Females (percent)*
Good housekeeper and mother	54	26
Faithful	40	55
Attentive to husband's needs	40	76
Obedient	51	32
Respectful	31	40
Considerate, compliant	20	37
Helpful	23	14
Loves husband	4	18
Does not deny (sexually)	3	7
Loyal	1	6
Other responses[b]	10	23
Number of respondents	(71)	(72)
Total responses	(197)	(242)

[a] Percentages are based on the number of respondents rather than responses. Since most respondents cited more than one characteristic, percentages total more than 100.

[b] "Other" responses of the males composed 6 percent of the total responses. Examples are, "Should go to the movies with her husband"; "Should not fight with the neighbors"; "Behaves well with his family." None of the responses in the "Other" category occurred more than once. "Other" responses of the females composed 11 percent of their total responses. Examples are, "Should be content with what her husband gives her"; "Is honest with husband"; "Asks permission when she goes out"; "Is considerate with his relatives." None of these responses occurred more than three times.

In general, the ideal wife is seen as submissive (obedient, respectful, compliant, and helpful) and faithful, and as a good housekeeper and mother. There is a high degree of concensus between the sexes on these values, although men put particular emphasis on obedience, helpfulness, and the good-housekeeper-mother role. Companionate or developmental responses are practically nonexistent. Only three males in the sample mentioned love as an ideal, and one more (in the "other" category) mentioned understanding. A few more wives than husbands mentioned love, and two mentioned understanding and encouragement. This represents the meager store of companionship conceptions as far as the role of the wife is concerned. Table 25 shows the wives' conceptions of the ideal husband.

TABLE 25

DEFINITION OF THE GOOD HUSBAND

Distribution of responses to Q.28,F

	Percent
Kind, considerate	68
Good provider	60
Faithful	52
Doesn't beat wife	32
Helpful to wife	31
Loves wife	18
Companionable	12
Has no vices	7
Other responses[a]	28
Number of respondents	(72)
Total responses	(241)

[a] "Other" responses composed 12 percent of the total number of responses. Examples are, "Stays at home"; "Has respectful companions"; "Takes his wife's advice"; "Is good to his wife's family." None of the responses in this category occurred more than three times.

Women, of course, do not ask that a husband be obedient, respectful, or attentive. In the main, they ask that he support them adequately, be faithful and kind to them. The same minority of women who saw the ideal wife as loving her husband see the ideal husband as loving the wife, but a new category of "companionability" arises. Actually, the responses subsumed under this title referred to such mundane ideals as taking the wife out occasionally and consulting her on important matters. Only one woman (in the "other" category) asked that a husband understand his wife, but a good number of women felt it necessary to include "not beating the wife" as a requirement of the ideal husband.

MARITAL ROLES

A number of questions were asked concerning the way in which decisions were made in different areas of family life. Three types of families can be delineated from the answers, varying according to the degree to which the wife enters into decisions. These types vary more in degree than in kind, and for this reason can most properly be given terms which reflect a continuum rather than three distinct types. "Traditional," "less traditional," and "least traditional" would be more suitable than the usual "traditional," "transitional" and "modern." All three groups are only variations on traditionalism, and in each the husband is unquestioned master. For this reason, the traditional group will be given more detailed discussion; the others, merely contrasted with it.

Traditional Families. In these families the wives appear to have no other responsibilities than satisfying their husbands needs, raising children, and keeping house. In some of the families we may delineate a type of wife who seems almost "rudderless." Unable or afraid to think or make decisions for themselves, such women rely almost completely on their husbands for directions. The "rudderless" woman describes herself as completely governed by her husband and rationalizes this by her belief in male superiority.

> I have no rights. He is the one who gives orders here. He is the man, so he has those rights. . . . That is the way it has always been in all places, man giving orders. (C2F)

> I can't have any (rights). He governs me; I do not govern myself. . . . I think it is better that way. (B4F)

Such women express fear in making a decision on their own, for a wrong decision would incur penalties from the husband. One woman even felt that if her husband did not so govern her it would indicate he did not care about her. In those instances in which a woman disagrees with the decision of the husband, she must remain silent and bear the decision without comment. In fact, the question, "How do you settle disagreements?" was meaningless to such women. They said they had no disagreements because they always agreed with their husbands. Such women feel that the only way to get any concessions from their husbands is by *not* arguing.

We never argue . . . because I obey him and accept all he says. (B5F)

The woman should always give up, always lose. Later, when they realize we are humble, they forget and are happy. (X7F)

Sometimes even being right [the woman should give in]. It is better to lose her rights and avoid trouble. (Y4F)

(And if she objects to your going out?) Well, she has never been opposed to what I have done, because I have taught her from the beginning that I am the one who gives orders. (A10M)

Unquestioning obedience appears to be the rule in this group. These women accept their new cloister, both as a prerogative of the male and for their own good.

Sometimes I have told him I want to go out, and he will say, "The woman's place is in the home," and I obey and am content. (A5F)

He forbids me to go out alone. I can't dance or anything like that. . . . I don't consider it so bad, because the woman must respect her husband and please him. (H20F)

I can't dance with other men and chatter in the neighbors' houses. . . . I think it's right, for women should always be at home. They, as men, can defend themselves better and should have more freedom. (Y3F)

In such families, the woman does not even shop or make the decisions on what shall be bought for the house. In one case, a woman was allowed to buy her own "personal things such as hairpins." The detailed remarks of one respondent show the degree to which a husband can actually control his wife.

If I want to buy something, I tell him, but he won't buy it soon. He brings it when he decides to do it. Everything that is done here is ordered by him, even when I am going to kill a hen he has to order it. . . . He even buys my own clothes and shoes. If I have money, as I sometimes do from washing clothes, I give it to him; he buys those things for me. (And if they don't please or fit you?) I never say a word. The last time I asked him for colored sandals, and he brought me brown oxfords. I don't dare say anything. . . . (C2F)

The Less Traditional. In this group, the wives share to a somewhat greater extent in the decisions of the family. For example, they frequently take over the purchasing of small and personal items. Although arguments are settled by the husband, the woman in this group appears capable of arguing. Again, while she does not share in making important decisions, the husband usually talks over the situation with his wife and makes up his own mind. Most decisions as to the children and their care and household matters are in her hands.

The Least Traditional. Only in this group is there a possible qualitative difference. Several women in this group are working, and in a few cases the husband is unemployed or incapacitated for work. In this group there is considerable interchange of opinion on important matters, including the husbands' work; and the wives appear to share in the eventual decisions. The wife is actively consulted in such matters and her advice taken seriously by the husband. The wife takes over the purchasing of small items and, on large items, either shops with her husband or occasionally does so alone. In those cases in which the woman is working, the remarks suggest that the situation was once traditional but has changed since the wife has taken over some of the economic responsibilities.

The respondents in this group, however, are hardly "least traditional" by continental American standards, but only in comparison with others in the sample. To illustrate that even the women in this group are traditional, a few illustrations will be provided. These are statements of women falling in the "least traditional" category.

> After you get married, the man is the one who rules. One has to do as he says. I think it is right that way. . . . (A12F)

> They do as they will, and one cannot order them. The man goes out when he wants to, and the woman has to ask permission and can't go to places he doesn't like. . . . Men may have affairs after they are married . . . but not women. (What do you think of that?) That's right. The woman must be for her husband, her children, and her house. (H12F)

Two women who work show that their allegiance is still to their husbands. Despite their participation in decision, it is ultimately the man who rules.

Although he is crippled, he still is the chief of the family. The head of the family is the husband. He is the one who decides, and without his consent the wife shouldn't do anything. (Z8F)

He is the one who gives orders in everything—in the house, to the wife and children, who must obey him. (What do you think of that?) That is correct. Men have to govern, to control. They can do it better than women. (C7F)

Comparison of the Three Types. An index of traditionalism, which divided the sample roughly into three equal groups along the continuum described above, was prepared.[4] These three groups were then compared on other characteristics. Perhaps the most significant finding here was that the *males* in the three groups show little difference in terms of attitudes or demographic characteristics. Age, education, residence, and birth place showed no correlations with the three types. When the three groups were compared by the husbands' conception of the ideal wife, again no differences appeared. Just as many husbands from the "least traditional" group mentioned obedience, respect, and attentiveness as important attributes of the ideal wife as did those in the more traditional groups.

There are differences, however, among the females on some of these characteristics.[5] While age and current residence of the wife made little difference, education and birthplace showed fairly large differences. Table 26 presents these differences.

Thus it is particularly the better educated women, but to some degree those women with town or urban backgrounds, who appear to be living more frequently in the least traditional family setups. This would seem to suggest that the crucial factors reside more with the females than with the males. It suggests, very tentatively of course, that education and urban life do not predispose men to loosen their desire or need to dominate women; but where the woman herself is exposed to these liberalizing forces, she either marries a more flexible male or forces on him, perhaps by her

[4] The index employed the various subdivisions of Q.20,F. See Appendix C for details of its construction.

[5] Very slight differences are seen on ideal roles for husband and wife as seen by the three different groups. The only striking differential occurs in the "shouldn't beat wife" category. Only 3 women in the least traditional group thought it necessary to mention this, while 19 women in the more traditional groups made their ideal explicit.

TABLE 26

BIRTHPLACE AND EDUCATION OF WOMEN, BY DEGREE OF TRADITIONALISM

	EDUCATION		BIRTHPLACE	
	Four Years or Less (percent)	*Five Years or More (percent)*	*Country (percent)*	*Other (percent)*
Traditional	43	8	36	21
Less traditional	31	50	40	33
Least traditional	26	42	24	46
	100	100	100	100
Number of respondents	(42)	(24)	(42)	(24)

superior ability to handle serious problems, a more liberal give-and-take situation in the family.

One other significant difference among the three groups is the type of marital union. Table 27 shows the distribution.

TABLE 27

TYPE OF MARITAL UNION, BY DEGREE OF TRADITIONALISM

	Civil and Religious Union (percent)	*Consensual Union (percent)*
Traditional	24	40
Less traditional	38	37
Least traditional	38	24
	100	101
Number of respondents	(37)	(29)

The fact that consensual unions appear to be characterized by more traditional types of marital relations would lend credence to the previously expressed hypothesis that such unions deprive the woman of more rights than they give her. It renders unlikely the hypothesis, implicit in the analyses of Mintz and Petrullo, that such unions are characterized by greater freedom for the woman.

ROLE TRANSITION IN MARRIAGE

The foregoing description of the unquestioned dominance of the male might appear somewhat inconsistent with the materials in the previous chapters which suggest that many males seek mother substitutes in marriage. If the latter is the case, it might be expected that the husband-wife relationship in the authority sphere would resemble that of the mother-son relationship, or that after marriage the male would remain subservient to his mother. This does not seem to be true. Mother love does not seem to involve mother dominance after marriage or lead to dominance or equality in relations with the wife even when the latter is a mother figure. Upon marriage, the male appears successfully to emancipate himself from whatever ties of submission bound him to his family of orientation. At the same time he assumes the new role of household chief, seemingly without conflict. What insures this smooth transition from the relatively submissive and worshipful son to the dominant and independent husband? Unfortunately, no systematic questions were directed toward this area, and we can only speculate as to the nature of the structures which assist the male in bridging the gap between the family of orientation and the family of procreation.

Well-Defined Status Ascription. Although the male child must be humble and obedient, he cannot help being aware that age and sex are criteria for differing rights and duties. At all times he can observe the subservience of his sisters to himself, and the subervience of his mother to his father. At the same time he is aware that increasing age brings increasing privileges, and that upon marriage the zenith of authority is reached—he is then his own master, as his father is his own. The very fact of his long period of servitude to his parents may give him additional motivation for anticipating the time when he can assume an adult role. This may encourage the testing out of the husband-father role in fantasy, so that, when the time comes for assumption of the role, the transition may not be severe.

Neo-local Residence and Elopement. The very fact of neo-local residence may force upon the male a degree of responsibility not possible in a family system of the matri-local or patri-local type.

Marriage dramatizes the passage of the youth into adulthood, and the new household compels and permits the exercising and reality testing of the adult role. This would be extremely difficult, and probably not necessary, were the new family to live with the parents of one of the couple.[6]

The family of orientation appears to encourage the independence of the new family. As we shall see in the following chapter, a good number of respondents, when asked about the duties of a son after marriage, emphasized the fact that his first duties are to his wife and children. A good son is seen as one who helps his parents, but only *after* he has provided sufficiently for his own family. This expectation of the independence of the newly married son must be communicated in many ways to him, and it encourages and perhaps compels him to assume his new role as authoritarian husband.

The elopement phenomenon is at once the initial and the most dramatic manifestation of the new independence and authority of the male. We have already noted that the male *steals* the female, often revenging himself against her parents—perhaps a kind of gesture of insecurely held authority. It is clear that the battle is between parents and son-in-law, while the daughter is only the commodity sought by both parties. By stealing the girl, the male demonstrates that he is a man and not a boy. One woman expressed this by saying, "He had to take me away to show me that he was a *macho*." Finally, we recall the ritualistic, almost game-playing quality of the elopement, the parents staging a mock kind of fury over the theft. This might suggest that they, too, dimly realize that the function of the act is to establish the adulthood of their son-in-law.

Counter Forces. Thus far we have speculated that even where dependency feelings are transferred to the wife, these feelings shall be *confined to the emotional sphere.* They insure that the mother role of the wife includes nothing of the authority of the real mother but only the pleasant emotional aspects of the previous relationship. There are, however, some signs in Puerto Rico that the mother-son

[6] The dominance of the mother-in-law in the traditional Chinese family is a case in point. Her authority over the new daughter-in-law is greater than that of her son, and hers is the responsibility for integrating the new family member into the household. See M. Levy, *The Family Revolution in Modern China* (London: Oxford University Press, 1949).

relationship is not always successfully broken, even if the husband-wife relationship is clearly hierarchized. Thus, two mothers in the present sample mentioned how humble their married sons still were with them, and in one case the son still allows himself to be beaten occasionally by the mother, saying, "Yes, *mamita,* you are right." The relationship appears to be a one-way dependency, for most mothers in the sample held that their married daughters helped them more than their married sons.

Other evidence indicates that the husband-wife bond in the lower class is relatively weak, perhaps the weakest of immediate family relationships. The suspicion, hostility, general marital dissatisfaction, and perhaps mother-dependency feelings which appear to characterize so much of lower-class marital relationships may be so powerful that they cannot always be offset by the authority structure outlined above. One of the most revealing and eloquent statements in the sample demonstrates that, to one woman at least, the husband-wife bond is much weaker than other family bonds: the husband is so suspect that he is viewed almost as a tangential family member—in the respondent's own words, as a loan.

> The father's love is greater than the husband's love. It is more constant. The husband is here today and may be gone tomorrow, but the father is always the father (*el padre es siempre*). The son is the same as the father. He will always work for his mother. The husband is like a loan, because the day he wants, he can leave and abandon his wife. (B8F)

We may have here a family constellation somewhat similar to the British West Indian or even Southern American Negro family, at least in terms of the function of the wife. Somewhat like the Negro mother, though of course not to the same extent, the Puerto Rican mother may be the backbone of her family by default. The frequent absence of the male from the household, his lack of participation in household details when present, and the ever-present threat of his desertion may be forcing on the lower-class mother a more strategic and responsible role in the family.[7] The children may per-

[7] K. Wolf, discussing a middle class group, notes that "in domestic crises men, in spite of their masculine assertiveness, fall into the role of rebellious but dependent children, while their wives take the role of irritated yet indulgent mothers" ("Growing up and Its Price in Three Puerto Rican Subcultures, *Psychiatry,* XV, No. 4 [Nov. 1952], 429).

ceive the ineffectiveness and the possible transiency of the father. As one respondent put it, "There is a saying that fathers there are many, but mother there is only one." Unfortunately, however, the wife appears to have responsibility and accountability *without authority,* and she must always operate in the name and as executrix of the husband. Such structure may in itself be in disequilibrium, for it tends to pull authority into line with responsibility and accountability.

Thus we may conclude that a very complex system of conflicting structures is operative in the Puerto Rican family. The solidarity systems are just strong enough to hold the majority of families together, but the high rate of desertions and the fragile nature of so many existing unions suggest that the equilibrium is precarious. This whole area of family relations is one which begs for detailed investigation. The above speculations could form a beginning.

SEX RELATIONS IN MARRIAGE

SEXUAL BEHAVIOR OF THE MARRIED FEMALE

The lower-class girl has been traumatized or left ignorant concerning what will happen to her when she marries. In several of the cases in our sample, the brides-to-be were given the facts of life only just before the wedding ceremony, and, as might be expected, their reaction was one of panic. As one of them said, "My heart dropped to my feet." In many cases, the wedding-night experience appeared to be traumatic.

> That was horrible! *Ay Jesús!* But I thought that it happened to all women and none of them die. (H6F)

> *Ay,* God, I don't like to talk about that! (Don't you like to remember?) No! (Z7F)

> That is one's most terrible night. . . . It seemed as if the whole world were coming over me. (X7F)

In several instances, the idea that one should sleep with a "strange" man proved so traumatic for the bride that intercourse had to be delayed for several days. We are given the impression here of the completely terrified bride who will not even let the husband come near her.

Imagine, five days after having eloped I was still a virgin. I refused to have sexual relations, and he threatened to take me back home. (TRC)

I did not let him do anything till five or six days after. Every time he approached, I started screaming. (TRE)

I took off my shoes, and put them on again. I didn't dare go to bed. Later I went to bed, and he approached, and I told him I would scream. . . . So I spent five nights refusing to have contact with him, and then he told me he would take me back home. (H35F)

In practically all cases the males displayed a somewhat surprising degree of consideration toward the bride, handling her with delicacy, tact, and patience.

He wanted to seize me, and I started to cry. He begged me not to cry and told me that it was nothing and happened to all married women, and that I should not be frightened. (A11F)

I didn't dare take off my clothes and lie in that bed with him. . . . But all that was over when he took me to the bed and made me feel at ease. He kissed me many times and told me nothing bad was going to happen. He was good to me, made me feel at ease and up in the clouds. . . . He is always considerate with me. (Y6F)

I began to cry. He sat by my side and with my forehead in his hands started telling me, "Look what I have done to marry you. I have had to work hard to get the money to buy all the things to get married. I have had to work even at night. . . . I have done all this because I love you so much!" He started kissing and caressing me until I felt sorry for him because of all the work he had because of me. Then I agreed to go to bed and give myself up to God's will and his. (C1F)

The aura of sanctity and goodness which surrounds the fiancée may account for the male's gentle treatment of her at this time. Indeed, he undoubtedly welcomes some degree of modesty and protestation as a sign that his spouse is pure and innocent. If she did not act in this fashion, he might suspect her of being a "bad" woman. Consequently, he understands and even approves of her horror of the first night, and treats her with particular consideration. As a few women said, however, one cannot protest too much or too long, or the husband will begin to be suspicious that his bride is not a virgin and is putting off the inevitable moment of discovery on his part.

Despite the consideration on the part of the male, however, in the majority of cases the wedding night was traumatic for the women. Trembling, weeping, and speechlessness were frequently reported throughout the interviews. It is quite probable that the sudden discovery of sex after so many years of sheltered existence has profound effects on the sexual psychology of the married woman. Turning our attention to the subsequent female attitudes toward sexual matters, we see that such may be the case.

Sex as Duty. Most of the women in the sample maintain that they do not enjoy sexual relations. Considering the premarital repression of sexual behavior and feelings which is typical for the girls, the lurid tales about men which they may have been told, and the final shock of the wedding night experience, it is not surprising that many women even after years of marriage find the sexual act most distasteful.

Now I don't feel ashamed any more, but I don't like it. I think it's disgusting, repulsive. (Y3F)

I don't enjoy anything. It's repulsive to me. (TRE)

I feel nausea for that [sexual relations]. (H35F)

In addition to the reasons expressed above, frigidity, or at least sexual apathy, seems based on the limited sex techniques of many Puerto Rican males. Since they tend to take it for granted that the wife will not greatly enjoy relations, and since they feel that "women are for the men" anyway, they are not overly concerned about satisfying their wives. The few women who knew what an orgasm was explained that their men "do not wait" for them, but they did not appear dissatisfied with this situation.

He is faster than I and doesn't wait for me. . . . (What do you think about that?) Nothing. At that moment one is anxious to finish, and I don't tell him anything. (X10F)

They come more quickly than women. When they get tired they leave one. . . . It is all right with me, for one gets more rest that way. (TRE)

. . . we women are slower, and they don't wait for us. (C8F)

To explain the allegedly greater sexual drive in men, women maintained that the male is stronger and superior in sexual as well as other matters. The male carries the semen, has the active agent of procreation, and is the true source of generation.[8] Women find this natural and right.

> . . . the man is stronger in sex than the woman. . . . This was sent by nature. The woman enjoys it, but not like the man. I think that is because of the sexual superiority of the man. (Y6F)

> He is the stronger sex, he engenders, he has the privilege. (Z3F)

> I think they enjoy it more, because they are stronger than we. I think it's right like that. (H17F)

With so much disinterest and such frequent revulsion from sex, fairly powerful forces must operate to insure compliance on the part of the women. The most important of these is duty. As one man put it, "As long as she gets married she is obliged to have sexual relations with him every time he feels like it." As we shall see, this does not work out so smoothly in practice, but in general women, too, feel that sexual relations are one of their most important obligations.

> I don't enjoy it at all. I do it because I have to do it. . . . Nearly every woman dislikes it. . . . They do it out of obligation. (A9F)

> It was always bad, but I had to do it . . . because I thought that it was my duty. (A5F)

> Man always enjoys it more, because the woman, being his own wife, accepts him without desire, just to comply with obligations. (Y5M)

This obligation appears to be so extensive that some women deceive their husbands into thinking they are enjoying the act. When asked whether men or women derived more pleasure from sexual relations, 24 percent of the males stated that women enjoyed it more, and another 20 percent thought the pleasure was equal for both. In answering the same question, only 15 percent of the women felt that the sexes enjoy the same pleasure, and none thought that the women enjoy it more. Thus, men are either deceiving themselves or being deceived by their wives. There is some evidence to support the latter notion, for two women in the

[8] One woman had an organic explanation for the fact that men have more orgasms. Like the extra sense which is one of the gifts of men, extra phosphorous in the brain of the male accounts for his greater orgastic potential.

sample, felt that to show no pleasure might cause the husband to suspect that his wife had another lover. A narrow course must be steered by the woman, however, for *too much* enjoyment would not be appropriate and would even result in the same suspicion.

She doesn't enjoy it as much as the man. . . . Sometimes the woman is timid because possibly she doesn't want to appear the same as the man. (Why?) She might get it into her head that the man might mistrust her if she tries to match him in sexual matters in marriage. (Y5M)

The final reason why women comply is that they may be compelled to do so. The delicacy with which the bride is treated may be tempered once the male patience is worn thin, and the general dominance of the male may be exercised toward this end. "One forces the woman to do it even if she does not feel like doing it," stated one male, and the following illustration, although treating mainly of a previous generation, shows to what lengths the male will occasionally go.

I remember my father acted in the same way as my husband. Mother resisted going to bed with him, and he threatened to cut her throat with a *machete*. I heard all these quarrels, and I went to the hammock where my mother was sleeping and asked her to go to bed with papa. In the same way I had to give in with my husband to avoid quarrels. (TRF)

Despite these forces impelling the woman to accede to the man's desires, a very considerable amount of sexual denial goes on. Of the 63 women from whom information was obtained, only 26, or four out of every ten, said they never denied their husbands. The remainder explained that they did so because they do not enjoy sexual activity, because they are usually too tired, or, as we shall see in the next chapter, because they desire to avoid pregnancy. However, they are very careful to practice denial in a fashion which will not offend the male. During menstruation, the pre- and post-partum period, and sickness the female is excused from sexual intercourse. Since the former two states do not lend themselves easily to simulation, the woman frequently relies on pretending sickness.

I make believe I'm asleep and I tell him I'm sick or that something aches, for that's too much for me. (Y3F)

I am careful not to do it persistently. . . . One can deny when one is sick, but only then. (A11F)

Sometimes when he wants to do it I make him believe I'm asleep or pretend I'm sick and that I can't do it. (H19F)

Moreover, as suggested by the first quote, women are careful not to practice denial too frequently. As far as could be ascertained, only four women denied their husbands "frequently." Stories of denying women who were severely beaten or killed by irate husbands are not infrequent, and there is always the fear that the husband will interpret denial as unfaithfulness. This is one of many manifestations of the underlying male suspicion concerning the fidelity of his wife and daughters.

The man may become jealous, thinking she has another husband. He might divorce her or even kill her because he thinks she loves another man. (B4F)

I don't deny myself to him, because he might think I have another man. (H23F)

She should not deny herself, because the husband might start thinking that she has another man. (A11F)

This is not fantasy on the part of the women. Men frequently give the same reasons.

When the woman doesn't want her husband, it's because she doesn't like her husband any more, or she likes someone else or has someone else in mind, or she may be sick. (B5M)

(What if the woman refused sexual relations without a reason such as menstruation?) Then the man should watch her to see if she has another man. (A9F)

It is also alleged that overly frequent denial drives the male to other women. Wives are so fearful that this will happen anyway that they desire to give no cause for encouragement.

. . . if the wife denies more than once he can go with other women. (A11F)

That's why so many marriages have been broken, for the husbands leave the house and search for other women. . . . (Y8F)

One woman saw the male sex drive as so powerful that any frustration might be dangerous. The interpretation given the story below by the storyteller shows how the community sided with the male and construed the woman's denial as the cause for his death.

A man from [a near-by *barrio*] went to his wife for intercourse, and she denied him. . . . Since he could not have intercourse, he got an infection, a very bad one, and died three days later. . . . The people said she denied because she had another man. That's the only thing that can be said of a woman who denies her husband. . . . That is very dangerous to the man. He can die. (B5F)

Sex as Desirable. Thus far we have concerned ourselves with one type of woman—the prevailing type which is indifferent to or repelled by sexual relations and which eschews them whenever it seems safe to do so. The predominance of this type seems explicable in the light of the cloistered premarital life of the average lower-class woman in the sample. But it should not be thought that all women fall into this category. The statement by one anthropologist working in Puerto Rico, that in his community "So much is intercourse considered in terms of obligation that one woman who enjoyed sexual intercourse 'for its own sake' was considered sick by the other women of the *barrio*,"[9] is completely misleading. It is probably true that modesty and the prevailing role conceptions of women forbid the admission of sexual pleasure to the female community. But the evidence from the present study leaves little doubt that there is a strong minority of women which genuinely enjoys sexual relationships. As one woman expressed it somewhat angrily, "It's hypocritical to say that the sexual act is bad, and that she doesn't like to do it. That's a lie, because I'm a woman, too, and I like to do it." Only one woman in the total sample said that the woman *never* derives any pleasure from sexual relations. Twenty-one women said they enjoyed such relations as much as their husbands, and two said they enjoyed them more than their husbands. The remarks of some women show that they experience real pleasure from the sexual act:

. . . that is something that drives you. (Do you think the woman needs that?) Yes, I think so. (Y2F)

[9] E. Wolf, "Culture Change and Culture Stability in a Puerto Rican Coffee Community" (unpublished Ph.D. dissertation, Columbia University, 1951), p. 94.

When a woman does that, she feels the same as they [the men] feel, for the real joy is when both do it at the same time. (X10F)

I am stronger than he. He says, "Well you are going to kill me one of these days," and he laughs and makes a joke of it. (X2F)

Men were particularly ready to admit that women enjoyed such relations. Several men admitted that they knew their wives were enjoying intercourse by the presence of secretions. Several had interesting explanations for their presumed pleasure in the act. Two men explained it as due to the fact that the woman retains the semen, another as due to a rut period occurring during Lent.

Moreover, there is the reported datum that a great number of women indulge in extramarital affairs. Given the general influence of the virginity cult, given the suspicion of husbands and the violence of their sanctions, the statements below, which suggest a good deal of female extramarital activity, might not have been expected.

(Are there any cases of unfaithfulness on the part of the woman?) There are a million cases. While the husband is working, they are giving food and money to the guy. (H7M)

There are thousands of women who are playing dirty tricks on their husbands, and the husbands look like fools. (H23F)

There are many cases of unfaithful wives around here. . . . I am acquainted with everybody in this town, and I know about eight or ten cases. (Y1M)

We recall, too, that a good number of men had their first sexual experiences with married women. There are several instances in the sample of males who claim to have been *enticed* by married women to have sexual relations with them. Again, given the cultural setting, such a seemingly frequent deviation from the norm is striking. What can account for it?

In the first place, the female is more accessible after marriage. In her family of orientation, brothers, sisters, and parents were present to insure that the girl would have no occasion to temptation. When married, especially in the early years, only the husband is present in the household, and his various duties keep him out of the house for a good share of the day.

Second, we mentioned previously that once a girl loses her virginity she is automatically classed in the "bad girl" category and provides "new flesh" for the men. This was with regard to the loss of virginity prior to marriage. Perhaps, however, the loss of virginity may be of considerable significance *per se,* irrespective of the condition (licit or illicit) under which it is lost. That is, there may be some tendency in the lower class to think of married women as sexually accessible since they are already experienced. This would be particularly true for consensually married women. Since there is always the possibility that they may abandon their husbands, they may be seen as special targets by the male.

SEXUAL BEHAVIOR OF THE MARRIED MALE

Desexualization of the Wife. Unlike the woman, the male enters marriage with a good deal of experience which has whetted his sexual appetite.[10] He has learned that sexual experience is enjoyable and has none of the fears and misconceptions which inhibit his bride. One woman expressed this situation quite clearly:

> Women have never had sexual contact before getting married and don't know. As men have already had it, they know about it and therefore enjoy it more. (H10F)

While the male is well aware that the woman is generally at his disposal whenever he should desire her, there is a good deal of evidence to indicate that the lower-class male is sexually frustrated as far as his wife is concerned. This might be due to his own psychological conflicts as well as to his wife's attitude toward sex.

We have already discussed the proposition that the lower-class wife is very frequently a mother projection for the male. If true, this fact could cause difficulties in marriage, where incestuous guilt might accompany sexual relations. At least two solutions would seem available to the male: (1) desexualizing the sexual act by keeping his actions and particularly his feelings as nonerotic as possible. (2) engaging in extramarital activity, using the "bad women" as vehicles of expression for his uninhibited sexual desires, while preserving his wife for reproductive and dutiful sexual activity.

[10] It should be emphasized, however, that the premarital experience with prostitutes and semiprofessionals is poor training for the kind of sexual problems the male will meet with his wife.

Of all the delicate questions on the interview schedule, the question which caused the most difficulty and resistance was, "With regard to sexual relations, did you find your wife different from the women you had known before you married? Were your feelings toward her different?" (Q.32A1,2,M). Several respondents were stunned by the question, one rose from his seat and threatened the interviewer. Male interviewers complained about this question and handled it so gingerly that, in general, it was not successful. Many men were insulted by the question, for it seemed to intimate that their wives were of the loose variety or "bad" women. When the question was answered, it showed that they made a sharp distinction between the type of sexual activity they experienced with their wives and that which they had with other women.

> The one I have now has the qualities of a good wife, while the others I had were not virgins. . . . My wife doesn't know of immoral acts while having relations, such as prostitutes know. (C2M)

> The man holds his own wife at a sacred level. He goes with other women, but with his own wife he has more consideration. (C3M)

> It is different with the wife. With her it is love, pure and good. (Y2M)

Not only may the attitude toward the wife be desexualized, but the sexual techniques appear to be of a more conventional type. For real sensuality, the "bad" women are preferred.

> We treat our wives with more consideration. . . . Prostitutes are more daring. Since she was going to be my wife, I had to treat her as a real companion. (B8M)

> With my wife I only have sexual intercourse to please her. I don't treat her too roughly. When a man gets a woman not his wife, he tries to satisfy himself fully. . . . With the wife, although he has intercourse with her, he treats her with a certain delicacy and respect. . . . With the other woman he kisses her passionately . . . bites her, would like to eat her up. (Y8M)

In two cases in which the men were gentle about their wives' denial, the wives described their husbands in familial terms. One said she loved her husband like a father, and the other said her husband could treat her as a sister. Two other men said that they did not enjoy sexual contact with their wives and preferred other women. This evidence, while slight, might support the hypothesis of a pattern of desexualizing the wife in lower-class society.

Extramarital Activity and Machismo. When asked which sex had greater sexual freedom in Puerto Rico, all the women agreed that the males were so favored, and two out of every three women approved of this. The reasons for such acquiescence should be clear from the previous discussions. Both men and women feel that this is inherent in the nature of things and that women are weak and cannot stand much freedom. In answer to this question, women spoke of themselves as "a weak arm" and as a "delicate crystal that breaks easily." Men occasionally described themselves as a self-sufficient world (*Nosotros somos un mundo*) and as made in the image of God. Whereas men can go to and from all places at all hours with impunity, woman's honor is so delicate that any independent activity outside the home may damage it.

After marriage a woman must be watched even more carefully than before. The community unites with the suspicious husband and disapproves of much outside contact.

> When single, she can always go to dances and movies, although she must be careful. But when she marries, she can't be seen talking with friends or other men. She can be discredited immediately. (H1F)

A woman who engages in extramarital activity becomes figuratively (and often literally) a prostitute. The man is merely seen as a *picaflor* (lady killer), and perhaps admired. Chapter II has shown that women expected filandering on the part of the male as a consequence of his sexual nature. Though there seems to be growing resentment at such activity, the ideal still seems to be that the woman should bear such behavior stoically. Two different women told how their fathers had had children by their mother's sisters, and that their mothers had to deliver and rear the children without complaint. Another reprimanded her daughter for complaining too much about her (the daughter's) husband's infidelity, saying, "If I have suffered it, she can too." Two women felt that such behavior was permissible if the husband spared them the suffering of knowing about it, but most preferred honesty on the part of their husbands.

> If he has an affair with another girl and tells her, she should let him, for he is a man. (H19F)

My husband takes married women. . . . I think that, as a male, if he likes her, he takes advantage of her, and it isn't bad. I don't think he would stop loving me because of that, for he always behaved in the same way with me. (A3F)

Of the 49 men for whom we have information, 26 admitted extramarital relations, and 23 denied them.[11] If so many were willing to admit this to the interviewer, we can probaly assume that even more than these had in reality indulged in illicit affairs. Even among those who claimed they did not indulge in extramarital relations, some said that they would if they had the chance. Their general feeling was that, while one should not actively seek such affairs, if the occasion arises, a man would be a fool not to take advantage of it.

If I find a woman that gives me the opportunity, I don't let her go. Opportunity comes only once in a lifetime. (C2M)

One would like to keep his word with his wife, but if the chance comes, one takes it just for pleasure. (C6M)

Well, I don't need to, but if the chance comes, I take it. (B3M)

. . . if the chance comes, one is not going to be too foolish and let it pass. (H4M)

While the culture permits extramarital activity on the part of men, there is some evidence indicating that social-psychological forces may *encourage* it. In a number of cases there appears to be a considerable degree of anxiety concerning virility. Several of the male respondents, (See Chapter II, Table 5) in discussing *machismo,* told of other men who when drunk would rant about their virile qualities. During intoxication the otherwise inhibited anxieties concerning manliness are expressed and show a kind of compulsive insistence that the man is truly a *macho*.

There are some men who get drunk and then think they are alone in the world, and you hear them shouting, "I am an *hombre macho!*" . . . [This is the type] who likes to make love to women and to fight with all the men in his path. (A11M)

[11] Kinsey estimates that about half of all married males have extra-marital relations at some point in marriage. A. Kinsey, W. Pomeroy, and C. Martin, *Sexual Behavior in the Human Male* (Philadelphia: Saunders, 1949), p. 585.

[The *hombre macho*] is what the drunken man talks about. (B4M)

When people are drunk they say "I am a complete *macho* . . ." They flirt with the girls and like to go with prostitutes. (C10M)

In this sense, the *hombre macho* is a braggart and has to show that he is more virile than others by conquering women and by fighting. But he fights chiefly those who are weaker, and the love making has a false, compulsive note.

He shows it by fighting and by being a woman chaser. . . . I think he does it *to prove that he is more man than the rest of men.* (A5M)

He is a man who *fights with the weak* and . . . has a woman wherever he goes. . . . I think they do it *in order to prove their machura.* (*Machura?*) Yes, to show he can make a woman have kids. (A10M)

The man boasts of his courage and brags every place he goes. He treats women badly. Sometimes he even beats them to get what he wants. (B5M)

They start using obscene language. They fight also, but *if they face a tough guy, they try to control themselves. . . .* They go with many women and show off, *trying to demonstrate they are superior to others.* (C6M)

Thus, the type of man described by the respondents seems to fit the picture of the insecure male, uncertain of his manhood, trying by ostentatious and transparent methods to prove his virility to himself and his fellows. In delineating this type, the men in the sample were of course always careful not to identify themselves with it.

Other men gave statements which may be interpreted as indicating that the male is "on edge" concerning his virility. This type of statement showed a very definite fear that the man would meet a woman sexually stronger than himself. In the male's inner world this may take the form of fantasy about being sexually conquered by a powerful female and merely be the expression of the fears concerning sexual inadequacy. Note, in the following statements, the conception that one should immediately take the proferred sexual opportunity, implicitly to prove one's sexual capacities, and that a man must either conquer a woman or leave her.

If she demands that stuff from you, you should never postpone it. *You should always be like the fighting cock.* (A8M)

If a man meets a fierce woman (*brava*), he should show her his manhood and try to dominate her . . . by giving her no rest during the night. *If one sees he cannot dominate her, he should abandon her.* (A9M)

If I go to the street and meet a girl, *I have to show her that I am an hombre completo.* If I have to make love to her, I do it. (H18M)

The man should take advantage of his opportunity and enjoy the woman. *If he does not, the man is put in a ridiculous position* with the woman. (A3M)

Other men spoke of the necessity of being sexually powerful with one's wife, for, if not, she would take another man, and a couple of wives said that their husbands had eloped with them to show that they were *macho*. Several men found themselves inexplicably attractive to women and told with delight of the way in which they deceived them and their husbands. One delighted in "humiliating them." Another told a tale of sexual bravado which resembles pure fantasy.

I took away the wife of a detective. One night he caught us. We jumped through a window. He shot at us and the bullets whistled. I went crawling under some houses and was almost naked. A woman called me and gave me some of her son's clothes. The woman hid in another house. . . . Women can't see my underwear. The minute I touch them they get pregnant. (H19M)

Perhaps promiscuity and serial consensual unions are means by which the male attempts to convince himself of his *machismo*. In the light of the fact that so many men think of their wives as mothers, it is also conceivable that the wives serve as successful mother substitutes but do not provide the kind of tangible proof that the male has established adult sexuality. This may be one fact which drives him to numerous promiscuous and consensual contacts. One woman seemed to express something of the sort when she said of her husband, "He tells me that a wife is as safe as a mother, and, as for the women in the streets, men have to run after them." On the other hand, the Don Juan type of search for the mother seems reflected in the words of a male respondent who spoke somewhat sadly of his fruitless quest: "I think it is very difficult to find a woman who is like a mother with a son. I don't think that woman exists. I have not found her."

MARITAL SOLIDARITY AND COMMUNICATION

Much of the data in the preceding chapters would lead us to suspect that the degree and depth of effective interspousal communication is not great among the lower class. Chapters II and III have shown the barriers of status which exist between men and women and between boys and girls. Chapter IV has shown how the norms of respect operate to insure that intimacy will never be too great between the sexes. Dominance patterns may also militate toward a minimum of communication; that is, the man tells and the woman listens. Additionally, girls do not generally appear to develop a great deal of affection or "closeness" for their fathers, a factor which may carry over into their relationship with their husbands. Finally, the unusual amount of mutual suspicion as regards sexual behavior could operate to limit effective communication. With fathers distrusting daughters, husbands distrusting wives, and wives distrusting husbands, we might expect a minimum of free-flowing communication. In the present section we shall attempt to see to what extent communication does seem limited, and expand upon the causes leading to this situation.

SEPARATE ACTIVITIES

In the lower class there seem to be relatively few common activities.[12] Though few outside means of entertainment are available, the local *cafetín,* or sleep after a hard day of toil, serves as escape for the male in the evenings. The woman is, of course, tied down by a large family, but even where she is not, she is expected to remain home and wait for her husband to return. Consequently, when women were asked what they did together with their husbands, many of their responses showed a very low level of common activity. Seven respondents said that they had no common activity whatsoever.

[12] Even in middle-class society, the uneasy relations between men and women can be observed. At parties women group in one part of the room, men in another, usually near the bar. The men discuss politics and swap stories, the women discuss children. The only common activity is almost purely physical—dancing—and even here most wives are nervous about dancing with men other than their husbands. In middle-class society, too, there is a strong tendency toward separate recreation, the man spending many evenings with "the boys," with whom he feels essentially more at home.

We almost never sit down to talk about anything for he comes so tired, drinks his coffee, goes fishing, comes late, and goes to bed. (X5F)

We never do anything together. . . . We are used to it that way and never go out together. (X10F)

We don't do anything but have sexual intercourse. (C8F)

He doesn't go out with me. He goes out alone. Every night he goes to the movies. He has never gone out with me. (X6F)

Another 26 cases have common activities in the home only. These respondents mentioned talking, listening to the radio, and being around the house together. Another 17 mentioned limited outside activities, such as attending church and visiting relatives and friends together. A final 20 cases cited common activities in public places, such as walking in parks, attending fiestas, visiting stores, and going to the movies. Thus, about half of the sample failed to mention any common activities outside of the home, and many of the remaining cases reported either infrequent or limited outside activities.

SUSPICION AND LACK OF RAPPORT

When asked what kinds of things they talked about with their husbands, four women reported that they never talked about anything. Of the remainder, most discussed the children and their economic situation.[18]

Based on the hypothesis that there was a considerable gulf between the sexes in marriage, and that this gulf would strongly affect communication, the questions, "Is there anything in his life that he does not discuss with you?" and "Is there anything in your life that you do not discuss with him?" were asked. Twenty-six women in the sample said that they told their husbands everything and that their husbands told everything to them. Twenty-three women said

[18] A striking evidence of the general lack of communication between the spouses was brought to light in reinterviews with a selected sample of the respondents. In only 2 out of 25 reinterviewed families had there been any detailed discussion about their interviews. In 8 cases there was none at all, and in the remaining 15 cases discussion was very limited. In most of these latter cases, the wife asked the husband about his interview and was rebuffed or put off by cryptic statements such as, "He asked simple things" or "We talked about many things." In a few cases the husband quizzed the wife about her interview but refused to tell her about his own. In most instances the chief topic of discussion was the personality of the interviewer.

they kept some things from their husbands, and 27 women said their husbands kept some things to themselves. The nature of the things concealed as well as the reason for their concealment show clearly the thread of mutual suspicion which characterizes the relation between the sexes. There is, first of all, a small group who claim that their husbands tell them nothing at all.

He doesn't tell me about what happens to him in his work, his outside life, nothing. (H1F)

He doesn't talk about anything with me. . . . Neither do I talk of anything with him. (X10F)

He tells me nothing, nothing that happens to him; and his problems he solves by himself. (Y2F)

Men were not asked this question, but the volunteered response of one man suggests that a man's business is his own, while his wife's business belongs to both:

She tells me everything, while I don't tell her anything of what I do. (Y4F)

Others felt that the light-headed nature of women did not enable them to keep information to themselves and that, consequently, they should not be apprised of important matters.

He says he knows things that he won't tell me because I tell everything. (Y7F)

Don't you know that women should not be told everything? There is the story of the man who gave three points of advice to his son: Not to rear another's child, not to plant a tree that bears no fruit, and never to tell secrets to your wife. (B5F)

For the woman's part, there is also the conception that men are evil-tempered and violent, and that telling them certain things might provoke them to violence.

The husband should not be told every little thing that is heard by the woman, so that there will be no arguments or bad temptations. . . . For example, "That fellow told me I was beautiful" or "Our son had a quarrel with another." . . . Men have a bad temperament and can become furious and kill someone. . . . That's why one should not confide in anyone, not even in one's wife. That's why not all that a husband knows should be told to his wife, nor the wife tell everything to the husband. (B5F)

If I had an argument or something like that, I wouldn't tell my husband, for he might lose his patience and could do something bad —either beat the person or kill [him]. (C8F)

If I know things, I don't tell him. I don't like to tell him to avoid trouble. . . . Crimes have occurred because of that. . . . For example, the husband has come home, and the wife tells him of some trouble with a neighbor and . . . he takes a machete and might even kill the neighbor. (B4F)

There are also those women who simply believe that one should not tell everything to a man, even if he is your husband. They seem to feel most directly the gulf between the sexes, and by their statements they show that there are many things which a woman should keep to herself, not only to avoid trouble but just because "it is better that way."

He never tells me about things he does outside. I don't tell him either. There are things you mustn't tell your husband. We are not used to telling each other [much]. (H4F)

I tell everything to other persons but . . . I never tell him anything. . . . I am the kind of person who doesn't like to tell personal things to men, not even to my husband—you know, I lack that feeling of intimacy with him. (C10F)

We scarcely talk about our own life. I am not used to doing it. . . . We are responsible for solving our own problems alone. . . . We know how to defend ourselves and how to behave. (Z6F)

I don't tell him about me either, almost nothing. What for? (H20F)

There are a few women who do not know whether or not their husbands keep anything from them. This kind of answer in itself is, of course, indicative of low communication. Three women, however, go even farther. They say that, whereas they do not know whether or not there are things their husbands do not tell them, they *suspect* that there are.

That's the thing I don't know. I think he doesn't tell me everything. (Z3F)

There must be something, because nearly always men have secrets they don't tell their wives about. (C6F)

Perhaps he has lots of things he doesn't tell me about. Perhaps he has another woman and I don't know it. (H16F)

The last quotation reveals the basis for such suspicions. A large number of women are fearful that their husbands are unfaithful to them and are concealing the affair. This is merely another evidence of the conception that man is rapacious and insatiable. If one cannot trust one's brothers and one's father, surely one cannot trust one's husband.

I don't know if he has them [women]. I don't think he does. But if he takes them, he is not going to tell me, because he doesn't want to make me suffer. (H18F)

. . . he goes out and doesn't tell his wife what he does. Men have sexual relations when single and married. (H14F)

If he has other women, he doesn't tell me. I know he's having an affair right now. Thank God I'm not jealous. (H5F)

Men go out and have experiences with other women and don't tell us. (C1F)

The whole complex of suspicion and its effects on communication are well exemplified by the remarks of a woman who felt most strongly that men had to have more than one woman.

He can't be faithful. . . . Every man needs more than one woman. *You confide in your husband, but you don't believe in him.* Man is never faithful. (B8F)

Two women show how far these fears and tensions can go. One of them had previously given the impression that she was married to the model husband.

(I thought he was a perfect husband?) Listen, I'm going to tell you the truth. I'm afraid of having sexual intercourse with him. He is so woman crazy I'm afraid he might infect me with a [venereal] disease. (H10F)

Another woman told how she lives in fear for the same reason.[14]

[14] Sex appears frequently to be used as a method of aggression by both sexes, but particularly by the male. A few wives mentioned denying their husbands (tactfully, of course) to punish them for filandering or for other matters. As we shall subsequently note, there are husbands who have impregnated their wives out of malice or revenge. Finally, one story was told which shows that deliberate infection of the wife is not beyond possibility: "A lady here refused her husband's [sexual] demands, and he went to some prostitutes and got gonorrhea. Then he gave his wife the infection. The people say he did it to take revenge on her because she had denied him." (C3M)

I live with him in distrust. I fear he may infect me any time. I never go out; I am always watching him. (X6F)

SEX-DISCUSSION TABUS

Unfortunately, on this very important topic the questions were not sufficiently specific, and probing was not well handled. The thinness of the material here makes interpretation somewhat difficult. Error, however, will probably be in the direction of assuming more discussion of sexual matters than actually occurs. Of the 64 women who answered the probe, "Do you ever discuss sexual matters with your husband?" (43B,F), 28 said yes, 28 said no, and 8 gave answers which suggested their discussion on the subject was limited. The difficulty of interpretation lies with those who replied in the affirmative, for when this response was given, little probing was done. Consequently, many of these cases may more properly belong in the "limited communication" category. At any rate we can examine the responses of those who denied having such discussions in order to assess the reasons for this behavior.

In this area it is not only the general lack of communication between spouses that keeps so many people away from the subject of sex, it is also the modesty patterns, early developed in the girl, combined with a sense of *respeto* of each partner for the other. In the case of modesty, it is clear, again, that the sexes never feel intimate enough to permit any great relaxation of the tabus. Even though he is your husband, such things should not be discussed with a man.

I would be ashamed to talk about such things. *I don't like to talk about that with anybody.* (Even with him?) No. I don't like to do it. (Z7F)

I tell him everything, but about sexual matters I don't tell him. (Why not?) I don't like that. *I think that the intimate life of a person shouldn't be told to anybody.* To you, all right, because it is for a study, as if it were told to a doctor. (Z3F)

Other women give evidence of the wall of status between the sexes when they talk about "respecting the man too much" to talk about sex with him. Sex talk is the prerogative of the man rather than the woman. For her to initiate such conversation would be stepping beyond the privileges of her status. Thus she respects him too much to do so.

I never talk about these matters with him, maybe because *I respect him.* . . . (H7F)

I never discuss such things. I'm ashamed to do it, and *I feel too much respect for him.* (TRE)

Another reason given for not discussing sexual matters is that the children might overhear. Apparently lower-class parents take the greatest of care to insure that their sexual activities go unnoticed by the children.[15] Conversation on sexual matters is one manifestation of the attempt to keep the children, and in particular the girls, in ignorance of such things.

We are not used to discussing such things. We don't do it to keep the children from knowing about it. As there are many children and the house is not very big, we don't discuss them. (X7M)

I would like to talk about them, but at home there is little space. The house is small. And even to do anything during the night [intercourse], one has to be very careful because the house is made of wood and zinc, and this material makes too much noise. (B8M)

MARITAL ADJUSTMENT

It might be well, finally, to attempt to assess the degree of marital adjustment within the sample.[16] However, it should be kept in mind that we are dealing with relatively well-adjusted couples, since they

[15] Given the crowded sleeping conditions in the average lower-class home (76 percent of the rural population sleep with three or more to a room, 39 percent with five or more: Roberts and Stefani, *Patterns of Living in Puerto Rican Families,* Río Piedras: University of Puerto Rico, 1949, p. 86), this ideal may not always be realized. K. Wolf (*op. cit.,* p. 414) concludes that such proximity breeds knowledge, while Landy concludes that "given the whole context of desire to keep the female in ignorance, she is more frightened by parental intercourse than informed" (personal communication). At any rate, the anxiety with which respondents expressed their precautions makes it clear at least that serious attempts are made to conceal intercourse from the children.

[16] A relationship between fertility and marital satisfaction has been found in studies in the United States, but little is known about the nature of the relationship. See R. Reed, "The Interrelationship of Marital Adjustment, Fertility Control, and Size of Family," in P. Whelpton and C. Kiser, eds., *Social and Psychological Factors Affecting Fertility* (New York: Milbank Memorial Fund, 1950), pp. 259–301.

have been married for a median of nine years. In order to derive an index of marital satisfaction, three questions were combined: "Many women tell us that they expected better things from marriage. How would you say yours has turned out?" (Q.39,F) "Has it turned out as well as you expected?" (Q.39A,F) "How would you rate your husband?" (Q.29,F) The last question included the reading of a five-point scale ranging from "extraordinarily good" to "very bad.' 'The marginals for these questions are presented in Table 28.

TABLE 28

MARITAL-SATISFACTION QUESTIONS AND COMPOSITE INDEX OF MARITAL SATISFACTION

	Good	*Fair*	*Bad*	*Better*	*Same*	*Worse*
Q.39,F	44	12	6			
Q.39A,F				14	19	10
Q.29,F	48	19	2			

Composite Index

Satisfied with marriage	44
Dissatisfied with marriage[a]	28

[a] Composition of the "dissatisfied-with-marriage" group: all women who said their marriage had turned out badly and/or worse than they expected; those who said it had turned out "fair" and gave no answer as to what they expected; plus those cases who rated their husbands as fair, bad, or very bad.

In combining these three questions in order to separate the well-adjusted from the maladjusted marriages, 28 cases, or 39 percent of the sample, fell in the maladjusted-marriage category. Thus, despite the already present bias in the direction of adjustment, a fairly high proportion of the sample expresses varying degrees of dissatisfaction with their current marriage.

CONCLUSIONS

The relations between the married man and woman in the lower class are characterized by male dominance and a double standard of sexual activity. All families in our sample appear "traditional" in the sense of male dominance, but they vary according to the degree to which the wife participates in the making of decisions. The difference between degrees of traditionalism appears to depend mainly on education and place of birth of the woman, suggesting the hypothesis that the female rather than the male is the key in the "liberalizing" of lower-class authority relationships.

The predisposition toward an aversion to sexual relations with which the woman enters marriage is frequently heightened by the trauma of the wedding night. Many wives report that they perform sexually out of a sense of duty to their husbands, but deny sexually as frequently as they can without incurring suspicion or wrath. A minority of the women report pleasurable sex relationships, and others are reputedly interested in extramarital relations. In general, however, this is the prerogative of the male, who is inclined to engage in such relations whenever the opportunity presents itself, partly as a demonstration of his virility.

The filial emotional attitude with which so many males regard their wives encourages a process of desexualization of the wife, a fact which may at once increase the males' interest in extramarital relations and sexually frustrate those wives who are capable of a satisfactory relationship.

A high degree of mutual suspicion appears to characterize the relation between many married couples of the lower class. Marital dissatisfaction, at least on the part of the women, also seems quite frequent. These factors, plus the differential statuses of the sexes and a dearth of common activities, help to account for the relative absence of communication between the spouses on sexual and other matters.

The total picture would lead one to conclude that married couples of the lower class are living in a fragile or brittle relationship which has a high potential for disintegration. One factor influential in preserving family solidarity is the role of the husband, who, despite seemingly conflicting attitudes of dependency toward the wife, is able to exert an unquestioned dominance in family relationships. But there is some evidence to indicate that the balance between the husband's authority and the wife's actual role in the family is a delicate one. Thus, both the propensity for consensual unions and the high turnover in such unions become more understandable and leave the implication that any powerful influence leading to the independence of women would lead to a greater number of desertions and delayed marriages and a higher incidence of nonmarriage.

All the foregoing factors probably have their influence on fertility, although, at this stage in research, the effects cannot be defined with any precision. It should be clear, however, that marital coital frequency may be limited by sexual incompatibility and marital dissatisfaction; and that serial unions and extramarital relations may reduce or raise total exposure to pregnancy. The general lack of communication between spouses, tabus on discussion of sexual matters, and the authoritarian role of the male in all family matters might be expected to affect the use of birth control. The remaining chapters will attempt to throw more light on these presumed relationships.

VII

Attitudes toward Fertility: The Fertility Belief System

> About three or four children [is ideal] for the poor people. . . . And for the rich, they can have all that God wants to give them.
>
> A MOTHER

SMALL-FAMILY IDEALS

In Chapter I we referred to the fertility belief system as the sum total of consciously held beliefs and attitudes, common to a group, which have explicit reference to fertility behavior. This would include the culturally approved number of children and the reasons for belief in this number. In many peasant cultures, barrenness is a disgrace, especially to the woman. Note in the following statement of a Sinhalese mother how the barren woman is pitied, scorned, and, in some cases, even ostracized.

I pity her. She will have no one to help her and care for her when she is ill. In old age she will have no one to sit with her and comfort her. If she does anything bad people say it is due to the fact that she is barren. They refer to her as the *vanda gani* (barren woman), a contemptuous term. They will not show her first to a girl who has attained puberty. We must not meet such a woman when we set out on an auspicious task like going to a wedding or pirith ceremony, or to see a bride and groom-to-be. She is unlucky, and it is believed that the business won't be a success. So she is avoided.[1]

But if barrenness is a disgrace, how *many* children should one

[1] B. Ryan, "Institutional Factors in Sinhalese Fertility," *Milbank Memorial Fund Quarterly,* XXX, No. 4 (Oct. 1952), 370.

have? In some cases there seems to be indifference, a fatalistic acceptance of the number that come;[2] in others, an ambivalence whereby one is very proud of and considers ideal the number one has, but wants no more;[3] in still others, a feeling of "the more the better" may be characteristic.[4] In Puerto Rico one hears frequently that the lower class will not limit its fertility because "children are the capital of the poor," and "where one can eat, so can many." However, the most recent evidence shows that, if such attitudes on the part of the lower class were ever universal, a revolution in family-size ideals has occurred.

Hatt has provided the most definitive data in this regard. About 75 percent of the men and 80 percent of the women in his sample gave a number less than four as their ideal. Only about 2 percent felt that this matter was "as God wills."[5] In the present survey, 56 percent of the males and 63 percent of the females mentioned a number less than four as their ideal.[6] When the 143 members of the sample were asked why they held *X* number of children to be ideal, all but 34 persons exclusively mentioned *disadvantages* of children.[7]

Respondents were particularly articulate on the question dealing with family size and showed that they had given some thought to the general problem. Many respondents were somewhat bitter at the different fates of the rich and the poor in this respect, maintaining

[2] Even in contemporary England about one third of a largely urban sample of married women thought it best to leave the number of children one has to chance. Mass Observation, *Britain and Her Birth Rate* (London: John Murray, 1945), p. 56.

[3] See, for example, M. J. Hagood, *Mothers of the South* (Chapel Hill: University of North Carolina Press, 1939), pp. 122–23.

[4] Despite cultural emphases on high fertility, however, it is likely that women the world over view the situation ambivalently. Ryan notes, for example, that in his sample "it was sharply evident to the interviewers that infinite numbers of children were an unqualified blessing in situations where several women were present;" while in private interviews a good number favored small families. Ryan, *op. cit.*, pp. 367–69.

[5] P. K. Hatt, *Backgrounds of Human Fertility in Puerto Rico* (Princeton: Princeton University Press, 1952), Table 37, p. 53.

[6] Seventy-six percent of the males and 91 percent of the females gave a number less than five as their ideal.

[7] When specifically asked about the *disadvantages* of a large family, only 2 of the 143 could think of none.

that to have "all the children God sends" is a luxury which only the rich can afford.

About three or four for the poor people . . . and for the rich, they can have all that God wants to give them. (C7F)

Two. There is no advantage in having more children. If one is poor one shouldn't have more than two. The rich can have more because they have money to educate them and are not sacrificed or even killed working as the poor do. For the rich, they are even a recreation, for the poor man they are always a burden. The rich care better for the sons, but it is great work for the poor to rear them, and the wife of the poor gets sick with many children because she can't feed herself well nor have the medicines if she needs them. So, two is enough. (B1F)

Other respondents specifically deny the aphorisms which are usually attributed to their class:

Although there is a saying that if you have enough for one you have enough for ten, that is a saying only. You can't have ten in the same way you have one. For three perhaps, but not for ten. (Y4F)

The reasons why small families are desirable have already been detailed by Hatt, and our own data add little to these. Most people say that it is economically difficult or impossible to rear a large family properly; but over a quarter of Hatt's respondents and about the same proportion from the present sample say that it is difficult to *educate* a large number of children. Greater educational opportunities and new emphases on social mobility may be encouraging many lower-class members to stress education for their children, both for its own sake and as a means for social mobility. The quotations below would suggest that such attitudes may not always have been present[8] and as yet may not have permeated the entire lower class.

[8] Analyzing his data by age, Hatt sees "the likelihood that there is a real and significant trend toward smaller ideal families in Puerto Rico." However, the correlation between age and ideal number of children may to a large extent be due to a tendency to rationalize the number of children one already has. Since older women have more children, they might be expected to express a larger ideal than younger women. This hypothesis is supported by the fact that a coefficient of correlation of .20 was found between ideal and actual number of children, and that actual number rises with ideal number in each date of marriage category. Hatt, *op. cit.*, Table 274, p. 321.

In other times, people did not care about that, since they brought up their children any old way. When there are more than three, they cannot be given as good an education as one would like. (Y8F)

There are many who don't aspire to give them a good education, but I would like mine to study something, for that is the only heritage a poor person can leave to his child. (H2F)

There are many other evidences from the interview materials backing up the impression that the lower class is in favor of smaller families. One of these is the apparent absence among women of fears of barrenness. It was previously hypothesized that such fears on the part of women would be a potent factor in encouraging high fertility. If this was ever true, social change appears to have occurred, at least to the extent that the fear is seldom verbalized. Fifty-six women were asked the following question: "Some women fear they might be called *machorras* (barren women). Has that got anything to do with having children early in marriage?" Although this question was loaded, only a dozen of the fifty-six women answered affirmatively. Forty-four disagreed with the suggestion, many of these expressing indifference to the idea of being called barren themselves. Five women said that a woman should be glad to be barren.

I have heard several friends saying, "I wish I were a *machorra,* so that I would not have to work so hard!" (A5F)

That has nothing to do with it. If the woman has no children, so much the better for her. (B4F)

As for me, it would have been better if they called me barren. I have never heard anyone say it is bad, or that they don't like it. (C2F)

One woman suggested that this conception is a new one, that in another generation women did fear barrenness.

In older times women were ashamed not to have children. Only those having children were of good fortune. Today science has changed the divine plan. Women of today even expose themselves to death trying to avoid children. Now they don't worry about not having any. (Z3F)

Indeed, one might guess that the high-fertility-minded fear of being *machorra* may be coming to be replaced by fear of being a *güira* (guinea pig) or *paridora* (woman who reproduces frequently). Among the women, at least, the great prestige of the large family appears to be dying, and women who have small families are now the ones to be envied.[9]

A striking evidence of the interest in small family size is the amount of sexual abstinence and denial which appears to occur.[10] In some cases, men appear deliberately to use other women rather than impregnate their wives. While the employment of this method of birth control may be a rationalization for extramarital relations, some of the statements below ring true.

One has to look for other women. That is the most suitable method, and the handiest one. (He laughs.) (H6M)

Sometimes I have stopped using my wife, afraid of making her pregnant. (What do you do then?) I go out. (H5M)

Sometimes I didn't use my wife and went with other women. But I didn't tell her anything, so that she would not know I was doing it to avoid intercourse with her. (H7M)

In the first case cited above, despite its appearance of rationalization, there seems to have been a plan which included the wife.

She became jealous, and I had to explain to her that we should not have more children. She made up her mind and agreed with me. (H6M)

[9] Such contemptuous attitudes toward the woman who bears "too frequently" are undoubtedly of crucial importance in bringing about behavioral conformity to a group's standard of appropriate family size. Such attitudes have been noted by other observers in areas of fertility decline. In describing the climate of opinion among Western European women in the earlier decades of the century, von Ungern-Sternberg writes, "Even a certain milieu of mental terror has developed which ridicules women with 3, 4, 5, or more children and creates in them a feeling of inferiority, backwardness and deficient education. Expressions like 'rabbit-hutch' have a strikingly suggestive effect upon most women and lead to the adoption of a prevailing norm which recognizes about 2 children, at the most, as advisable." Roderich von Ungern-Sternberg, *The Causes of the Decline in Birth-Rate within the European Sphere of Civilization,* tr. by Hilda H. Wullen (Cold Spring Harbor, Long Island, N.Y.: Eugenics Research Association Monograph Series, No. IV, 1931), p. 43. A public opinion survey in Great Britain disclosed that "The old social attitude which considered it immoral to restrict families is giving place to an attitude which considers it immoral *not* to restrict them. . . . Large families today are considered old-fashioned at best, at worst somehow indecent" (Mass Observation, *op. cit.*, p. 75).

[10] The use of other birth-control methods will be considered in Chapter IX. The frequency of their use (especially the method of sterilization) is additional evidence of the small-family mentality.

In some cases this reduces the fertility in one family but compensates for it by raising it in another.

I avoid having contact with my wife and look for other women outside. That way I avoid having more children. (What kind of women?) Married women, because if they get pregnant there is no danger. (Z6M)

In most cases, however, it is the woman who is more interested in reducing fertility, and a frequent recourse is sexual denial.[11] Since many women do not see sex as pleasurable anyway, this is an easy expedient and may even be a rationalization used to discourage sexual contact.

You know what I do? I hit him with my legs and throw him out of the bed. We have quarreled about it for nine years and he even threatened to kill me. But I got pregnant of the last two anyway. (And after that?) Well, sometimes when I am waiting for menstruation or after it, I get angry with him and don't talk to him, so he can't come to bother me. (C10F)

He needs me more than I need him. . . . In that way we have fewer children. Because if we both wanted each other, then we would be full of children. (A8F)

There are two such cases as illustrated by the first quotation above, in which the woman practices rhythm surreptitiously by means of denial.[12] A circular process may occur, an emotional constellation productive of considerable marital strife. Pregnancy fears may breed frigidity, frigidity lead to denial, denial create marital tensions and further frigidity.

I feel tired of that business, and I don't like it . . . because if we go on doing that, we go on having children. . . . (A9F)

I did it in the first years of marriage, but I'm already tired. (Don't you enjoy it now?) Sometimes I enjoy it, but not others. Perhaps it is because I am afraid of getting pregnant again. *How could I enjoy*

[11] Brief summaries of "rather typical attitudes" of thirteen women in a study by King in Puerto Rico disclosed that two had prompted their husbands to seek other women to avoid pregnancy, another had left her husband to avoid more pregnancies, and another's husband was threatening abandonment because of the wife's denial. M. King, "Cultural Aspects of Birth Control in Puerto Rico," *Human Biology,* XX, No. 1 (Feb. 1948), 26–27.

[12] There are two other cases in which jelly was used surreptitiously, the women "not daring" to tell their husbands.

it, thinking of what would become of me if I have another child? (Y5F)

There are also several stories of fights between husbands and wives over the issue of birth control. "We were always fighting about that," "I threatened to leave him," "I told him we couldn't go on this way," and the like, are typical comments volunteered by women, but never by men, to show how they, rather than their husbands, wanted to do something about their fertility. The most extreme cases are those of two women who claim they chose their husbands on the basis of their apparent sterility!

(But you came to live with another man, didn't you?) Yes, but I knew this one had no children; that's why I went with him. I came to live with him conscious of that, otherwise I wouldn't have lived with him; one can't have any more children. (X6F)

No, I never thought of having children, because his sister told me he had no children. She said we were going to be happy because we weren't going to have children. Because he had another wife and never had had children. (Why did you think of that?) I thought it was better for me because when one has no children one is happy. (H7F)

About a dozen respondents voiced an age-old belief—that conception is the product of joint orgasm.[13] Thus if joint orgasm is eschewed, birth control is achieved. That the belief is not the exclusive property of the uneducated is demonstrated by the quotation below:

Dr. X told me that in order to become pregnant both man and wife have to have an orgasm at the same time. . . . I have reached the conclusion that this is wrong. (H16F)

It is conceivable that at one time this belief reinforced both fertility and sexual pleasure in marriage. In societies requiring high

[13] This conception has been noted as far back as 100 B.C. in Islam (Himes, *Medical History of Contraception*, London, George Allen and Unwin, 1936, p. 142); in contemporary urban England (Mass Observation, *op. cit.*, p. 59); and in the southern rural United States (Hagood, *op. cit.*, p. 118). Stone and Himes, in noting its prevalence among American women a generation ago, suggest that ". . . the practice is probably based on the belief that during the orgasm the woman, too, discharges a fluid comparable to male emission, and that if this fluid is not discharged, conception cannot occur" (*Planned Parenthood: A Practical Guide to Birth Control Methods*, New York, Viking Press, 1951, p. 136.

fertility it may have legitimized and encouraged sexual pleasure for the female, thus prompting high fertility by means of more frequent intercourse.[14] Among the small-family-minded lower class of Puerto Rico, however, it has the opposite effect. Since most women want few children, it *rationalizes their frigidity.* As a cheap and simple method of birth control, repression of the orgasm may be quite popular among those women who are already predisposed toward sexual indifference or revulsion. Thus a folk belief which may once have encouraged both fertility and pleasure may now have the contrary effect.

With so much evidence pointing in the direction of small-family ideals, we might expect that these ideals are carried out in practice. Yet the demographic evidence indicates that there has been little decline in fertility over the last half century.[15] The average rural Puerto Rican woman has borne 6.8 children by the completion of the child-bearing period, and urban women have borne 4.8.[16] According to Hatt's data, the average number of children surviving to at least age twelve is 4.8 per family for all married women age fifty and over.[17] These statistics show that Puerto Ricans have families larger than they consider ideal. In the present small sample, in which the median age of women is only 29.5, the women have already had an average of four pregnancies. Even when dead chil-

[14] On the other hand, in Christian societies the enjoyment of passionate coitus has long been frowned on as evil. See Himes, *op. cit.*, p. 184.

[15] Although the crude birth rate has remained roughly at 40 per thousand for the past half century (see J. Janer, "Population Growth in Puerto Rico and Its Relation to Time Changes in Vital Statistics," *Human Biology,* Dec. 1945, pp. 267–313), it has recently shown signs of decline, dropping to 35.9 in 1952. This may, however, be due only to the emigration of individuals in the fertile age period. Marital fertility appears to be dropping somewhat but has been compensated for by increases in the proportion of the population marrying. See C. Tietze, "Human Fertility in Puerto Rico," *American Journal of Sociology,* (July 1947), pp. 34–40, and Robert Osborn's chapter in Hatt, *op. cit.*). Hatt found sizable differences in fertility among different income, educational, and residence groups. Since these occur mainly after 1920, a trend in birth reduction for the more secularized groups seems to be apparent. From an analysis of the fluctuations in the marriage rate and in first- and second-order births, Combs and Davis conclude that "Puerto Rican fertility is beginning to be sensitive to economic conditions in a modern way" ("The Pattern of Puerto Rican Fertility," *Population Studies,* IV [March 1951] 379).

[16] Bureau of the Census Series PC-14, No. 21, June 24, 1954.

[17] Hatt, *op. cit,* p. 54.

dren are excluded from the computations, Table 29 shows that many families have *already* exceeded their family size ideals.

TABLE 29

DISCREPANCIES BETWEEN IDEAL SIZE OF FAMILY AND ACTUAL NUMBER OF LIVING CHILDREN, BY SEX

	Males	*Females*
Same as ideal number or less	37	37
One more than ideal number	4	10
Two or three more than ideal number	12	11
Four or more than ideal	17	13
Number of respondents	(70)	(71)

We now have the difficult task of reconciling the small-family ideals with the practice of having large families. Two major hypotheses will be investigated throughout the remainder of the report: (1) that small-family ideals are vitiated by poor communication and/or conflicting attitudes toward fertility; (2) that the means of realizing small-family ideals either are not known or are known and objected to.

COMMUNICATION OF FAMILY IDEALS

Although in general both husbands and wives have small-family ideals, lack of communication between the sexes often obstructs the awareness of a common ideal. That is, the general lack of communication, which we have described as typical of many lower-class families, and the specific lack of communication on sexual matters often result in the peculiar situation where both adults want few children but neither is aware that the other feels this way.[18]

Thus, when women were asked how many children their husbands wanted, nine showed a complete lack of knowledge of their husbands' ideals, saying, "He never says anything about that" or,

[18] Fifteen percent of the married women in Hatt's sample said they did not know how many children their husbands wanted. The percentage was considerably higher among the older couples. Hatt, *op. cit.*, Table 276, p. 325.

"He has never talked with me about that."[19] A check on the husbands' interviews shows that all but one of the nine husbands wanted the same number of children as their wives or fewer children.

Of those women who ventured an estimate of their husbands' family-size ideals, over half estimated incorrectly, as judged by their husbands' own stated ideals. Table 30 shows the extent to which wives are aware of the ideal number desired by their husbands.

TABLE 30

AWARENESS ON PART OF WIFE OF HUSBAND'S IDEAL NUMBER OF CHILDREN

Wife Thinks Husband Wants	HUSBAND ACTUALLY WANTS		
	Same as Wife	*More than Wife*	*Less than Wife*
Same as she	17	3	1
More than she	11	3	2
Less than she	6	1	1
Number of families	(34)	(7)	(4)

For those families for which information is available for both sexes, only 21 wives attributed the same ideal number of children to their husbands as the husbands themselves gave the interviewer. Roughly five out of every ten wives who ventured an opinion did not correctly reflect the husbands' opinions. This figure is particularly striking when we consider that the median and modal ideal

[19] Whelpton and Kiser, in their study of urban, largely middle-class families describe a case which illustrates the problem: "Although there were two children in this family the husband and wife had never talked about the number of children they desired. During recent years, the wife had come to think that the husband did not want a third child, hence that they would not have another even though she herself wanted it. The husband, on his part, had formed a similar opinion. As a result of being interviewed, however, the couple talked over some of the questions that had been asked, and discovered that each was mistaken as to the other's attitude. When last seen they were planning to have a third child" (P. Whelpton, and C. Kiser, "Developing the Schedules, and Choosing the Type of Couples and the Area to Be Studied," in *Social and Psychological Factors Affecting Fertility,* New York, Milbank Memorial Fund, 1950, p. 152).

number of children is three for *both* sexes. Thus, even by chance, a woman would be likely to guess correctly for her spouse.

More men have the same ideals as their wives than the latter realize. A total of seventeen men have the same ideals as their wives, whereas their wives believe that the ideals vary. Thus it may be concluded that whereas both sexes prefer small families, these preferences may not become sufficiently verbalized within the family to allow for concerted action. Table 31 shows that lack of correct knowledge of the husband's ideal family size has some relation to a general lack of communication between the spouses.

TABLE 31

DEGREE OF GENERAL COMMUNICATION BETWEEN SPOUSES, BY WIFE'S AWARENESS OF HUSBAND'S IDEAL FAMILY SIZE

	High Communication (percent)	*Medium Communication (percent)*	*Low Communication (percent)*
Wife guesses correctly	69	23	31
Wife guesses incorrectly	25	45	63
Wife does not know	6	32	6
	100	100	100
Number of families	(16)	(22)	(16)

While lack of information on one or the other of the indices[20] makes the number of cases awkwardly few, those cases tend in the expected direction. Only in the high communication group does a large proportion of the women appear to be accurately aware of their husbands' fertility ideals. The largest proportion of incorrect evaluations was given by women in the least-communication families, although, if the "Don't Know's" are considered, those with medium communication have even larger discrepancies. If this statistic reflects reality, it would suggest that effective communication on ideal family size occurs *only* when general communication is quite high between the married couple of the lower class.

[20] See Appendix C for details on the communication index construction.

CONFLICTING FERTILITY IDEALS

Despite the fact that the bulk of the evidence suggests an interest in small families, there are present a number of contrary beliefs more characteristic of large-family mentalities. That such can exist side by side with modern ideals concerning the small family may be an evidence of cultural lag, or it may represent genuine ambivalence. The present research cannot determine which of these alternatives seems more prominent, but the considerable indications of large-family mentality will be presented. These may be subsumed under three broad categories: (1) the hope that children will be of assistance in one's old age; (2) the belief in immediate impregnation following marriage; (3) the tendency on the part of males to identify a large family with *machismo*.

CHILDREN AND OLD AGE

When respondents were asked why they held *X* to be the ideal number of children, only 34 out of 143 men and women answered in terms of the advantages of children. However, when asked the more leading question, "What are the advantages of a large family?" about half of the males and a quarter of the females mentioned unqualified advantages.

Thus, while the small family may be said to be a general ideal, a good proportion also think there are advantages to large families.[21] That such exist may well cause a certain amount of ambivalence

[21] There is some evidence that feelings of small-family-mindedness do not resemble those more typical of the United States. Most of the reasons given by the sample for preferring a small family are in terms of the *children* rather than in terms of the parents. The health, rearing, and education of the chlidren are seen to be jeopardized in the large family more frequently than are the interests, health, and goals of the parents. (In response to the question, "What do you think are the main reasons why couples do not have more children?" 20 percent of a cross section of Americans said, "Interference with one's freedom." H. Cantril and M. Strunk, *Public Opinion 1935–1946* (Princeton: Princeton University Press, 1951), p. 43. Possibly the ideals in Puerto Rico are in transition, midway between the large-family-mindedness of truly underdeveloped areas and the more hedonistic and individualistic small-family-mindedness of modern society. This hypothesis is also lent credence by the fact that, of the 42 women who were asked whether they would want more children "if they had money," 17 replied in the affirmative.

with respect to family-size ideals. What are the advantages of the large family as seen by lower-class respondents?

The principal advantage appears to be a hope that children will help in one's old age. Of the 34 respondents who think in terms of the advantages of children when giving an ideal number of children for a family, half cited help in old age as their reason. When Hatt's respondents were asked why they did not choose a lower number for their ideal family size, about half of the 13,000 gave this same reason.[22]

In the present survey, however, there is a good deal of contrary evidence on this score. There are, first of all, respondents who deny that children help their parents in the latter's old age.

Sons don't help their parents. . . . I have seen so many cases in which the father has worked hard supporting his sons, and later on, when they were men, they helped nobody. (B5M)

The son is rare who helps his parents. (H9F)

Some can see certain advantages but feel that these are outweighed by the disadvantage of having to struggle to support a large family. The physical and economic pains of bringing them up are not worth the dubious prospect of security in one's old age.

All of them can help to support the family. (Then why do you prefer a small family?) Because my earnings are not enough to support them. (A8M)

Some say it is more profitable to have a lot of children because in the future they will help, but the wife is the one who has to give birth to them, exposing herself to death, so she doesn't like it. (H19F)

A frequently held attitude was that one's real obligation is to his wife and children. To help one's parents as well is commendable and noble if money is available, but it is a luxury which many respondents do not really expect.

If he is a good son, he helps his parents, but he is not obliged to do it, because he belongs to his wife and sons. (Y5F)

If he is a good son he always remembers his parents, but not because it's his duty. After he gets married, his obligation is to his wife and children. (H19F)

[22] Hatt, *op. cit.*, Table 42, p. 59.

The logical conclusion to the foregoing reasoning was well stated by one respondent.

If they are going to help, few will help as well as many, so it is preferable to have few. (H7F)

But despite such arguments we are still left with a not inconsiderable number of respondents who are looking forward to help in old age. One might conclude that social change has been such as to make many lower-class individuals dubious about economic help on the part of their children. Landlessness, minimum-age laws for working, and the popularity of formal education make the son's contribution minimal and of short duration. Increasing physical mobility, the breakdown of extended family obligations, and the increasing isolation of the nuclear family make subsequent help less likely than in the past. Yet some parents still hope that children are an investment which pays good dividends when these are needed most. Such parents may not cherish such hopes for long in Puerto Rico's rapidly industrializing economy, but the fact that many still do suggests that family-size ideals, while predominantly in the direction of the small family, are not unequivocally so.

THE DESIRE FOR A RAPID FIRST PREGNANCY

Most Puerto Ricans, despite small-family ideals, want to start their families immediately. Slightly over half of Hatt's sample wanted their first child "as soon as possible" after marriage, and another third wanted it between the first and second years of marriage. Hatt concluded that "the importance of beginning a family soon, then, is a value rather more generally accepted throughout the society than are any principles with regard to either the size of the family or the acceptability of planning the family."[23] In our own sample, 49 percent of the males and 36 percent of the females felt that the ideal time for the first birth was "as soon as possible."

Let us consider the reasons for desiring an immediate pregnancy. The reason most frequently stated by the wives, and one of the more frequent for the husbands, is the argument, frequently heard in our own society, that one should get childbearing and child rearing over

[23] Hatt, *op. cit.*, p. 185.

as quickly as possible. There is, first of all, the belief, voiced by nine women, that the "sooner you start the sooner you finish." Wanting to get child rearing over with quickly may lead many women to behavior which has the opposite effect, for the sooner they start, the more children ultimately will be born, barring contraception.

The second reason for believing in an early start is that "you see them grown up sooner." This kind of reason, stated by eight women and six men, means that the parents will still be young when the children are grown. The advantage to this, as seen by the respondents, are several. Most of the men and some of the women in this group wanted to put the children on their feet before the death of their parents. While still young and in the labor force, the parents can assist their growing children. This attitude may stem partly from a low life-expectancy outlook. (Life expectancy in 1940 was only forty-five years for all of Puerto Rico.) It probably also takes into account the difficulties which the aged have in continuing to support themselves, not to mention their children.

For the males particularly, however, other reasons are equally important. One of these is that a marriage without children is not really a marriage, and that the sooner one can establish himself as a *padre de familia,* the sooner does his prestige go up—that is, the sooner does he become a real adult.[24]

Closely related to this is the already-mentioned hypothesis that men tend to be uncertain about their virility. One way of proving virility is to be a *conquistador de mujeres;* but, since impregnation of other women is tabued, the man will either not father children of these illicit partners or not take credit for them. Consequently, he still has to prove his virility in the sense of being able to procreate.

> I was anxious to have my first child to see if I was sterile or not, because one has to avoid children with other women before marriage. (B4M)

The sooner the male can prove this, the sooner his anxiety is relieved and the sooner is he accepted into the male adult world. Of

[24] "[Because] working people here do not regard a marriage as truly consummated before the birth of the first child, consensually married couples will seek to have a child . . . within a year of their union" S. Mintz, "Cañamelar: The Contemporary Culture of a Rural Puerto Rican Proletariat," unpublished Ph.D. dissertation, Columbia University, 1951, Chap. VI, p. 21.

the 39 men who answered "Immediately" to the question as to the ideal time after marriage to have the first child, 8 gave the reason, "To show that the man is not sterile." In answer to the question, "Is a man anxious to have his first child?" all but five males replied in the affirmative. When asked why, no less than 31 of the 63 men replied, "In order to prove that one is a man," or "To show that one is not sterile." Some of these responses are illustrated below.

That business of being married and having no children looks bad. One likes to have them to prove he is not *machorro* (barren). (Z7M)

. . . a man feels more virile when he knows he can make a child. (Z3M)

A man is anxious to have his son early to prove his *hombría* (manliness). . . . I mean that he wants his first child in order to prove that he can make sons, that he is not barren. (A11M)

One of the interesting aspects of this anxiety is that much of its motive power comes from the adult male community. A number of men expressed the fear of being laughed at and ridiculed by their fellows if they did not have a child. Perhaps there is a tendency to assume that a man is not a man unless proven to be one. From the safety of their offspring, fathers build up their own sense of virility by mocking those who have not yet been proven. Note in the quotations below how strong the community pressure appears to be.

If one is not *un hombre completo,* he can't live in town. The people talk about him. (What do they say?) Well, that he is not a real man because he doesn't have children. . . . When I had my children, I felt happy. (Why?) Because I knew that I could have children, that I am not sterile. (Y8M)

One wants to have a child so that people don't talk about him. (How is that?) Yes, man, if you don't have children, people say that you're sterile and make fun of you. That's why when I had my first child I was all happy inside. (Y4M)

. . . that proves if one is sterile or not, and if you are sterile you are worthless in the public eye. (What do you mean?) If a man is not *completo* here, he would be the laughing stock of everyone around here, and that is very painful for a man. (X8M)

We have seen that women are not especially concerned about proving their fertility, but many of them recognize that such is not the case with men. Several women expressed disdain that the man should feel this way, one woman phrasing it particularly effectively.

Men want children soon. They say they are an entertainment and they go crazy for the first-born; but it is really that they want to be sure they can have children. (A13F)

In one case, a young man uses his children to convince his fellows that he is a man.

My husband's brother, who is sixteen, got married and has a child, and his wife is now pregnant again. When he fights with other men, people tell him he is not a man, he is only sixteen. He tells them, "Well, I have children, I am *un hombre completo.*" (C6F)

There is a final factor encouraging the early inception of fertility which merits some discussion. This is the suspicion of infidelity with which each sex tends to regard the other. The first manifestation of this is the fear that a late pregnancy may be interpreted by the male as a sign of infidelity. As one woman put it, "If she gets pregnant too late, the man may say that she is pregnant of another man and not of him." While this is a logical consequence of the infidelity phobias on the part of the male, it is infrequently mentioned. The more usual attitude on the part of both sexes, but particularly of the male, is that children tie down the spouse and make it much more difficult for her to desert.[25]

He told me the more kids I have, the more tied to him I was . . . that with so many kids I could not abandon him to go with another man or return to my family. (TRC)

[Men want children soon] so as to have their women tied to the home. (C6F)

[25] Carried to its extreme, suspicion becomes hostility, and impregnation may even be used as an instrument of revenge or hostility on the part of the male. One unhappily married woman, for example, says that the only thing her husband can do to her now is to get her pregnant again; but that she is "being shrewd and not letting him touch me." In another case, a woman told of a man who impregnated his wife out of pure malice. They had agreed to use condoms, but the male tricked her by tearing them before having intercourse. Her subsequent comment might suggest that the practice may not be unique: "That's why the nurses always advise us to examine the condoms very carefully, because some men make tiny holes in them, just to get the wife pregnant. I am always very careful of that." (B8F)

In one case this was carried out quite methodically. The story was told independently by both husband and wife. The husband told the interviewer that he wanted no children at all.

> (Then why did you have a child?) Because I got angry with my wife. Her mother took her to town and got her work as a servant. Later she came back to me full of love, and I forgave her, so she stopped working. I had that child so that she couldn't go away any more. Having a child, she was bound to stay. (B5M)

One woman opined that men wanted children soon so that they could secure their wives in the home while they themselves were able to seek other conquests.

> When they have children and like to go out alone, they can do it, because they know that their wives are obliged to stay at home while they go after other women. (H23F)

With some women suspicion has the contrary effect, however. They are so uncertain that their marriages will last that they want pregnancy *delayed,* so that separation will be easier if they do not get along. The majority of women in our sample wanted a delayed pregnancy (although not put off for long), and one of the most frequent reasons given for this was "to see if the marriage will turn out all right"—an expression clearly manifesting the misgivings with which many women face marriage.[26]

THE LARGE FAMILY AND *machismo*

As we have already suggested, women are not greatly concerned with proving their fecundity, but the situation is quite different with men. When asked whether men in general wanted to have many or few children, 20 out of the 51 mothers who answered said that men wanted many, or that men didn't care how many they had. As seen by the women, the principal reason for this was that

[26] An even more frequently given reason for delayed pregnancy may indicate new conceptions of husband-wife relations. Twenty-nine women said they preferred a delayed pregnancy because they wanted more freedom and more opportunity to enjoy their honeymoons and subsequent husband-wife relationships. This would suggest both a growing sense of independence on the part of the women and the beginning of a tendency toward marriages resembling the companionate type.

the men only "make" the children, the women must bear and rear them.

> The kind of man who likes to have many children is the sort who says that it's the women who bear the children and raise them. The man doesn't have to care for them. That's why he doesn't object to having many. (H12F)

> They don't care because they only care about making them. They don't have troubles with them. They like making a lot of them. (X7F)

> I say to my husband, "When you don't expect it, you are going to have two or three more kids." And he says, "When did you ever see a man giving birth to child? It is your concern." And I say, "But you make them." (Z6F)

If it is the husband who "makes" the children, we would expect more anxiety on his part about this function, and indeed this is true. We have already discussed the sterility fears which encourage the male to produce a rapid first birth, but there may be other forces which encourage him to keep producing. One of these is *machismo*.[27] Women realize this male motivation and contrast males with themselves in this regard.

> Some women feel sad not having any children, but that is because they like children and not because they don't want to be called *machorras*. (And what about the husbands?) Men care more about having them; they want to know that they can have them. (X8F)

> Men feel bad if they are called *machorros*. Mine likes it when another baby is coming, for he feels more *macho* if he has many. . . . He feels more of a man having many. (X3F)

> Many husbands like them because there is more happiness having children. I believe sometimes they like to have children in order to prove that they are *machos*. (Z4F)

Although many men said that at least one child was needed to prove one's virility, few of them said explicitly that many were

[27] This point would not appear to merit the importance it was given in the original design, where it was supposed that the need to prove one's *machismo* drove men to have large families. This does drive some men to have at least one child, but not necessarily to have many. Several men said that one or two children were enough to demonstrate that one is not sterile. The weight of the emphasis here is on *sterility* rather than on general virility or the ability to produce a large number of sons.

needed for this reason. A large family helps the ego in other ways, however. There are very few ways in which a lower-class male can gain prestige in a community, for he has neither the economic nor the educational capital to improve himself.[28] Completely frustrated in the economic sphere, it is all a man can do to obtain enough food to allow himself and his family to exist.[29] It is virtually impossible to purchase articles of the conspicuous-consumption variety which might gain him prestige among his peers. Children become a major showpiece. The folk saying, that "Children are the capital of the poor," may no longer reflect economic reality, but it may still reflect the function of children as evidences of conspicuous consumption. Many men, when they said that a large family gives a man prestige, appeared to mean the prestige of being able to *support* such a large family rather than that of being able to *produce* one.

It is my opinion that in order to be an *hombre completo* a man should have a wife and children, and that these should be well fed and have clothes to wear and the necessary things to live well. (Y4M)

A large family helps to prove the *hombría* of a man. (How?) Because it takes a real man to maintain and educate a large family. (B4M)

Thus, despite his lowly status and inability to advance in life, a man can prove that he is a real man after all, by showing his ability to support a large family. The female has no such motivation. Economically derived prestige is not normally part of the feminine world. She is not expected to provide sustenance for the children. The good mother is she who takes care of the goods, including

[28] The extraordinary amount of internal and external migration which occurs on the part of the lower class is one of the manifestations of the desire to improve one's self. Although the individual is unable to do so in the home environment, recent developments have made it possible for him to "leave the scene" and seek prestige by achievements outside the community. For an excellent account of internal migration, see R. Parke, "Internal Migration in Puerto Rico" (unpublished Master's essay, Columbia University, 1952).

[29] "Sixty-two percent [of the population] have less than the amount needed to buy a minimum adequate diet [$140 per year]" L. J. Roberts and R. L. Stefani, *Patterns of Living in Puerto Rican Families,* (Río Piedras, University of Puerto Rico, 1949, p. 13). Standards of living, however, have improved substantially in the past decade. Whereas the median annual income of wage earners' families was $360 in 1941, it rose to $919 by 1952, a 68-percent increase in real income. Puerto Rico Department of Labor, Preliminary Release No. 1, August 1953.

children, which are provided by the husband. Moreover, since the male "makes the children," it is the male more than the female who fears sterility. Thus, *the burden of proof both in an economic and sexual sense lies with the male.*

There are several other reasons encouraging the male to high fertility, but these need only be mentioned. There are men who say that the more children one has, the surer one is of the wife's fidelity and of her inability to abandon her husband. This has already been explored in the discussion of immediate pregnancy. There are also a fair number of men who hold that children give stability and responsibility to the male—"something to fight for." Perhaps this attitude mitigates the sense of hopelessness about the economic world. There is really no point in trying, since only luck can produce fortune.[30] But if one has children, one has to strive—at least to the point of providing them with food and clothing. This much can be done, and it gives the male a sense of purpose and responsibility which he otherwise would not have.

One minor factor in encouraging fertility is the requirement that the husband should have at least one male offspring. This is probably universally true of patriarchal societies, where a male is required to carry on the family line. In the lower-class society of Puerto Rico, however, the relative absence of clans, the relative isolation of the nuclear family, and the lack of land or possessions for inheritance might be expected to weaken the emphasis on the continuation of the family line. More detailed study is needed before reaching any conclusions on this point, but there is considerable evidence from the interview materials suggesting that *other* factors play a role in the desire for a male son.

One of these has already been mentioned. Since the male is the symbol of virility, male offspring are one indication of one's *machismo.* More accurately, at least one male heir is a *sine qua non* of manliness, and the producer of girls is seen as laughable. With all

[30] See Padilla's discussion of gambling in the lower class: "Nocora: An Agrarian Reform Sugar Community in Puerto Rico" (unpublished Ph.D. dissertation, Columbia University, 1951), Chap. VII, pp. 10–16. The legal and illegal lottery is of immense popularity in the lower class, for it is practically the only way in which a lower-class man can amass capital in his own community.

the predispositions toward anxiety concerning his *hombría* which we have described, the married male is particularly concerned lest he fall into the luckless group of fathers known as *chancleteros*. Moreover, since the man is seen as the "maker" of children, the production of too many *chancletas* reflects upon him.

We men want the other men to see that we can have male sons. (What about the women?) The women, too, so they can't gossip about us, saying that we make only *chancletas*. (A5M)

I wanted a male son . . . so as to know I was a *macho*. (A *macho?*) Yes, to show that I am not like the men that only have females. (B5M)

Other men desire male offspring narcissistically. No women gave such reasons for desiring girls. Perhaps their own self-images are too unfavorable to allow such explicit narcissistic preferences.

I hope for boys because I like the males better, *like I am* . . . for my own self love and pride. (Y8M)

The father prefers boys, so they will *grow up like him*. So that they learn his occupation, play an instrument like him, go out and have a good time like him, and *so that they will be machos like him*. (Y4F)

I would have liked to have had my first child later, but my husband wanted a son soon. He said he was eager *to see whom he* [*the child*] *resembled*. (B1F)

Such desires could affect fertility by encouraging a rapid succession of births until at least one male offspring occurs. At each *chancleta,* a man's anxieties about his virility and his need for narcissistic fulfillment might encourage him to "keep trying" until a male son dissipates his fears.[31] How frequently this occurs we do not know. That it does occur, however, we can conclude from the statements below.

Out there lives a man who has five daughters and doesn't want to have his wife operated on until they have a son—so she goes on having children. (Z1F)

He didn't want to avoid children because he wanted a son. After the third girl he decided to have no more, but only because I begged him

[31] One son may not be enough. High-mortality-mindedness in the lower class may lead a man to require more than one for the sake of security. See Chap. I, note 30.

so much that I convinced him. . . . He said he wouldn't let me be sterilized until I had a boy. (H4F)

This attitude, of course, also leads to various difficulties in marital relations. There is no way of ascertaining how many lower-class women have been abandoned for this reason, but several statements from female respondents would suggest that this, too, occurs.

When I had a still birth on the first one, he told me was going to abandon me. Soon after I became pregnant again and had a boy, and he was glad. (C2F)

[He threatened to leave me], but after we had the male son he behaved better. (Why would that be?) He said that he would stay living with the woman who gave him a son. (H1F)

[After the first one was born a girl] he used to say that if he didn't get a boy this time he would leave me, as he didn't want any more women. (A12F)

SUMMARY

In this chapter we have examined some of the major components of our sample's fertility belief system. While small-family ideals are almost unanimously verbalized, these are seldom reflected in practice, at least as judged by actual family size. One explanation of this discrepancy might be found in the poor communication which exists between husbands and wives. Ideals held individually are seldom aired and, consequently, seldom held in common.

Perhaps more important are other components of the fertility belief system which vitiate desires for the small family, or at least render many families ambivalent about action. Although hopes appear to be to some degree diminishing, the wish that a large number of children will serve as social security for one's old age may still be strong enough to dampen concern over family size for many couples. There are also several factors impelling couples to start their families soon and to have their births in rapid succession. On the part of the women, the notion that "the sooner you start the sooner you finish" and the fear that their early deaths may leave young children helpless serve as blocks to action on family size.

In the case of the males, the belief system seems even more ambivalent. Hypotheses from previous chapters suggested that male character structure is such as to render men more positively oriented but less self-confident in the sphere of sexual relations than women. Since the burden of proof for sexuality and fecundity seems to fall on the male, he is especially concerned to disprove his sterility by rapid impregnation after marriage and, to a lesser extent, to continue to prove his virility by continued impregnations. He also wants to prove that he can produce male offspring and that he is enough of a man to rear, support, and educate a large family—a kind of conspicuous consumption where other avenues of prestige-getting are blocked. Finally, as a product of the suspicions and hostility between husbands and wives, there appears to be a tendency on the part of the male to view pregnancy and children as a means of tying the wife securely to the home and, occasionally, a tendency to use impregnation as an act of hostility.

Such values are inconsistent with the small-family mentality. For many lower-class families these values will have to assume less importance before the small-family ideology can be realized. The following chapter will, in part, be devoted to examining other factors in the fertility belief system—more specifically, attitudes toward birth-control techniques—and to determine what part these factors play in frustrating small-family ideals.

VIII

Attitudes toward Birth Control

> The Catholic religion says it's a sin to use birth control, but I think it's a greater sin if [those children] have nothing to eat.
>
> A CATHOLIC RESPONDENT

> After a mountain clinic performed a dozen or so sterilizations, it was attacked in a pastoral letter. The reading of the letter in the rural churches was followed by a wave of inquiries at public health clinics and to private doctors as to the availability of the operation which had been denounced by the bishop.
>
> CLARENCE SENIOR

KNOWLEDGE OF BIRTH CONTROL METHODS

In Chapter I we observed that the degree to which birth controls are employed depends in part upon the diffusion of knowledge of birth-control technology, and that this in turn depends upon the form and content of the communications system, the availability of methods, and the predispositions of the audience. In Puerto Rico, good roads and cheap transportation make the small island area (35 by 100 miles) fairly accessible to a large proportion of the population; and exposure to the mass media is greater than might be supposed, considering existing income and educational levels. According to the island-wide survey of Roberts, and Stefani in 1947, even in the lower economic half of the population, about a third of the families are exposed to a newspaper in the home at least weekly,[1] and about a quarter are exposed to the radio more or less regularly.[2]

The source of the second quotation at the head of this chapter is Clarence Senior, "An Approach to Research in Overcoming Cultural Barriers to Family Limitation," in G. Mair, ed., *Studies in Population* (Proceedings of the Annual Meeting of the Population Association of America; Princeton: Princeton University Press, 1949), p. 150.

[1] L. J. Roberts and R. L. Stefani, *Patterns of Living in Puerto Rican Families* (Río Piedras: University of Puerto Rico, 1949), Table 222, p. 402.

[2] *Ibid.*, Table 230, p. 406.

With reference to the diffusion of birth-control technology, not only are methods available in the usual retail outlets, but free supplies are available to most of the population. Throughout the following pages, we shall discuss in greater detail the degree of diffusion of such free materials, the content of the mass media which have relevance to birth control, the degree of awareness of methods on the part of our sample, and the predisposition of the sample toward various methods.

THE BIRTH-CONTROL PROGRAM

Birth-control clinics are not new in Puerto Rico. Attempts by private groups were stifled as far back as 1925, but in 1935 an island-wide program was initiated by a federal agency, the Puerto Rican Emergency Relief Administration. Mobile units with a physician and social worker visited all the towns on the island several times a month, and considerable publicity in the way of leaflets and public meetings attracted lower-class Puerto Ricans into the clinics. Pressure from the Catholic hierarchy on the continent, however, rapidly brought this program to a close.

Private funds continued the program until a court decision in 1939 legalized the distribution of birth-control materials by physicians for medical reasons. On the strength of this case 160 prematernal clinics were established. These were authorized to give free contraceptive materials to all individuals who desired them and who met broadly interpreted medical criteria. Although the private facilities were in some ways expanded, the publicity given the clinics was discontinued. In the opinion of local observers, the birth-control program "went underground" as far as promotion was concerned. Nevertheless, the fact that there are 160 well-located clinics and that these have been in operation for well over a decade would suggest that information must be trickling down to the lower classes.[8]

PROPAGANDA, INDIRECT AND DIRECT

It is the opinion of the writer that one of the most important elements in alerting the population to the possibilities of controlling birth by modern means has been the highly publicized battle

[8] See Chapter IX for the extent to which the clinics are used.

between the spokesmen for the Church and those who favor birth control. From the beginning of 1949 to the end of 1951, close to two hundred articles dealing with different aspects of the population problem have appeared in the Puerto Rican newspapers. This is an average of about one article for every five days of publication. Of these articles, slightly over half discussed birth control, a quarter sterilization, and the remainder the population problem in general. A breakdown of three San Juan newspapers shows definite leanings. In the case of *El Diario,* a progovernment paper, over half the articles were in favor of birth control or at least recognized the existence of a population problem, while only a quarter were opposed.[4] Over three fourths of the articles in the opposition paper, *El Imparcial,* were classified as negative regarding birth control or the existence of a population problem, while only 6 percent of the articles could be classified as positive.[5] *El Mundo,* generally considered to be the best and most impartial newspaper, was favorable in a third of its articles, unfavorable in about 40 percent, and neutral in about a quarter.

The clergy and their spokesmen are the most frequently represented of any group, their statements counting for over a quarter of the total. Columnists are next, with professionals and government officials composing the third largest group. Those opposing birth control outweighed those favoring it. Of the total number of articles, close to half opposed it, a little less than a third favored it, and the remaining articles were neutral. Regardless of their stand on the issues, it is clear that such a heavy amount of newspaper coverage on population, birth control, and sterilization is sure to alert some readers to the fact that there are means available to limit conception.

At least one private organization directs some of its efforts toward education for birth control. The Asociación de Estudios Poblacionales de Puerto Rico was founded a few years ago to arouse

[4] *El Diario* carried very few articles on sterilization; *El Imparcial,* a great many.

[5] When the *Imparcial's* inquiring photographer asked six young Puerto Ricans how many children they would like to have when they married, however, four of them wanted only two, and the remainder three. *Imparcial,* Oct. 1, 1952.

public discussion of the population problem. Composed of close to two hundred professionals, largely from the metropolitan area, it not only attempts to reach and influence community leaders but has made some efforts to reach the people themselves. Over 200,000 simply written and well-illustrated "throw-aways" have been distributed, with the purpose of informing the lower-class population of the existence of birth-control facilities.[6]

Public forums have frequently been held by the Population Association on the problem of population in Puerto Rico, and a few other groups have sponsored such public meetings. In 1952, for example, the Seventh Convention of Social Workers of Puerto Rico devoted its conference to the population problem. Approximately two dozen papers were read by leading academic, governmental, and religious representatives. The entire program (including several papers on birth control) was broadcast by radio, and considerable newspaper publicity was devoted to the content of the speeches. In sum, the mass media of Puerto Rico have presented many opportunities for learning about birth control, at the very least for those who are exposed to these media.

THE KNOWLEDGE OF SPECIFIC METHODS

With this background of action over the past decade, and with rising levels of living and education, we would not expect the degree of ignorance of modern methods of birth control which characterizes the populations of underdeveloped nations. In our present sample, no family evidenced complete ignorance of birth-control methods. All men and all but three women in the sample knew about sterilization as a means of birth control, and Table 32 shows that a good proportion of husbands and wives knew other modern methods as well. Unfortunately, the flexible nature of the interview method produced a high number of "no informations" in this area, but within the number for whom information is available there appears to be more knowledge than might have been expected for such a poorly educated and impoverished group.

[6] In March, 1954, the Association changed its name to Asociación Pro-Bienestar de la Familia, elected Dr. Emilio Cofresí as full-time executive secretary, and laid plans for a much more extensive program.

TABLE 32

KNOWLEDGE OF BIRTH-CONTROL METHODS, BY SEX

Percentage of respondents who know the particular method

	MALES		FEMALES	
	Percent	*Base*[a]	*Percent*	*Base*
Condom	100	(71)	84	(69)
Diaphragm	28	(39)	46	(59)
Jelly	20	(40)	38	(58)
Douche	48	(42)	41	(54)

[a] Percentages are calculated on the basis of all for whom there is adequate information. A respondent was placed in the "does not know" category if he met either of two criteria: (1) denying knowledge of a method mentioned specifically by an interviewer; (2) denying that he knew any methods other than those he had already mentioned in answer to the question, "What methods do you know?" Thus, "No information" is a residual category, *probably composed mainly of individuals who do not know the method.* However, since it could not be assumed that because a respondent did not mention a method he did not know it, all such cases were put in the "No information" category.

The condom is known by all but ten women in the sample, and the diaphragm is known by close to half of those women for whom information was secured. Of the other methods, there is less knowledge, but this result may be partly due to the high proportion of women who were not specifically asked about these methods. Only eight women in the sample claimed they knew no methods at all, but of these, all but three knew about sterilization.

Knowledge of birth-control methods would appear to have some relation to education and current residence of women.[7]

Although awareness of modern methods is unusually high, there are still a large number of men and women who do not know such methods as the diaphragm, jelly, and douche. One of the major factors that keep women from becoming informed appears to be modesty. The long-term effects of the complex of virginity perhaps reinforced by unsatisfactory sexual experience in marriage, lead to a high degree of squeamishness on the part of women concerning the seeking of information on birth control. Most women know

[7] Birthplace, age, and degree of traditionalism show no or very slight differences.

TABLE 33

KNOWLEDGE OF BIRTH-CONTROL METHODS, BY EDUCATION AND RESIDENCE OF WIVES

	Knows no Methods or Condom and/or Withdrawal only (percent)	*Knows Other Methods (Diaphragm, Douche, etc.) (percent)*
Education		
Four years and under	74	56
Five years and over	26	44
	100	100
Residence		
Country	48	17
Other	52	83
	100	100
Number of respondents	(35)	(36)

about the Public Health Units as sources of information, but many are too modest to attend the clinics. The principal reason for this is that they are afraid of being examined by a male physician. As one woman said, after five years of marriage she could neither undress in front of her husband nor look at him naked. How then could she let a doctor see her? The quotations below express the same feeling.

If we go there, they have to look you all over, and I am ashamed. I have had five kids and nobody has seen me. I had two babies in the hospital with nurses and three at home with my mother; the midwife came only to cut the umbilical cord. (Y2F)

I never went to the Health Unit, even when I was pregnant. I didn't like to be examined by a doctor. . . . I have never been examined by a doctor. (Y4F)

I know about the Public Health Unit, and once they wanted to give me methods but I refused to ask for them because I was ashamed of being examined by a doctor. (TRC)

A few women were so modest that they could not bring themselves to ask for the information, to say nothing of an examination.

I am ashamed of asking for them, and that's why I never go to the Health Unit. Some of my friends asked me to do it as they are going, but I am ashamed. (Of what?) Of asking them. (C2F)

I don't want to go to anybody to ask for that. (Why?) Because I don't like to. Those are matters which, ever since I was a little girl, I've never discussed with anybody. (B6F)

Other women are ashamed of being *seen* at prematernal clinics. Such clinics are regularly held one afternoon a week in most places on the island, and it is not unlikely that many women are ashamed of being seen attending these clinics because the other women know they concern birth control.[8]

Many friends of mine invited me to the Health Unit, and I didn't dare to go. (Why?) Because it was known by everyone that in town on Tuesday they give prophylactics in the Health Unit. Women are seen coming out of the unit with their package, and everybody knows what they have gone there for. (C6F)

I know the Public Health Unit, but I don't let the people see me there because they start talking; and for that reason I have not allowed my wife to go there. The people always talk and interfere with the lives of others. (C10M)

This last quotation brings up an interesting fact. There are even a few men who are embarrassed about procuring birth-control materials.[9] They object to going into the drug stores to ask for condoms.

I don't dare go to a drug store to buy those. I feel too embarrassed. (H12M)

The truth is that I don't dare go to a drug store to buy them. Sometimes I abstain from using my wife, even when I desire her. I don't like that, but I cannot do anything else. (H17M)

[8] King notes that many women stated, "Neighbors may think that venereal disease treatments are being taken. A number of women expressed horror at the prospect of being subjected to a vaginal examination, particularly by a male physician. . . . [Concerning childbirth] several women declared that they preferred a midwife, even though inadequately trained, to a male doctor whose services might be obtained free of charge, specifically because of shame at being seen by a man" (M. King, "Cultural Aspects of Birth Control in Puerto Rico," *Human Biology,* XX, No. 1 [Feb. 1948], p. 32).

[9] A total of 15 women gave such modesty references as are illustrated above, a high proportion in a sample of 72. These 15 women tended to be somewhat older, less educated, and more traditional, but the differences are not great.

If modesty keeps many individuals from seeking information and materials in public sources, modesty and general barriers against communication have the same effect *within the family*.

From Table 32 it is clear that there is a sizable discrepancy between the sexes in their knowledge of specific methods of birth control.[10] Whereas all husbands know the condom, ten wives do not. A higher proportion of men than women do not know about the diaphragm and jelly. This is brought out more clearly by Table 34 in which husbands and wives were matched and compared by knowledge.

TABLE 34

DISCREPANCY IN KNOWLEDGE OF FOUR BIRTH-CONTROL METHODS BETWEEN HUSBANDS AND WIVES

	One Method	*Two or More Methods*	*Total*
Wife knows, husband does not know	9	6	15
Wife knows, husband probably[a] does not know	7	9	16
Husband knows, wife does not know	16	3	19
Husband knows, wife probably does not know	10	1	11
Total	(42)	(19)	(61)

[a] The "Probably does not know" categories include the "No answers" on knowledge about a particular method, on the assumption that it is *likely* that if a respondent did not voluntarily mention a method he did not know about it.

The table clearly shows the lack of communication between husbands and wives. In 34 cases there is definite information indicating

[10] The Indianapolis study found that fairly wide discrepancies in knowledge of birth control exist between men and women prior to marriage. Once married, however, women learn quickly, and by the second pregnancy they are about as knowledgeable as their husbands. P. Whelpton and C. Kiser, eds., *Social and Psychological Factors Affecting Fertility* (New York: Milbank Memorial Fund, 1950).

that one member of the marriage knows one or more methods that the other member does not know, and in another 27 cases this situation is probable. Thus, it is likely that in 57 families out of 72[11] the information possessed on birth control is somewhat vitiated by the fact that some of this information is not shared, i.e., is not the common property of both spouses. Such a pattern does not at this stage in research appear dependent on such factors as education, traditionalism, marital satisfaction, or age, the discrepancies appearing equally frequently among better educated, least traditional, maritally satisfied, and younger couples as in others.

We have already seen that suspicion and status are definite barriers to communication between husband and wife, particularly in matters of sex. We can now see how this directly affects the use of birth control. Note in the following two illustrations that both women know about the condom but that neither has mentioned it to her husband, in one case despite the fact that she felt that his knowledge was inadequate.

He doesn't know of those things as other men do. He talks with me about that, and he doesn't know about using the condom with his wife. He says that is for bad women of the sort found in cabarets. I know that it is used with the wife. . . . (B1F)

I have heard other women speak of the condom. I have never spoken to my husband about it, and he has never mentioned it to me. That is why I believe he doesn't like it. (H4F)

Respect for the status of the husband, and the modesty which is so much a part of the female role appear to play the principal part in blocking communication. The following quotations show the way in which these complexes can directly result in the frustration of birth-control knowledge.

We were just married, and I didn't dare tell him to avoid children, so I became pregnant. (A3F)

I don't know what he thinks about that. I don't like to hear or talk

[11] In Table 34 there are four duplications, i.e., four cases in which *X* knew a method that *Y* did not know while *Y* knew a method which *X* did not know.

about certain things. I don't speak of those things with my husband. I feel ashamed. (H15F)

I went to the Health Unit without telling him. I didn't tell him about it for three days, when I finally got up enough courage. (H1F)

I feel much respect for him. I have heard some of my friends talking about rubbers, and I like the idea. (Did you tell your husband?) *No, I did not dare to.* I never speak of those things with him. I get ashamed. (C2F)

A few men gave similar reasons for not discussing birth control with their wives. To discuss such sordid matters with their wives would be almost sacrilegious to these men.

(Why don't you ask your wife what she prefers?) Me, talk about these things to my wife? Look, man, I couldn't even try. . . . I am not accustomed to talk about these things with my wife. (C4M)

The wife will be offended if one uses the condom. (But have you ever talked it over with your wife?) No never. *I would not dare to do it.* (Y2M)

To other men, not modesty but authority blocks communication. Since the man is the maker of important decisions, it does not occur to him to discuss such matters with his wife unless he has made up his mind to use such methods.

(From whom came the idea of birth control?) Well from me, who else? (X9M)

(What about contraceptives for women?) I have never asked her about them. (And about having children, what do you ask her?) Nothing. (Why?) Because it has never occurred to me to ask her. (A10M)

Thus the discrepancies in the knowledge of birth-control methods which appear to exist between husbands and wives become understandable when the dynamics of communication between husband and wife are understood.

CATHOLICISM AND BIRTH CONTROL

In many of the underdeveloped countries of the world, religion is a potent force in discouraging infertility, if not in directly encouraging a high birth rate. Catholicism is, of course, the outstanding example of a religion which has been outspoken and unyielding on the use of any other than "natural" means to control population growth. Since about 85 percent of Puerto Rico's population consider themselves Roman Catholic, and since the Church is as well-entrenched in Puerto Rico as in the rest of Latin America, it should be of considerable interest to examine briefly the clergy's tactics and the effect which these have had on the general public in Puerto Rico.

THE PUBLIC CAMPAIGN

As far as can be determined, official Church criticism went underground along with the birth-control program, at least for several years. For the past few years, however, the Church, along with the Independentistas,[12] has been highly vocal in attacking the present administration for its alleged "neo-Malthusian policies." The Independentistas have attempted to make political hay out of the birth control issue, particularly the government's alleged sterilization program. A few years ago an offhand and half-facetious remark by the Commissioner of Health concerning male sterilization appeared to trip off the opposition. On the following day the Independentista newspaper carried headlines concerning sterilization and castration of males. From this point on, the Independentistas and Catholic spokesmen have lost little opportunity to attack the government on birth control and sterilization.

The most interesting recent development has been the establishment of a Catholic lay group devoted to pressuring the government on the subject of birth control. Organized in 1951 in order to "combat the violations of natural law in Puerto Rico," the Unión pro Defensa de Moral Natural is headed by four professional men.[13] In their manifesto of September 7, 1951, they showed clearly their interest in legislation.

> When civil laws and practices contradict fundamental rights and duties, such laws . . . become abuses of power. Unfortunately, in our legis-

[12] The major opposition party in Puerto Rico, standing for complete independence from the United States.

[13] The leader of the group is also a high ranking board member in the Independentista party.

lation we have laws of this type: the three so-called eugenic laws of 1937, the divorce law, the clause in the Organic Act which removes the right of parents to educate their children according to their conscience, and others.[14]

A month later the group sent an open letter to the committee on the Bill of Rights for the Constitution. This letter indicated that the Union's interests ran beyond birth control. The following were among the things which the Union wanted the constitution to prohibit: divorce; artificial insemination; teaching and propaganda on birth control; the diffusion and sale of literature or methods pertaining to birth control; sterilization; and premarital medical examinations. Under the general slogan, "El aborto es un crimen! La contracepción es impureza! La esterilización es una mutilación!" the Union has received considerable newspaper space in its frequent criticisms of birth control.

The clergy itself has not been silent but, as evidenced by the newspapers at least,[15] has been considerably less vociferous and demanding than the lay groups. It has, however, frequently threatened political pressure. A convention of priests published a statement in 1951, for example, holding that "No Catholic can give his vote to those who defend those [birth-control] practices. Catholics, fight to save our Christian morals."[16] A week before the 1952 elections in Puerto Rico, one of the strongest statements made by high church officials was issued by the bishop of Ponce, attacking the administration for its neo-Malthusian policies. The statement brought a storm of controversy on the eve of the elections, but although the Independentista party doubled its relatively small vote, the Popular party received the largest number of votes and the strongest majority in its three terms in power.

From the pulpits, of course, comes much of the propaganda against birth control. While we have no evidence at hand concerning

[14] *Mundo* (San Juan), September 7, 1951.

[15] The clergy, however, has something of a newspaper of its own. *Luz y Verdad* (Light and Truth) is a two sheet publication issued weekly in Catholic Churches throughout the island. It frequently contains polemics against birth control.

[16] *Imparcial* (San Juan), August 25, 1951.

the frequency of such attacks, one respondent related a story showing that in her parish the priests are not employing subtle techniques.[17]

> We went to Mass, and the priest asked that everyone who practiced birth control raise their hands. We raised ours, and he called us apart, one by one, and told us it was a very great sin to avoid children who wanted to come into this world. (H24F)

Before proceeding to examine the opinions of the members of our sample, it would seem of importance to elaborate somewhat the content of the arguments advanced by the articulate minority. This will be done for two reasons. First, to see subsequently to what extent the attitudes of the lower class appear to be based on the propaganda arguments they have seen in the newspapers. Second, the arguments which appear in the Puerto Rican newspapers will undoubtedly be repeated in Latin America as population-control programs get under way.

The first group of criticisms comes from individuals who see in population control an issue with which to cudgel the party in power. They are eager to demonstrate that the government's impressive industrialization program is really a failure. Thus, when the government complains that population is outstripping available and growing resources, they cite this as evidence that the industrialization program is a failure. Having failed to cope with the great increments to the labor force as a result of the staggering natural increase, the government is seen as "desperately" having to resort to birth control to cover their inadequacies.

> The Economic Development Administration, having failed until now in whatever industrial experiments it has begun, also fosters birth control.[18]

[17] In general, the major Protestant denominations in Puerto Rico are favorable to birth control, and several articles have appeared in the newspapers by Protestant leaders to this effect. However, there are two or three Protestant sects in Puerto Rico which, if not officially opposing birth control, have enough ministers who take this stand to have some effect on their adherents. Judging by one comment in our sample, the sect techniques are even less subtle than those employed by the Catholic clergy: "I don't use contraceptives because it is forbidden by our church. (What does the church do?) They put discipline on them and don't let them use the veil or preach in the congregation, and seat them in the last row of benches in the church." (Z5F)

[18] *Día* (Ponce), February 16, 1949.

Though much praise is given to the industrial experiments of the government, Puerto Rico has not yet begun a serious industrial program to absorb the abundance of workers.[19]

The opponents of the government then brand its attempts to "salvage the failing program of industrialization" as despotic, as "a monstruous method taken from Hitlerism";[20] ". . . what Hitler sanctioned by force [they try] to legalize here."[21]

The government is accused of all sorts of nefarious and diabolically clever schemes to foster population control. Public housing is one of these methods: ". . . they have built and continue to build thousands of houses so enormously small that no family that has two or three children can live in them."[22]

Others hint darkly that the government is conducting "clandestine experiments" in order to achieve its ends, using or trying to use human beings like animals.

The government of Muñoz Marín has been collaborating secretly in a so-called scientific experiment in which hundreds of Puerto Rican women are being used to test a new contraceptive. Hundreds of poor women, suffering and humble, whom the government alleges to defend in their social and human dignity, have been submitted like guinea pigs to an experiment contrary to the most elementary demands of public morality.[23]

Another type of argument expresses fears of race or class genocide, and, if sincere, may represent the anxieties of a community rapidly changing from high to low mortality. For centuries, Puerto Rico's values encouraging a high birth rate have been consistent with and functional to a society with a high death rate. These values cannot be expected to change as rapidly as the rate of mortality, and the anxiety-filled articulations of the representatives of the *status quo* give eloquent testimony to the fear that the new low-fertility values will imperil the society.

Unfortunately, it is difficult to tell whether such arguments are mere rationalizations for a religious or political line or whether they

[19] Nemesio de Toledo, *Día* (Ponce), February 12, 1949.

[20] *Imparcial* (San Juan), February 15, 1949.

[21] Nemesio de Toledo, in *Día* (Ponce), February 15, 1949.

[22] Advertisement by the Unión pro Defensa de Moral Natural in the *Imparcial* (San Juan), September 19, 1951.

[23] Concepción de Gracia, in *Mundo* (San Juan), October 24, 1951.

also represent genuine conservative fears. It seems possible, however, that many of the individuals opposing birth control are convinced of the social dangers of this practice, and for this reason their arguments are presented.

There is, first, a group which charges the government with an attempt at class genocide—that is, the extinction of the poor and the destruction of their means to reproduce. According to this group, the government program "is a plan to put an end to the reproductive capacity of the Puerto Rican."[24]

> The desire to have or not have children is the base upon which the life of our country has rested. If nobody wanted to continue his life through the birth of children, within a short time the Puerto Rican people would be extinguished. . . . The population of France became stagnant when they resorted to the practice of sterilization. As a result, France grew weaker, and its decadence and failure in the Second World War were caused by this.[25]

> The government faces the problem of poverty in Puerto Rico with the absurd theory that in order to have less poverty it is necessary to eliminate the poor.[26]

Most interesting of all is the contention that birth control will bring down social and moral ruin on the island. A Catholic philosopher charges the government with adopting means which will destroy the family:

> . . . we are destroying the family by gigantic steps, in fomenting, on the part of a group of maniacs who occupy key posts in our government, the sterilization of our women, and by neo-Malthusian practices which are undermining the roots of family life.[27]

Another professional, president of the Defenders of the Faith in Puerto Rico, fears the corruption of Puerto Rican womanhood: "The spread of information on birth control has silently continued corrupting good women who once felt the noble desire of becoming mothers."[28] A leading government official feels that birth control will destroy society in general: "I believe that the spread of contra-

[24] *Imparcial* (San Juan), February 15, 1949.
[25] Ibern Fleytas, Speech to Lions Club of San Juan, March 17, 1949.
[26] Concepción de Gracia, in *Imparcial* (San Juan), August 25, 1951.
[27] José Lazaro, in *Mundo* (San Juan), October 3, 1949.
[28] J. F. Rodríguez, in *Diario* (San Juan), March 3, 1949.

ceptive methods can only bring forth the degeneration of society."[29] A female Catholic leader agrees that population control would result in the complete degeneration of her sex:

We would be sinning if we did not protest against the dishonor which they are bringing to the Puerto Rican woman, against those who try to corrupt and degrade her, taking away the crown of the Christian mother, and making of her the worst which can be said of any woman.[30]

A Catholic physician is at once the most eloquent and the most pessimistic concerning the deteriorating effects of birth control:

Only enjoying pleasure [i.e., by using birth control], we would find innocent creatures rushing into free love; prostitution would acquire the force of a whirlwind; and an infinite number of homes would tremble, fearing infidelity. . . . Unbridled instinct would become a beast trying to satiate its appetite on virtue. The veil of innocence would be rent, leaving latent avarice uncovered; and the human beast would begin to show his tragic head and to devour life's spirituality. Who could ever revive the morals of Puerto Rico after they had been torn to pieces?[31]

The same speaker, in dealing with sterilization, ventures medical opinion along with social:

Nobody could prove that a sterilized person would afterwards be in normal health. Frequently, sterilization results in flatulence, idiocy, premature senility, and a change of sex. It also involves the danger of free sexual love, corruption, the destruction of homes, and other social calamities.[32]

THE LOWER CLASS AND CATHOLICISM

The preceding section has made it clear that a formidable amount of propaganda against birth control is being issued from the various

[29] *Mundo* (San Juan), October 15, 1951.

[30] Leonora Agrait de Barea, in *Mundo* (San Juan), September 11, 1951.

[31] Ibern Fleytas, in *Diario* (San Juan), March 29, 1949.

[32] Ibern Fleytas, in *Mundo* (San Juan), March 17, 1949. Very few of his colleagues agree. Of 453 Puerto Rican physicians who responded to a questionnaire, only 13 believed that sterilization has undesirable effects on the mental or physical health of women. Only 7 maintained that contraceptives have this effect. Sixty-six percent believed sterilization to be justified in cases of poverty, and 81 percent felt that birth control methods were justified for such reasons. J. Belaval, E. Cofresí, and J. Janer, "Opinión de la clase médica de Puerto Rico sobre el uso de la esterilización y los contraceptivos" (mimeographed report, July 1953).

mass media on the island. We now face the crucial question: to what extent does it reflect, or to what extent has it affected, the attitudes of the general population of Puerto Rico, i.e., of the lower class? Is it true, as the Catholics claim, that ". . . economists or sociologists . . . encourage mortal sin for over 90 percent of the people of Puerto Rico?"[33] How does the presumably Catholic population react to the threat of "mortal sin?"

There are several factors which mitigate the seemingly overwhelming Catholicism in Puerto Rico. In the first place, it is a very different type from that seen in the United States. It is true that it is much more a part of life in the sense that it is integrated into other, particularly recreational, institutions in Puerto Rico, but at the same time it is much more secular and less concerned with dogma. Particularly for the lower classes it is a cult of saints often hardly distinguishable from magic, in which various sorts of rituals are performed in order to propitiate the supernatural forces. A great number of Puerto Ricans realize the difference between the dogmatic and the ritualistic aspect of Catholicism and classify themselves as *Católico a mi manera*—"Catholic in my own way." This usually means that they do not feel bound by all the dogmas of the Church, but that they believe in God and participate occasionally in Catholic rituals and feasts. Thirty-eight percent of the males and 23 percent of the females in Hatt's sample so classified themselves when asked about the importance of religion in their lives.[34]

Men often remark that religion *es cosa de mujer* (a thing for women), and observation of church attendance readily confirms this. Male attendance appears to drop off sharply at or around adolescence, suggesting that part of the conception of the adult male is not to put too much emphasis on religious and, by implication, girlish matters.

Actually, however, by continental standards, neither men nor women attend church frequently. Catholic teaching holds that the Catholic must attend church every Sunday "under pain of mortal sin," but only about 10 percent of the island's males and 19 percent

[33] M. Taylor, "Neo-Malthusianism in Puerto Rico," *Review of Social Economy*, X (March, 1952), 52.

[34] Hatt, *op. cit.*, Table 24, p. 41.

of its females attend services at least four times per month. Eighty percent of the males and 70 percent of the females never attend, or attend "occasionally."[35]

Thus, we should not expect rigid adherence to the Catholic Church's teaching concerning birth control. Indeed, from all indications, the weight of the Church in this matter is rarely felt on the individual conscience. There are several sources of evidence for this conclusion. When, for example, Hatt's respondents were asked when they considered birth control acceptable, only about 12 percent of the population believed that "no couple has the right to limit the size of its family." Another 20 percent held that only those whose health is in danger have this right, and the remainder of the sample felt that all couples or those with economic problems have the right to practice birth control.[36] Cofresí, in a study of 2,125 women who attend various Public Health Clinics, found that only 5.8 percent of this group gave religious or moral reasons for not using birth control.[37] In our own sample of 143 men and women, only 13 individuals mentioned religious factors in their lengthy discussions of birth control. Thus, either the general population does not know about the Church teaching or, knowing, discounts it. The latter hypothesis would seem more likely because of the great amount of literature and the number of sermons which the Church has devoted to the issue. On the other hand, a quarter of the population over ten years of age is illiterate, and many more do not go to church. Thus, it is conceivable that once such individuals knew about the Church position, they would follow it.

In order to see to what extent this might be true, a subsample of 46 Catholics within the larger sample were directly queried as to whether or not they knew what the Catholic Church had to say about birth control. Of this group, 30 knew and 16 did not. Of those who knew, only three agreed with the Church position (all three had practiced birth control, however), and the remainder disagreed. The 16 cases which did not know the Church stand were

[35] *Ibid.*, Table 23, p. 39.

[36] *Ibid.*, Table 60, p. 79.

[37] E. Cofresí, *Realidad poblacional de Puerto Rico* (San Juan, 1951), Table 36, p. 95.

asked what they would do if the Church were opposed to birth control. All 16 said it would make no difference to them. To demonstrate the fact that their replies were not merely "offhand answers," and to highlight the phenomenon of the Catholic "in his own way," a number of the replies are given below. There are, first of all, those cases who know the Catholic position. A good deal of cynicism toward the Church can be seen.

They forbid it. (What do you think of that?) It is good to use birth control. The priest isn't going to support the children. (H24M)

The Church does not like that business because the baptisms represent an income to the Church. (And you?) I would use them. (H18M)

The Catholic religion says it's a sin to avoid having children, but I think it is a greater sin if they have nothing to eat. (H11F)

It forbids it, but I think it should be, because if one has many children the Church is not going to support them. (H21F)

The Church says it is a sin, that as God provides for one he provides for a dozen, but it is not the same to have one as to have many. For the rich it is no sin, and they do it. They are sterilized, those who can afford having them and can give them all they need. . . . I think it is a worse sin to bring children into the world to suffer than to avoid them. (H45F)

Those who did not know the Church position are equally resistant to it. They maintain that although it may be sin for those who can afford children, God himself knows that they themselves cannot afford children, and consequently no sin is committed. While it may be a sin for the rich, God is wise enough to know it can be no sin for the poor.

God will punish those who don't have children and who avoid them. But not a mother with many, like me. I don't think that's a sin. (H1F)

(If the Church were against it?) I would go on doing it. I am not too fanatic about religion. God has to forgive me because he knows why I do it. (H9F)

(Suppose the Church told you not to practice birth control?) I would do it anyway. The poor cannot pay attention to that. (H14M)

Possibly they are right, but inasmuch as the poor are not able to support many children, they have to disregard the position of the

Church and make their own decision to use birth control. . . . Personally, I think it is not a sin. (H11M)

. . . the poor have to use them anyhow. The rich use them, and they do not need them. (H9M)

But what of the thirteen cases who presented religious objections? It is conceivable that these cases represent the small minority of Catholics who take their religion very strictly. A detailed examination of these cases, however, shows that this is probably not the case. The first point of interest is that of the 13, only 8 are Catholics. The remainder are members of small emotional sects (Pentecostal and Christ of the Antilles). These small sects, which thrive on fervid faith, are much better able than the Catholic Church to control the lives of their adherents. Their members do not drink, smoke, etc., and in addition are not supposed to use birth control. This group presented the most inflexible stand against birth control encountered in the sample.

The second point of interest is that the families in this group of 13 are relatively small. Six of the couples have had only one or two children, two have had only three, three have had four children, and the remaining two have had six and twelve. Thus, more than half of this group had had no real need to practice birth control. Let us now look more closely at those cases having more than three children to see how strong religious sentiment is here.

Case A11F, a 28-year-old Protestant woman, with four children, is already sterilized. While she presents strong religious arguments against birth control, she states that her husband practiced withdrawal for several months, and that after a difficult delivery she decided to be sterilized. She feels that in her case there was good justification for this (having had four children and a difficult delivery) and that she committed no sin.

Case H16F, a 28-year-old Catholic with four children, is also already sterilized. Her religious objections were brought out only upon probing, her spontaneous reasons being a fear of disease brought on by contraceptives.

Case Y2F, a 27-year-old woman with six children, no religion. Her religious arguments are directed only at sterilization, and even here she shows that her real objections involve fear of the operation. She states that she would use birth control but is ashamed of being examined at the health center.

Case H7F, a 19-year-old Catholic woman with three children, now pregnant. This woman does not know that the Catholic Church is opposed to birth control but feels that it is a sin and that God punishes those who use it. She says if she had to she would use only sterilization because it is much easier.

Case Z6F, a 40-year-old Catholic woman who has had twelve pregnancies. This, possibly along with the case above, appears to be the only case basing objections primarily on religious grounds. Even in this case, subsidiary fears of disease are expressed.

In sum, then, religious objections are infrequent and often appear to be rationalizations for other objections or the comfortable articulations of individuals who as yet feel no need to use birth control. We may conclude that the extensive anti-birth-control propaganda has had no appreciable effect on the lower class and that religion is no real impediment to the realization of low-fertility ideals.

OBJECTIONS TO BIRTH CONTROL

If ignorance of birth control methods and religious objections to their use are not of the significance which might have been anticipated, this does not leave the way completely clear for birth control. One of the striking results of the study is the overwhelming number of objections to modern birth-control methods for other than religious reasons. Table 35 below shows that those individuals who know about modern methods are almost invariably opposed to them.

Although the cases where information was obtained are so few in some categories as to render them almost useless, all the groups manifest the same pattern—an unusual number of objections to the various methods of birth control. With the possible exception of the condom method, there was little difference between the objections raised by men and those raised by women. Among other methods, only sterilization shows a high proportion of individuals of both sexes approving. The preponderance of objections makes a more detailed examination of these essential. What, first of all, are the objections? Table 36 summarizes the more frequently cited objections according to the specific method which was cited.

TABLE 35

ATTITUDES TOWARD BIRTH-CONTROL METHODS OF THOSE WHO KNOW THESE METHODS, BY SEX[a]

	CONDOM		DIAPHRAGM	
	Males (percent)	*Females (percent)*	*Males (percent)*	*Females (percent)*
Objects	91	75	86	91
Approves[b]	9	25	14	9
No information[c]	3	22	36	15
Number of respondents	(71)	(58)	(11)	(27)

	DOUCHE		STERILIZATION	
	Males (percent)	*Females (percent)*	*Males (percent)*	*Females (percent)*
Objects	78	87	43	42
Approves[b]	22	13	57	58
No information[c]	55	32	14	23
Number of respondents	(20)	(22)	(65)	(65)

[a] Table 35 has added to the objections of both sexes all those objections to each method which were attributed to one spouse by the other. While this did not affect the female table (only four husbands mentioned their wives' objections) it greatly added to the objections of the husbands, for many wives gave their spouses' objections along with their own. However, it should be understood that the husband's objections as stated by the wife were not included in Table 35 as part of *her* objections. If this had been done, it would have raised the wives' objections to sterilization, condom, and jelly by about 10 percent each.

[b] Approval ranged from "It's a good method" to "They're all right."

[c] Percentages are calculated on the basis of all for whom there is adequate information. "No information" is calculated as a percentage of the total number of respondents. Many respondents did not volunteer an attitude on a particular method, and were not properly probed.

The table is a detailed one, and its major components will be analyzed in detail in the following pages. A few general points about it should be noted, however. First of all, over half the women in the sample cite their husbands' objections to the various methods, whereas only four men (included in the "other" category) cite their wives' objections. This is, of course, most revealing of the authority structure, for it probably shows that males do not take their wives' objections seriously into account. Although many of them have the

TABLE 36

OBJECTIONS TO BIRTH-CONTROL METHODS, BY SEX

	Sterili-zation	*Condom*	*Dia-phragm*	*Jelly*	*Douche*	*With-drawal*	*All Methods*	*Total Objec-tions*	*Total Objec-tors*
FEMALES									
Harmful	14	22	10	2	3	—	4	55	37
Spouse objects	10	24	4	4	—	8	2	52	36
Trouble	—	1	5	4	4	1	1	16	10
Religion	5	4	2	1	—	1	3	16	8
Modesty	—	7	5	1	1	—	5	20	15
Other	3	12	4	6	4	2	—	31	20
Total objections	32	70	30	19[a]	14[a]	12	15	192	—
									126[b]
Total objectors	27	45	23	12	13	12	11	—	143
MALES									
Unpleasurable	—	40	—	1	—	14	—	55	41
Harmful	22	16	4	—	1	—	3	46	32
Dirty or for prostitutes	—	21	—	1	—	3	—	25	22
Trouble	—	2	5	3	2	—	1	13	11
Religion	2	4	—	—	—	—	5	11	5
Other	6	3	1	2	4	1	3	20	10
Total objections	30	86	10	7	7	20[a]	12	172	—
									121[b]
Total objectors	30	64	9	6	3	20	11	—	143

[a] Cases of objections to a particular method but no answer as to why (e.g., "I don't like it") are included in "Total objections" categories.

[b] Respondents gave the *same* reason for objecting to different methods more often than they gave different reasons for objecting to a single method. For this reason, the total number of objectors to the various methods exceeds the total number of

same objections as their wives, it does not occur to them to quote their wives' feelings on the subject. The implication is that, if they had no objections to the methods, they would be used regardless of the wives' feelings in the matter. On the other hand, one might draw the conclusion from the wives that, if their husbands so desired, they might use the methods perhaps despite their own objections. This conclusion is made likely by Cofresí's findings, which indicated that a quarter of the 2,125 women in his sample said that they did not practice birth control because of their husbands' objections.[38] There is also the possibility that men do not know their wives' opinions on this subject. In line with the conclusions on communication, it would be expected that men have more rights and freedom concerning the initiation of "discussion" of birth control. The wives may be expected to listen but not to contribute their own opinions. Thus, where communication occurs, it may tend to be one-sided.

The second major difference between the tables is that men have two major objections which are not cited by women. These refer mainly to the condom, but to some extent also to withdrawal. Both methods are seen as unpleasurable for the male, the former being viewed as dirty and/or for prostitutes.

Religious objections have already been discussed and were seen to be of minor importance. Modesty objections referred to reluctance to attend birth control clinics out of fear of being examined by a male physician; to ask or answer questions about the methods in the clinics; in one case, to be seen in the clinics; and, in another, for fear of being observed douching by the children.[39]

The "Other" category may be considered briefly. For the males, the principal objection is the fear of infidelity on the part of the wife. This will be given more attention below. Other objections in this category are that the methods are unreliable (all the various methods except sterilization are mentioned), and that they are too

[38] *Ibid.*, Table 36, p. 95. Cofresí's table lists the *principal* reasons for not using birth control. The objections contained in the tables above, however, present *all* the reasons for not liking the various methods.

[39] The low number of objections to douche, jelly, withdrawal, and diaphragm should not, of course, be interpreted as indicating greater acceptance of these methods. From previous tables it should be recalled that these methods were less frequently known or discussed, and a low proportion of answers on attitudes toward them is present even when they are known.

expensive (only two cases). For the women, the chief objection in the "Other" category was also unreliability of the methods, as well as that they are dirty (mainly directed at jelly). We may now consider the more important and more frequently cited objections in some detail.

INFIDELITY AND MALE CONTROL OF CONTRACEPTIVES

When males are asked about birth control methods in general, they almost invariably talk about the condom. When asked specifically about other methods, they show a surprising ignorance of these, particularly when it is realized that many of their own wives are aware of them. Moreover, those who know about them generally do not approve of female contraceptive methods except, in some cases, sterilization. A principal reason for this may be that men want to control conception and dislike putting this power in the hands of the women. Men, as we have seen, are the source of authority and important decisions in the family. Moreover, they consider the sexual sphere to be almost exclusively their own, since the woman is not supposed to be concerned with such matters. We have also suggested that men, because of their frequent feelings of inferiority in the sexual sphere, are anxious lest women overpower them in sexual matters. It is possible that the wife's use of birth control presents a threat to the male sense of superiority in this area. We would not expect, of course, that this should frequently be articulated, and the fact that it was articulated at all would seem significant. Note in the following statements the anxiety lest the women usurp the male prerogative and, in one case, the male "secret."

Those are used by high-class girls *when they are allowed too much freedom.* (What problems do such methods bring?) That women do as they please with their husbands. *I don't like to be governed by my wife.* If she tries to do it, I'll leave her. (H20M)

(And what will you do if he stops using contraceptives?) Well then I'll continue having children because *if he stops using them, it's probably due to the fact that he wants to have more children.* (But you told me you don't want any more. Why don't you use contraceptives yourself?) Oh, I wouldn't dare. *He is the one who decides those things, and if he doesn't want to use them, I wouldn't dare,* because he could get mad at me. (C2F)

I am the one who avoids them. She doesn't know the secret of avoiding children. *Women get pregnant if the men want them to.* (B5M)

Not only does the husband refuse "on principle" to have such control wrested from him, but he also fears that such power would be abused. The tensions, anxieties, and mutual suspicion which exist between the sexes cause the male to fear that control over conception on the part of the woman could lead to his being cuckolded; for once the fear of the visible effects of illicit relations are removed, the woman would "make a fool of the husband" by having relations with other men. This fear is most frequently expressed concerning sterilization, for this method is not only the most popular, but the most foolproof in terms of conception.

If a woman has an operation, her husband mistrusts her. He thinks the wife is unfaithful. You must keep all those things in mind. (Z1F)

There are a lot of women around here who are being operated on, but they are not doing it so much to prevent children. *They do it to protect themselves.* (In what way?) *Sleeping around with other men.* There are lots of such women around. The majority of them do it for that purpose. (Y3M)

(Are you against having the wife operated?) Yes, that is against natural laws and could give way to corruption, because *that would give the wife an opportunity to be unfaithful to the husband.* (X3M)

One man, when asked about sterilization, suggested that male sterilization would be preferable. Then both control for the male and visible consequences for the female are possible.

I think it is better to have the man sterilized, because if the woman gets pregnant you know it's not from you. It has been from somebody else. Don't you think that's better? (H9M)

Other female methods, while mentioned less frequently, are greeted with the same anxieties. In the following case, the respondent claims a failure of contraception almost led to a separation, showing that in term of male behavior, the womens' fears are not without basis.

I heard of a woman here who used the diaphragm. . . . Later she became pregnant, and the husband said the child was not his. . . . *They almost separated because, as they were using the method, the husband thought she was pregnant of another man.* (Z1F)

The phobia reaches its zenith in the case cited below, in which the intricacy of the logic is noteworthy. Not only has the suspicion been applied to the condom, but, after ten children, the respondent is so afraid of her husband's suspicions that she will not use the condom until she menstruates.

I brought [the condoms] home from the Health Center, and he accepted them and used them for about two years. After I had my last child four months ago I looked for prophylactics again at the Health Unit, but I *haven't used them yet because I haven't seen menstruation and if I use them and then I find out that I am pregnant again, my husband might think I had contact with other men;* so I can't use them until I know whether I am pregnant or not. (B3F)

This, too, is one more factor which impedes successful communication between husband and wife on birth control matters. Some wives have been so well inculcated with the phobic logic of their husbands that they do not dare suggest a female method for fear it will incur the suspicion of their husbands. For example, the author's research assistant engaged a young lady in conversation while waiting in a doctor's office. The latter explained that although she wanted to be sterilized, she could not suggest it to her husband. He was soon embarking for Korea and might suspect intentions of infidelity during his absence. A similar case is taken from the study.

Everybody advises him to have me operated on, because otherwise we are going to have too many children. . . . (How did you feel about his idea?) I was delighted, because I was willing to be operated on, but *I didn't dare tell him.* (Why didn't you dare?) Because many men don't like their wives to be operated on, because they think they are unfaithful to them, that the women want this in order to have contact with other men. (C6F)

THE CONDOM AND DIMINISHED PLEASURE

By far the most frequently cited male objection to the condom was that this method of birth control reduces male sensation during the sexual act. Thirty-five men (and three others, according to their wives) raised this objection. There is, of course, an objective basis for this complaint,[40] but this fact has not greatly impeded the use of the condom in certain cultures. Therefore, there may be something in Puerto Rican culture which aggravates the slight physical diminution in pleasure brought about by the condom so that it assumes a greater importance than might be expected.

While it appears true that many men mean literally what they say—that the condom is less pleasurable in a strictly physical sense because of interference with direct contact, there is some evidence which would suggest that a minority of the males are referring to diminished *psychological* pleasure. There are several sources of evidence leading to this conclusion. Our first clue comes from a group of eleven men who say that the condom is *dirty.*

They are filthy . . . repulsive . . . (In what way?) *Because when I take the condom off I feel sick to my stomach.* (A10M)

I never liked them. They give too much trouble. One gets disappointed removing them because *they look dirty.* (C3M)

I consider them filthy because of *the disgust they give after one finishes the sexual act.* (X8M)

(Do you feel disgust when you are removing them?) Yes. (What causes disgust to you?) When I have to remove that dirty thing. (H18M)

But why should a poverty-stricken lower-class male who lives in a shack without running water and without the most elementary hygienic essentials be so concerned about the alleged "filthiness" of the condom? Part of the answer may lie in the fact that lower-class Puerto Ricans are said to be almost phobic about body dirt.[41] Careless about their homes and environs, the lower-class individuals are fastidious about personal cleanliness, particularly concerning bodily secretions or products. Retention of the semen next to a bodily organ[42] may consequently evoke disgust from the male.

[40] "Rubber is a poor conductor of body warmth. Someone has said that the condom is a 'spider web against danger and an armor against pleasure.'" A. Stone, and N. Himes, *Planned Parenthood: A Practical Guide to Birth Control Methods* (New York: Viking Press, 1951), p. 132.

[41] See D. Landy's discussion of this tendency and of the manner in which it is transmitted to children, "Childrearing Patterns in a Puerto Rican Lower Class Community" (unpublished manuscript, University of Puerto Rico, 1952).

[42] Landy notes that the tendency is to "get rid of the dirt"—that is, to get it away from the person as quickly as possible. Garbage, faeces, and so forth are usually found away from the body but surprisingly close to the house.

My husband says that men do not feel the same pleasure because the semen stays inside the condom and doesn't fall inside the woman. (H9F)

This general propensity toward coprophobia is heightened by the fact that the organ concerned is the penis—an object of considerable reverence for the male anxious to prove his virility. We recall the citations from Chapter III indicating the adulation of the infant penis by adult males and females, and the evidence from other chapters indicating the manifestations of felt sexual inferiority which require "machistic" or phallic behavior. Thus, when dealing with this special object of reverence, indeed with the symbol of male strength and ego, any hint of "dirt" almost becomes profanation. At the same time there may be a sense of fettering masculinity by covering and confining the penis. That the symbol of masculinity must not be shrouded is evidenced by the frequently mentioned term, *la espuela limpia*—"the clean spur." In this phrase there seem coupled both the fear of dirt and of impeding or containing the "machistic" symbol.[43]

It is so good with a clean spur. (Y8M)

He never used the condom because he said he got more pleasure with a clean spur. (X10F)

A final factor which may be associated with diminished psychological pleasure is the conception that the condom is for prostitutes and consequently should not be used for one's wife. Seven men made this explicit.

The condom is for the prostitutes. . . . I don't use those things with my wife, because *it debases my wife to use something that is used with prostitutes.* (A5M)

I don't dare use that with my wife. (Why?) *Well that is only used with prostitutes, and my wife is an honest woman.* (Y4M)

He said he wouldn't use that filthy thing, that he may use it with women of the street to protect himself against infection, but not in

[43] The etymology of the *espuela limpia* is significant. It refers to the fighting cock which uses it own or natural spurs, in contrast to the artificial spur or *espuela postiza.* Thus the spur has a double connotation. It comes from the fighting cock—a well known phallic or masculine symbol—and from the organ of the cock which is most aggressive and punishing.

his home. He said, *'I am clean and my wife is clean so we don't need to use that.'* (H35F)

Even communication on the subject is blocked by the fear of degrading the wife.

That is used when one goes with prostitutes, and the wife would be offended if one used that. (Have you talked about it with your wife?) No, never, I would not dare do that. (Y2M)

Thus, while many men object to the condom on grounds of sheer sensation, it is possible that a number of men receive diminished pleasure from its use with their wives because of the complex of attitudes involving filth and the obscene.

FEARS CONCERNING THE PHYSICAL EFFECTS OF BIRTH CONTROL

There appears to be an extremely powerful prejudice against modern birth-control methods running through the lower class, based on the fear that condoms, diaphragms, jellies, sponges, douches, and sterilizations are dangerous to the health of women. As seen in Table 36, such fears are by far the most frequently cited personal objection of women.[44] Fewer men, but still a significantly high proportion, give the same reason. When men give such reasons, however, they always cite the danger for their wives, never for themselves.

It should not be thought that such fears are monopolized by ignorant old women. In fact, women expressing various superstitious fears about birth control have had a somewhat higher education and are neither older nor more traditional than the rest of the sample. Males who voice such fears have had about the same education as the rest of the sample but are somewhat older.

The specific nature of the fears is varied. The douche, for example, can be harmful to general health and to the sexual organs.

I've heard of it, but they say it weakens the uterus. . . . Women around here say it. (H11F)

[44] Cofresí found that such fears represented only 7 percent of the objections given by the 2,125 women in his sample. This sample, however, is strongly biased by the fact that it is chosen exclusively from clinic cases. Such women would be expected to evidence fewer superstitious fears. *Op. cit.,* Table 36, p. 95.

. . . they said it was harmful to the womb, that one might get sick there. (H19F)

I have heard about vinegar irrigations . . . but that is dangerous because vinegar causes loss in weight. (H14F)

The dread diseases, however, cancer and tuberculosis, are the principal feared outcomes of birth control. Cancer was the most frequently cited specific disease.

I don't know any methods. At the Public Health Unit they give instructions, but I fear them because *people say it causes cancer.* (Y3F)

Some women talk always about those things. That's why I heard about jelly, but I tell those persons, why do you use that? The talcum which those things have remains in your uterus and *you could get a cancer.* (Z6F)

Another frequent objection which is made against all mechanical devices is that the object may stay inside the woman. Extraordinary means are then seen as required to remove the object (one man even told that an operation had been required to remove a condom in a case he knew), and often the inability to remove the object is the cause of cancer and other disorders.[45]

I have never used prophylactics with my wife nor will I. . . . That is dangerous because, *if it breaks, the woman may die if that stays inside her womb.* (H13M)

It might hurt me inside. They told me so many stories and once I was told that something happened to a woman. *It stayed inside and went into her bladder.* (Y8F)

I heard about the sponge in the Public Health Unit, but people scared me, saying that *it may stay inside, and the doctor has to pull it out.* (B4F)

There [at the Public Health Center] I heard of a rubber diaphragm for the woman, but I didn't take it because other women scared me. One woman told me *that thing stayed inside the womb and the doctor had to pull it out.* (X6F)

Sterilization is the most widely known method and the method least objected to. Practically all the objections to sterilization, how-

[45] There is no evidence from our sample that such old-fashioned and truly harmful contraceptives as intra-uterine stems are known or used.

ever, are based on the conception that the woman's health suffers from it. Specific diseases are rarely mentioned here—only that the woman will feel sick, tired, and unable to do her housework properly. The latter is a frequent fear of the husbands.

I don't want to have her sterilized because she may get useless. (H7M)

One isn't good anymore after sterilization. Many women have told me they cannot do hard work after it. (Z6F)

Such fears were articulated so frequently that they probaly represent one of the major blocks in the way of acceptance of birth-control methods. The importance of this would suggest the desirability of some speculation as to the roots of such fears.

There are, first, the effects of poorly informed or biased physicians. Medical schools on the continent offer very little in the way of training students in birth-control methods, and most of Puerto Rico's physicians have received their training in the United States.[46] Although public health officers on the island have an opportunity to learn a great deal through practice in the clinics (*if* they so desire), private physicians may remain in relative ignorance. Because of the weight of medical authority and the predisposition of the lower classes to believe in the harmful effects of contraceptives, one physician can wield considerable influence. There is one excellent example of this taken from the present sample. A woman from a small town told the interviewer that a gynecologist had diagnosed her pelvic pains as due to the use of the condom. Two other respondents from the same town used this medical authority to back up their fears of the condom.

There is a woman here who used condoms and got sick. The doctor told her not to use them any more because she could get cancer. (Y6F)

We can't use birth control. A doctor said that the use of condoms

[46] "More than a few patients of an obstetrician living in Boston have told her that their specialists or surgeons have warned them that 'pessaries lead to cancer.'" Dorothy Dunbar Bromley, *Birth Control: Its Use and Misuse,* New York: Harper, 1934, p. 192. This volume contains a good discussion of the ignorance of many physicians concerning birth control. While somewhat dated, as judged from the amount of curriculum time spent in all American medical schools on birth control, the situation may not have changed greatly.

affects the uterus of the woman . . . the doctor forbade her to use them because it would harm her. (Y8M)

There is some evidence, too, indicating that Catholic lay groups may be propagandizing the lower classes concerning the "dangers of birth control." The following news item, for example, appeared in *El Mundo* of September 11, 1951.

La Pia Unión de Esposas y Madres Cristianas of San Germán . . . is currently active in carrying out orientation programs among the country women of that region, trying to prevent these women from being deceived and trying to convince them of the immorality of sterilization and neo-Malthusian methods, which, in addition to being a most grievous sin, *usually are causes of many diseases.*

It is interesting that coitus interruptus was never mentioned as dangerous but only as unpleasant. The uneducated may distrust the application of mechanical contrivances or gadgets to the body—particularly when that part of the body happens to be so important and so surrounded by tabus. One woman in speaking of sterilization phrased these fears well.

I was very afraid of sterilization because they cut something there that you probably need. When God provided you with that, it is because you need it, just as he gave you two hands. (A11F)

Thus, anything which interferes with the natural, rather than being conceived of as detrimental to morals, is seen as detrimental to health.

Finally, there are primitive conceptions of causality, which, given a predisposition to believe, often encourage the lower-class Puerto Rican to conclude that birth control is harmful. There is a good chance for some sort of pelvic disturbance in the lower-class woman sooner or later. Given the background of suspicion toward birth control, it is a short step to putting together a cause-and-effect relationship. That this is frequently done is evidenced by the quotations below.

I have seen cases of women who got sterilized and then died of TB.[47] (C1M)

[47] Since sterilizations are usually performed post partum, and since women are released from the hospital quickly (because of bed-space shortages) and take up household duties almost immediately, it is quite possible that disturbances do occur, *seemingly* the result of the sterilization.

I quit using condoms because my wife got sick in the ovaries . . . when we quit using them she didn't feel sick any more. (Did the doctor tell her that?) No, we supposed it.

Condoms can cause cancer or hemorrhage. I have seen many cases in which the woman almost died from cancer caused by the rubbers. They rub the skin and that causes a cancer. (Y6M)

Sterilization might kill her or harm her permanently as other cases I have seen. . . . I know a young lady who afterward became fat and listless. (Y3M)

SUMMARY

By and large, the lower-class population is aware of means of limiting family size. However, many individuals are not aware of all the methods available, and within any one family communication is frequently so poor between husband and wife that information on contraception is not shared. As a result, it is frequently the case that one spouse, usually the wife, is in ignorance of methods about which the other spouse is informed. This again would seem to be an impediment to action on family ideals.

Although over 85 percent of the population is Roman Catholic, and although the Church along with a major political party has made vigorous campaigns against birth control, religious or political ties have had little appreciable effect on attitudes toward birth control. Those few respondents who presented religious objections in our sample had the smallest families, and in other cases religious objections appeared to be rationalizations for more deep-seated objections to contraception.

The absence of religious tabus does not leave the path completely open to birth control, however. Practically all the individuals in the sample had other objections to the various contraceptives. Women resist chemical and mechanical methods through fear of disease and fear that their husbands will suspect them of infidelity. Moreover, even where they are willing to use these methods, many women are too modest to secure supplies at public centers. Some men object to female methods as they desire control over conception, and most men object to the condom because they find it unpleasurable, dirty, and associated with prostitutes. Sterilization is the method most favorably viewed, since most of the objections do not apply to it. However, fears of health and fidelity are also voiced by the respondents about this method.

Now that we have a picture of attitudes toward fertility and birth control, we can move to an examination of the dynamics of use, to determine when and how birth control is used.

IX

The Dynamics of Birth-Control Use

> Sometimes they are desperate, unemployed, and with many children. That is the Puerto Rican problem. Sometimes they have many children and give them to their relatives. They distribute four and keep two, because they aren't able to support them all.
>
> There are also men who leave their wives after they have four children. It is because they are not able to support them. They think they can solve the problem by leaving the wife.
>
> Many have the saying that where one eats, many can eat, but that is not true. Some would like to avoid having children, but they do not do it because they are lazy. They stay in bed, and because they don't want the trouble of getting up for a while, they do not avoid children. When the wife gets pregnant, they don't know what to do.
>
> A MALE RESPONDENT

THE EXTENT OF BIRTH-CONTROL PRACTICES

One source of information on birth-control use in Puerto Rico is the data on numbers attending the prematernal clinics. In 1945 the total number of active cases (defined as those which return more or less regularly for supplies) was 14,120. In 1950 this figure was 22,055, an increase of 56 percent. Table 37 shows the number of contraceptives distributed for these years.[1]

The five-year period has brought about an increase of about 50 percent in total contraceptive units distributed. Whereas the number of condoms has increased by only 13.6 percent, diaphragms show an increase of 274.0 percent, and jelly, not distributed in 1945, was the second most popular method in 1950.[2]

[1] From *Annual Reports of the Commissioner of Health,* San Juan, Puerto Rico.

[2] Actually, the proportions of different methods distributed may reflect department policy as much as "popularity" of method. Diaphragms and jelly (especially Preceptin in 1950) have received special emphasis in the clinics.

TABLE 37

CONTRACEPTIVES DISTRIBUTED BY PREMATERNAL CLINICS, 1945 AND 1950

	1945	*1950*
Condoms (dozens)	39,563	46,931
Jelly	—	12,406
Cream	2,138	2,491
Diaphragms	703	2,631
Foam powder	365	—
Sponges	345	—

Such figures, of course, underestimate the use of birth control by the population in general. To determine this, other kinds of data are needed. Within the past decade in Puerto Rico, three statistical studies containing data on the frequency of birth-control use have been conducted. Unfortunately, the largest of these, conducted by Hatt, does not report the findings on this subject, explaining that ". . . no accurate data on the use of contraception can be obtained, since its reported use on the island was so low . . ."[3]

The remaining two studies are of clinical populations, and are of course subject to the usual biases. The first, conducted in 1942, used as its source of data the responses of several thousand women who sought birth-control information at Public Health Clinics.

[3] P. K. Hatt, *Backgrounds of Human Fertility in Puerto Rico: A Sociological Survey* (Princeton: Princeton University Press, 1952), p. 443. It is the writer's opinion that the failure of Hatt's study to uncover a substantial degree of contraceptive practice was due to inadequate interviewer training. Since writing, two further studies conducted at the University of Puerto Rico's Social Science Research Center have indicated a high incidence of birth-control practice. The first found that of 3,000 married individuals who attended any of eight of the island's general medical-care centers between August and October of 1953, 53 percent had used a birth-control method at some point in their marriage. See J. M. Stycos, "The Pattern of Birth Control in Puerto Rico," *Eugenics Quarterly,* I, No. 3 (Sept. 1954), 176–81. The other study used a stratified sample of 1,000 families chosen in such a way as to be representative of the island as a whole. Preliminary tabulations indicate that in 40 percent of current marital unions birth control has been practiced at some point during the union. In the rural area the percentage ranges from 25.3 among those whose heads of household had no education, to 64.6 among those whose heads had nine or more years of education. In the urban areas the range is from 36.4 percent to 67.8 percent.

Thirty-four percent of the sample had practiced birth-control methods before their attendance at the clinic.[4] The second study, conducted in 1948, obtained interview data on 2,125 women who had attended *any* of the numerous Public Health Clinics. Curiously enough, this study also found that 34 percent of the women had practiced birth control.[5]

The present study, dealing with a small but presumably more typical population, found that 72 percent of the families had at some time practiced some method of birth control. The figure is probably excessively high and throws some doubt on the representativeness of the sample. Possibly, the fact that the sample was drawn from areas more conveniently situated with respect to transportation facilities than is true for most of Puerto Rico accounts for some of the difference. However, in the light of the interviewing methodology used in the present study, it is possible that the sample more nearly reflects reality than would at first appear likely. In contrast with the other studies, the interviewers on the present project exercised great care to establish rapport with their respondents, used a very flexible and relatively nonthreatening kind of questionnaire, and discussed birth control only after two or three hours of interviewing on other subjects. Moreover, *both* male and female were interviewed independently, and birth control histories were elicited from both. The husbands frequently gave information which the wives failed to report.[6]

Regardless of the absolute degree of birth-control practice, three out of four of the studies indicate that birth control is being practiced by a substantial proportion of the population in Puerto Rico. Is it possible, however, that this practice is limited largely to the upper classes? The two clinical studies demonstrate that while class

[4] G. Beebe, and J. Belaval, "Fertility and Contraception in Puerto Rico," *Puerto Rico Journal of Public Health and Tropical Medicine* (Sept. 1942), p. 13.

[5] E. Cofresí, *Realidad poblacional de Puerto Rico* (San Juan: Imprenta Venezuela, 1951), Table 33, p. 88.

[6] Wherever one spouse mentioned having used methods not mentioned by the other spouse, these were added to the total number of methods used by the family, on the assumption that an individual would be more likely to conceal birth control information than to fabricate it. By this assumption, withdrawal was the most frequently concealed method.

and residence strongly affect birth-control use, the latter is by no means limited to the well-educated or the urban dweller.

TABLE 38

INCIDENCE OF BIRTH-CONTROL PRACTICE, BY RESIDENCE AND EDUCATION

Percentages of respondents who have used birth control

	Cofresí[a] (*percent*)	*Beebe and Belaval*[b] (*percent*)
Rural	29	26
Urban	39	52
Highest-education group[c]	100	59
Lowest-education group	25	21

[a] E. Cofresí, *Realidad poblacional de Puerto Rico* (San Juan: Imprenta Venezuela), Table 32, p. 87.

[b] G. Beebe and J. Belaval, "Fertility and Contraception in Puerto Rico," *Puerto Rico Journal of Public Health and Tropical Medicine,* VII (Sept. 1942), 65.

[c] Cofresí's highest-education group was composed of college women, whereas Beebe's was composed of women with eight years or more of schooling. Lowest-education groups were "None" and "Three years and less," respectively.

If birth control is so frequently used by the lower class, it appears peculiar that its effects are so slight in terms of mass statistics. Since we have already dealt generally with a good number of the attitudinal factors which appear to inhibit birth control use, it would now seem profitable to examine how these factors operate in practice. Three general questions areas may be blocked out: When and under what conditions is birth control initiated? Once birth control is initiated, what degree of success is achieved? What patterns of use are found which help to explain success or failure?

THE NONPRACTITIONERS OF BIRTH CONTROL

The major question here is, how do families which have initiated birth control differ from those which have not? We might expect, for example, that within the lower class age, residence, religion and birthplace might distinguish users from non-users. To determine this, the characteristics of the 20 families which have never practiced birth control were compared with the characteristics of the remaining 52 families which have. While there were virtually no differences in age, religion, residence, or birthplace of husband, several other factors showed interesting differences. These are summarized in Table 39.

TABLE 39

BIRTH-CONTROL USE, BY DOMINANCE RELATIONS, BIRTHPLACE OF WIFE, NUMBER OF LIVING CHILDREN, AND NUMBER OF MALE MARITAL UNIONS

Percentages of those in each category who have ever used birth-control in their current unions

		Percent	*Base*
A.	Traditional families	55	(20)
	Other	76	(46)
B.	Wife born in country	66	(44)
	Other	82	(28)
C.	Less than four living children	59	(42)
	Four or more living children	90	(30)
D.	Males with two or more unions	55	(23)
	Males with one union only	73	(48)

Parts A and B of the table are along expected lines. The traditional families and those in which the wife was born in the country are heavily weighted with nonusers. Of greater interest, however, are parts C and D. First of all, the nonusers are primarily from families which have few children and which perhaps have felt less need to practice birth control. Of the 20 nonusers, 13 have three children or less.[7] Their comments back up the "lack of concern" hypothesis.

We want another girl. (A10F)

If we have one more, I will have her sterilized. (A8M)

[7] Some of the strongest religious objections to birth control came from respondents in this group, suggesting that religious objections tend to disappear when necessity requires it.

We've been lucky. If I had to, I'd use something. (C4M)

I want more children, and I can't seem to have them. (X7F)

If she gets pregnant again, I will have her sterilized. (H23M)

I haven't needed to use birth control. (H31F)

But what of the 7 cases which have more than three children? Part D of Table 39 provides some interesting data in this regard. It shows that men with more than one union are less likely to have used birth control in their current union. The explanation for this might in part be that a man who has had several unions feels obliged, or at least free, to start reproducing afresh in each new union. Men who have had children of other women can avoid financial responsibility for these by means of desertion.[8] More important, however, is the tendency on the part of the male to desire "his own" children, that is, children of his current wife, since his other children usually live with their mothers. Of the 7 nonusers with four or more children, 4 women have children of previous unions living in the household; but since these are not their current husband's biological offspring, the males may desire to have a few of "their own."

This is only my second child *by him*. I'll speak to him about it after this one is born. (Seven children in household—H20F)

We have not used them because *we* want three kids. (Six children by previous unions, two of whom live at home—B6F)

Of the remaining 3 cases in the group of 7 "deviants," 2 have only four children, the final case, five. All three of these mothers mention that they are entering menopause and have no need for birth control.

Thus, what appeared to be deviant cases are only a variation of the cases which have few children. Of the 20 families never having used birth control in their present union, 16 have three children or less *from their current unions,* even though more children may be living in the household. The remaining cases appear relatively infertile and are beyond the period of danger of further impregnation.

[8] Although males are largely responsible for support of their children by other women, few lower-class women take the opportunity to press their cases, perhaps because they do not know their legal rights.

SUCCESS

Fifty-two families in the sample have tried some form of birth control. How successful have they been? There are several ways by which the success of birth-control practices might be gauged. Unfortunately, our cases are too few and the data themselves too variable to apply the usual measures of exposure and fertility. Consequently, we are compelled to employ a broader and more subjective criterion of success—the discrepancy between the family's stated ideal size and its actual size. We would expect that the larger the discrepancy, the less likely that birth control would have been used. Table 40 shows that the contrary is true.

TABLE 40

DISCREPANCY BETWEEN IDEAL AND ACHIEVED NUMBER OF CHILDREN, BY BIRTH-CONTROL USE

Percentages of families having over 1.5 children more than their ideal

	HUSBANDS		WIVES	
	Percent	*Base*	*Percent*	*Base*
Never used birth-control	10	(20)	10	(20)
Used, but discontinued	27	(11)	36	(11)
Currently use birth control	34	(41)	37	(41)

This somewhat paradoxical finding has been partially explained above. We found that nonusers did not feel the need to practice birth control, since their families were relatively small. Now it also appears, however, that those who do feel a need to practice family limitation act inefficiently or too late. While our data are not sufficiently refined to yield precise measures of the care with which birth-control methods are used, an examination of the types of methods used and the order of their use can supply us with helpful information.

PATTERNS OF USE

Once a family decides to limit its size, there are many alternative techniques available. Methods can be secured for male or female;

they can be relatively expensive or cheap; mechanical, chemical, organic, or "natural"; temporary or permanent; troublesome or simple. Particularly in the lower class, what a family decides to use will depend largely on what is available to them. Folk techniques, if known, are always available, cheap, and "natural", but usually unpleasant. Mechanical and chemical methods are available at the Public Health Centers gratis; but various methods, such as the condom and the sponge, are frequently discouraged by them. Sterilization is also available, but only under certain conditions.

METHODS OF BIRTH CONTROL

It might be expected that the lower-class groups are primarily using folk methods of contraception. This proposition is negated by the findings both of the present study and of Cofresí's. In Cofresí's lower-class group (less than $500 annual family income), the condom was the most frequently used method (51 percent of the total methods used), sterilization the second most frequently used (23 percent),[9] and jelly third (6.5 percent). The only striking differences found in the upper class were more frequent use of the diaphragm (lower class, 4 percent, upper class, 18 percent) and somewhat less reliance on the condom.[10] The findings of Beebe and Belaval are somewhat contradictory. Withdrawal was the most fre-

[9] Sterilizations can be obtained free in many of Puerto Rico's public hospitals if the examining physician feels it is indicated for reasons of health. The signatures of both husband and wife are required, and some hospitals require that a pint or two of blood be donated by the family in return for the service. Sterilization is becoming so popular among the lower class that securing bed space for it in the hospitals has become a plum dispensed by local politicians. According to private information received, many officials have complained that the demand far exceeds the available supply of beds. As to the incidence of sterilization, according to an investigation by Dr. José Belaval, 17.8 percent of all hospital deliveries in 1950 were followed by sterilization. In Hatt's sample, about 8 percent of the upper-rental-group mothers and 3 percent of the lower-rental-group mothers had already been sterilized. Hatt, *op. cit.*, Table 318, p. 444. Recent evidence indicates that the incidence may be considerably higher. In the sample of 3,000 described in footnote 3, 20 percent of the wives had been sterilized. See J. M. Stycos, "Female Sterilization in Puerto Rico," *Eugenics Quarterly*, I (June 1954), 3–9. In the representative sample referred to in footnote 3, 16.7 percent of the married or consensually married women were found to be sterilized, the incidence ranging from 6.5 percent of the rural residents whose family heads had no education, to 30 percent of those with nine or more years of education in both rural and urban areas.

[10] Cofresí, *op. cit.*, Table 34, p. 90.

quently used single method (46 percent), with the condom second (17 percent) and douches third (6 percent).[11]

The discrepancies between the two studies are understandable in the light of the different populations from which they were drawn. Beebe's group was comprised entirely of women who were seeking birth-control information. This would automatically remove all sterilizations from his sample and make likely a high proportion of ineffective methods. Since Cofresí's sample was drawn from a much broader population, we would expect such ineffective methods as withdrawal to be cited with less frequency.

In our own sample, the ranking of methods ever used resembles Cofresí's more closely than Beebe's, but several differences are apparent. Table 41 presents the total of methods ever used, separating current from past methods as well.

TABLE 41

CURRENT AND PAST METHODS OF CURRENT AND PAST BIRTH-CONTROL USERS

	Current Methods of Current Users	*Past Methods of Current Users*	*Past Methods of Past Users*	*Total Methods Ever Used*	
	(number)	*(number)*	*(number)*	*(number)*	*(percent)*
Condom	8	16	6	30	26
Sterilization	20	—	—	20	18
Withdrawal	6	9	5	20	18
Abstinence	9	5	2	16	14
Diaphragm	—	3	3	6	5
Douche	1	4	—	5	4
Rhythm	—	5	—	5	4
Sponge	—	4	—	4	4
Folk	3	1	—	4	4
Jelly	—	1	2	3	3
Number of methods	(47)	(48)	(18)	(113)	100
Number of families	(42)	(42)	(10)	(52)	(52)

[11] Beebe and Belaval, *op. cit.*, Table 4, p. 66.

There are several points to be noted. (1) A wide range of birth-control methods have been used by the families over the years. On the average, each family in the table has used two different methods. (2) Despite this fact, female methods other than sterilization are employed relatively infrequently and are even more infrequently continued. Better to ascertain the direction of birth-control use over time, a more dynamic table is presented below.

TABLE 42

PRESENT BIRTH-CONTROL METHODS, BY METHODS USED IN THE PAST

PRESENT METHODS	PAST METHODS		
	None	*Folk, Abst., Withdr., Rhythm*	*Chem.-Mechan.*
None	20	2	8
Folk, abstinence, withdrawal, rhythm	—	9	6
Chemical-mechanical	—	3	5
Sterilization	6	3	10
Number of families	(26)	(17)	(29)

Relatively few who have used folk or "natural" methods have discontinued them or changed to sterilization or to mechanical-chemical methods. On the other hand, a good number have moved from chemical-mechanical to folk methods, sterilization, or "nothing." It would seem that sterilization has a particularly powerful "pull," whereas chemical and mechanical methods have considerable "push" toward other methods or toward discontinuance.

Both the high turnover of methods and the popularity of folk methods might help to explain the frustration of the small-family ideals of birth-control users. However, the frequency of sterilization might be thought to counteract this. Table 43 shows, as might be expected, that sterilization is more effective than other methods in bringing family-size ideals and achievement into line, but that it by no means guarantees this result.

TABLE 43

ACHIEVEMENT OF FAMILY IDEALS, BY METHOD OF BIRTH-CONTROL USED

	Have More than Ideal (percent)	*Have Same or Less than Ideal (percent)*
Sterilization	29	45
Other	71	55
	100	100
Number of families	(21)	(31)

At least one more factor will help in explaining the ineffectiveness of birth control—the time of initiation of birth-control measures. Obviously, if birth control methods, even sterilization, are initiated after the ideal number has been achieved, they can only reduce the discrepancy between ideals and achievement. Table 44 shows the extent to which methods were started "too late."

TABLE 44

TIME OF INITIATION OF BIRTH-CONTROL METHODS, BY BIRTH-CONTROL METHOD

	Started before Ideal Number of Children	*Started after Ideal Number of Children*	*No Information*
Sterilization	8	11	1
Other	14	13	5
Number of families	(22)	(24)	(6)

It is clear that there is no great tendency for users to start their methods before they "have to," as regards either sterilization or other methods. As far as sterilization is concerned, however, other data are available which suggest that in general it is initiated at a late date. In Hatts' large sample, the median birth after which sterilization was performed for women married between 1920 and 1929 was 5; for those married in the next ten-year period, 4.[12]

We now have several hypotheses concerning birth-control practices on the part of the lower class. (1) Birth control tends not to be initiated until several births have already occurred. (2) Once birth control is initiated, various methods are tried but presumably are not practiced methodically.[13] (3) Judging by the histories of turnover of methods, sterilization appears to be the most attractive method, and chemical-mechanical techniques the least attractive.

We shall in the following section attempt to bring together our information into a hypothetical paradigm, which will then be illustrated by selected family case studies.

A PARADIGM OF BIRTH-CONTROL USE

We are concerned here with unraveling the elements basic to decision making in regard to birth control—that is, with delineating the general factors which determine why family *A*'s ideals are translated into action of one type, as opposed to family *B*, which resorts to another type, or to family *C*, which does nothing at all or which tries and gives up. Looking at it from the point of view of an individual husband or wife, three elements are integral to decision making and action: (1) concern over ends, i.e., over having "too many" children; (2) knowledge of means, i.e., of methods of birth control; and (3) attitude toward means, i.e., the degree of ac-

[12] Hatt, *op. cit.*, Table 320, p. 446. It is probable that this trend is largely the result of earlier *upper-class* sterilizations. The lower class must rely on public services, and most hospitals and public-health physicians have rules of thumb about the appropriate time to sterilize. It is my impression that most hospitals hesitate to sterilize until the woman has had four or five children.

[13] Beebe and Belaval found much evidence for this hypothesis. "The beginnings of a contraceptive effort evident in the experience of the sample before admission to the service, the fact of enlistment, the demonstrated capacity to learn modern contraceptive techniques, and the effort made to secure protection, all unite in evidence that a portion of the population of lowest social and economic position is ready for contraception *without knowing what to do about it. . . . The high risk of conception after admission to the contraceptive service and its significance for discontinuance of the prescribed* methods constitute major problems" (*op. cit.*, p. 50, italics mine).

ceptance or resistance to birth-control methods. Each of these factors varies in intensity and in time.

Concern over Ends. Assuming that in general the lower-class population believes that three children are ideal, families will vary in the intensity with which they hold this belief. The range will be from those who would do "anything" to keep their numbers to that size, to those for whom it "would be nice" to have three children. Not only do families vary in their intensity of concern over the ideal family size, but in the time at which this concern begins. Some individuals will hold their ideals early in marriage, others become concerned only when it is "too late." Some will have relatively little concern early in marriage and change to intense concern later; others may do the opposite. Obviously we must learn more about what kind of people develop which kind of concern at what time.

Knowledge of Means. Concern cannot be translated into action unless it is accompanied by a knowledge of channels for action. A woman may be greatly concerned over having too many children, but ignorance of means inhibits action. However, a high concern may in many cases encourage *knowledge seeking,* which may or may not result in knowledge, depending on the social milieu. Knowledge varies in degree. For example, a person may know about male methods of birth control but not about female methods. Knowledge also varies in time. Information supplied at a time when concern is low may be forgotten, or at best not acted upon. Information also may occur "too late" and would, for example, be of no use after a woman has completed her childbearing period.

Attitude toward Means. Even if means are known, an adverse attitude toward some or all of them may inhibit birth-control use. Religious or superstitious objections, for example, can inhibit the utilization of known means. These objections may be strongly or weakly felt. For example, we have seen that religious objections are frequently rationalizations for lack of concern over family size, whereas fears about the physical effects of birth control are more likely to be genuine and intense. Obviously, too, the objections can vary over time. For example, religious reasons are frequently forgotten, once concern over family size becomes strong. Let us assume, however, that objections are constant over time, and schematize the various categories of the three major elements outlined above.

TABLE 45

SUMMARY OF THREE MAJOR ELEMENTS IN INDIVIDUAL MOTIVATION TOWARD BIRTH CONTROL

	CONCERN		KNOWLEDGE		ATTITUDE (RESISTANCE)	
	Intense	*Weak*	*Complete*	*Incomplete*	*Intense*	*Weak*
Early	a	b	e	f	—	—
Late	c	d	g	h	—	—
Early or late	—	—	—	—	i	j

The possible combinations of the three factors and their variables of intensity and time, even simplified as they are, are 32. However, even this number does not express the full range of combinations, since we have been describing individuals rather than families. In reality, both husband and wife must be represented in each of the elements and their variables, since they are seldom in agreement on all three. This multiplies the possible combinations of husband and wife to a formidable number.

Fortunately, these hypothetical combinations can be somewhat reduced in number by two further considerations. (1) Class and cultural patterns: Certain combinations are much more frequent in lower-class Puerto Rican society than others. For practical purposes, a good number of the hypothetical combinations can be ignored. We shall subsequently suggest some of the more frequent patterns. (2) Types of interpersonal relationships between spouses: We have so far treated husbands and wives as independently functioning individuals. In reality, they are interacting units, and for our present purposes two types of interaction are pertinent—dominance and communication.

In a marital relationship "completely" dominated by either husband or wife, the position of the subordinate spouse on the three basic factors is of no significance in terms of action; action will be determined regardless of the concern, knowledge, and attitude of the subordinate spouse. On the other hand, should the relationship be less traditional, the attitudes of both spouses must be taken into consideration.

Communication is another interpersonal factor of some importance in predicting action. It is possible, for example, for a husband and wife to have the same combinations of concern, knowledge, and attitude toward means, but without mutual awareness of this. A family which is characterized by commonly realized, rather than individualized, concurrence on ideals is more likely to act. It is also possible for one family member to withhold information which would be of assistance to the other.

One further factor helps to determine whether or not birth control will be initiated. We shall call this a catalyst. Often when a family is more or less ready to try something, a word of advice from a relative or the suggestion of a nurse or doctor will "trip off" the action.

Once birth control is initiated, the consistency and care with which it is used again depends upon all the factors described above. If concern is not great, it may be used carelessly. If objections are strong, the method may soon be abandoned. If knowledge is inadequate, it may be used improperly. If the method then fails because of improper or inconsistent use, the family may become discouraged with the method. If their concern is high, they may change to drastic techniques such as sterilization[14] or even desertion. If their concern is low, they will simply use nothing.

Better to grasp the number of variables we have described, a paradigm is presented below, followed by case histories which illustrate some of the major variables.

[14] Sterilization is "drastic" in the sense that it is an irreversible operation.

Under "Drastic measures" are subsumed such patterns as abortion, sterilization, desertion, and child dispersal. The studies of Hatt and Cofresí have not found abortion to be of any significance in Puerto Rico. We have already suggested that male desertion due to the pressures of fertility may be a frequent pattern, but, since we have dealt with intact families only, this remains a matter of some speculation.

Child dispersal is a common phenomenon in Puerto Rico, as suggested by the leading quotation to this chapter. Six and a half percent of Puerto Rico's households have one or more informally adopted children (*hijos de crianza*), and, despite neo-local residence patterns, 13.4 percent have grandchildren living in the home. L. J. Roberts and R. L. Stefani, *Patterns of Living in Puerto Rican Families* (Rio Piedras, University of Puerto Rico, 1949), Table 17, p. 279. While this phenomenon was not covered in the present study, it has received more detailed attention in the author's "Family and Fertility in Puerto Rico," *American Sociological Review,* XVII (Oct. 1952), 572–80, and merits further study.

SEVEN FAMILY HISTORIES OF BIRTH CONTROL

While it is not possible to illustrate even a significant portion of the possible combinations of the variables in the paradigm, we have selected seven typical cases, each of which contains fairly complete information on most of the strategic variables. Each case is labeled according to the variable which appears of greatest significance in the birth-control history. However, as a reading of the cases quickly shows, the particular variable exerts its influence in a context of the others, and the end product can be understood only in this total context.

B7: Late Concern on the Part of the Husband. In twenty-nine years of marriage this couple has had eight children. Birth control was started late in the marital history, despite small-family ideals. Communication: medium. Communication on sexual matters is poor. Dominance: traditional. Family ideals: both have small-family ideals, but at least in the case of the husband these came at a fairly late date.

History: The husband says he would have liked two or three

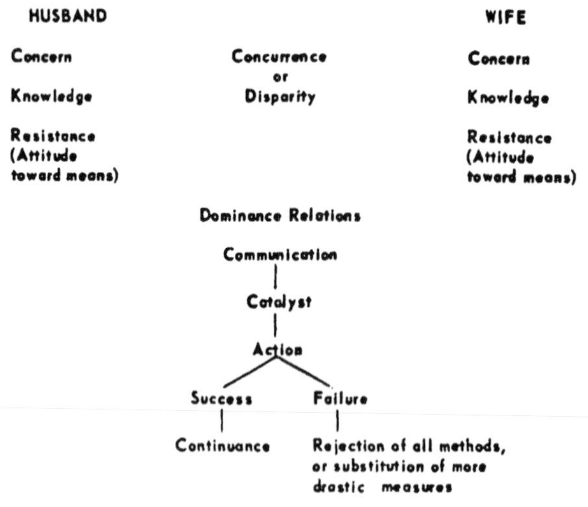

FIGURE II

A PARADIGM OF VARIABLES DETERMINING ACTION ON FAMILY LIMITATION

children but that he had not enough foresight. "I didn't think about the matter until it was too late." Moreover, he knew nothing about birth control until quite recently. He claims he would have used it, but "in the old times there was nothing of that." Even now, although he knows the "hospitals" offer birth-control materials, he seems to have only a hazy notion of what they are. The wife, too, was ignorant of birth-control methods until recently, when her aunt told her about withdrawal. She told her husband about this, and they started to use the method immediately.

Discussion: In this case we note a combination of ignorance and late concern, but additionally of poor communication. Though neither of the couple knew of birth-control methods, and the man was not concerned until late, the woman never discussed the matter with him nor urged him to seek means to control their growing family size. When she finally was advised of a folk method, she did communicate this piece of information to her husband, and he, by now concerned over family size, immediately adopted it.

C3: An Unconcerned Husband. In five years of marriage this couple has had two children. Birth control was started after the second child, but stopped. Communication: low. Dominance: traditional. Family ideals: both large, but ambivalent.

History: The wife is afraid of pregnancy and wants no more children. She says her husband wants no more, but that "men don't like to avoid them." A shy woman, she will not go to the health unit about an abdominal pain because she does not want a man to see her. However, after her last child her neighbors told her about methods of birth control, and her mother advised her to go to the prematernal clinic and "not to be foolish about it." She picked up a supply of condoms at the clinic, and her husband used them regularly for six months. He then grew "tired of them," complaining that they were dirty and too much trouble. The wife then secured a diaphragm and jelly, but after five months she began to work outside the home and now has no time to pick up her supply of jelly. She also resists going back to the condom because "it might stay inside and hurt." Consequently, they are currently using no birth-control method. The husband says that if the wife has another child, he will have to do something. "If I realize I cannot support more children than I have, that will force me to use a method."

Discussion: Fears of pregnancy caused the wife's concern to start early, and, prompted by public opinion, she conquered her feelings of embarrassment and went to the health unit. Her husband, however, was not so concerned, resisted the use of the condom, and soon abandoned it. Although the diaphragm was substituted to the satisfaction of both, the wife's work has interfered with her trips to the health unit. The husband is not yet sufficiently concerned to perform this chore himself, but he realizes that, if they continue reproducing, he will have to take some action. To this family with a low tolerance to birth control, interference with supply meant complete abandonment of birth control methods.

B8: A Case of Late Concern in Both Spouses. This couple has ten living children and has been married for twenty-one years. Birth control has been started only recently but is used regularly. Communication: low. Dominance: least traditional. Family ideals: both are now small-family-minded, but both were previously large-family-minded.

History: The wife's ideal number of children is now two or three, but this appears to be a recent development. Originally, she regarded a large family "as the most natural thing in the world," and even now she is very proud of her large family. She says that if her husband had his way, they would still be having children, although after the twelfth he "seemed satisfied." The husband says he is proud of his large family and of the fact that he has been able to support them, but, looking back, he thinks that a small family might have been preferable. After the fourth child, a nurse from the health unit came to the home and advised the wife to visit the clinic. The latter discussed the matter with her husband, but they decided that as they were young and healthy they preferred a large family. After each birth the nurse came to the house to talk to the wife, but without effect. Finally, after the twelfth pregnancy, friends and relatives advised the couple to practice birth control. The wife then realized she was "tired and weak" from so many children and went to the health unit and acquired a sponge. She developed "nausea" soon after, and both attributed this to use of the sponge. They decided to use condoms and have been using them religiously ever since. The husband, although he dislikes them, says, "I am using them because I don't want more children. . . . I do not go a single time without them." The wife is so convinced of their usefulness that she gives them to their friends and even offered the interviewer a package.

Discussion: Both members of this family started with large-family ideals. The visit of the nurse, so frequently a catalyst, had no effect, even though repeated after each pregnancy. Public opinion did precipitate action, but only after a dozen pregnancies. In retrospect, both husband and wife see a smaller number as ideal, but their own awakening came too late for them to activate their new ideals. Now that they have reached the stage where further pregnancies would jeopardize both health and economic stability, birth control is used, and used rigorously.

Y3: A Resistant Husband. This couple has had five girls in eleven years of married life, and the wife is again pregnant. Abstinence is occasionally practiced. Communication: low. Dominance: least traditional. Family ideals: both small.

History: Both spouses see the ideal number of children as three, but neither appears to have held this ideal very strongly. The husband wants a male child (communication is so bad that the wife says, "He says nothing to me, but others tell me he wants this one to be a boy"), and the wife knows only sterilization as a method. She objects to this method and gives both religious and superstitious reasons. She says she will never be sterilized but that she would have liked to use something else, had she known what to use. Asked why she did not go to the Public Health Unit, she replied that she would be too embarrassed, never having been seen by a doctor. She claims that her husband is not concerned with how many children he has. The husband denies this and says that he tried to persuade her to be sterilized, but without success. When asked about other methods, he says that the condom is for prostitutes and that he would never dare to suggest it to his wife. He claims that he tries to practice abstinence, but that, when he does, his wife accuses him of having another woman, and he has to give in to allay her suspicions.

Discussion: This is a family in which both parties exercise a fair amount of control, but prejudices and poor communication have resulted in ineffective action on birth control. Too modest to go to the Health Unit for information, the woman believes that sterilization and sexual continence are the only ways out. She fears the first method and does not trust her husband when he uses the second. The husband, anxious to have a male child, is not too concerned as yet over family limitation, although he did initiate discussion concerning sterilization. His own resistance toward the condom makes him reluctant even to mention this method to his wife. As a consequence, they continue reproducing.

H39: A Resistant Couple. In twelve years of marriage this couple has had six children. Birth control was started early, but discontinued, and a sterilization performed. Communication: medium. Dominance: traditional. Family Ideals: the wife's ideal number is smaller than the husband's. The husband's concern appears to have occurred late and was never as intense as that of the wife.

History: The husband has never done anything to control the number of births. Although he knows the condom and sterilization and has "thought about the matter," he has done nothing, because he feared his wife might get sick. He has been told that condoms cause infections in the woman. The wife has consistently tried to avoid children since the second child. She washed after intercourse and avoided simultaneous orgasm. Advised by a nurse to go to the Public Health Clinic, she attended, despite strong feelings of shame. Before seeing the physician she talked with some women in the waiting room. They told her about the diaphragm, and, frightened, she left. She reports that her husband says condoms are for prostitutes, and she is a clean woman. After her fifth child everyone told her to try to be sterilized. She went to the Municipal Hospital and arranged for the operation, but the baby came too rapidly and was delivered in the home. For the next three years she tried to deny her husband, but this was not always successful, and she again became pregnant. Her husband finally agreed to put up the money to buy blood, and the sterilization was effected.

Discussion: The husband's lack of concern and resistance to birth control put the onus on the wife. Ashamed and frightened by the Health Center and its methods, she used folk techniques. Unsuccessful, she tried sterilization. After six children the husband felt sufficiently concerned to pay for the required blood.

C6: A Case of Poor Communication and Suspicion. This family has had a total of five children in eight years of marriage. Birth control was started early, but stopped. Communication: medium. Sex is never discussed. Dominance: traditional. A very submissive woman who cannot recall any disagreement with her husband. Family ideals: both have small-family ideals, but these appear to have occurred rather late and have never been very strong.

History: When married, neither knew anything about birth control. The husband had heard about the condom, but his friends had told him it was for prostitutes. He claims that if he had known more about it, he would have less children now. After three difficult pregnancies, a visiting nurse urged the wife to visit the Public Health Clinic. She, however, is ashamed to go. She has never been examined by a doctor and is also ashamed of being seen in the clinic. Consequently, the husband went to the clinic and was given condoms, but used these for two months only. He claims that the supply was not sufficient, that he was told their use would cause his wife to become ill, and that they were a lot of trouble to use. After two more pregnancies his wife will still not visit the health unit, despite a strong fear of dying in childbirth. She says, however, that after her last child her husband suggested sterilization. She was delighted at the idea, but did not dare tell him this, since he might suspect that her interest was based on a desire to cuckold him. Everyone is talking to her husband, telling him to have her sterilized, and she feels confident that this will be done in the near future.

Discussion: This is a case of a very modest and submissive wife. Therefore, the onus of birth control falls on the husband. His objections to the condom caused its use to be erratic and short-lived.

His wife's bad health occasioned public opinion (friends, nurse, and in-laws) to pressure the husband to do something. He sees sterilization as the only way out. His wife is eager to be sterilized, but infidelity fears cause her to remain silent on the subject. Sterilization will probably occur, but much later than would have been the case if the wife had felt free to discuss such matters with her husband.

H45: A Dominant Wife. In nine years of marriage this couple has had four pregnancies. However, birth control was started after the first child, and the couple now plans sterilization. Communication: very low. Marital satisfaction is also very low, and suspicion very high. The wife married only to escape from home and planned to leave her husband shortly after. The husband has many extramarital affairs known to his wife, and sexual relations with the wife are infrequent. Dominance: household was rated as "less traditional," but the woman appears to be able to have her way on important decisions by threatening abandonment. Family ideals: the wife's ideal number of children is three, the husband's four. Her concern over children appears to have occurred before the husband's, however, and appears to be somewhat stronger.

History: The first pregnancy, which occurred almost immediately after marriage, came as something of a shock to the wife, who knew nothing of birth control and who expected that children would not come so soon. Also, she was still thinking of leaving her husband. Consequently, she sought information at the health unit and was given prophylactics. Her husband had used them premaritally and agreed to try them. They continued their use for four years, but then the husband decided he wanted a boy; their use was discontinued, and another pregnancy ensued. Later, having no one with whom to leave the child, she could not make the trip to the health unit to maintain the supply of condoms. The husband, apparently, only knew that his wife stopped going to the health unit. Communication appears so poor that he never inquired, nor was he told, the reason why. Since his wife did not supply the materials, and he felt they were too expensive to purchase, withdrawal was practiced. He dislikes this method but his wife compels him to use it, holding out the threat of desertion if he does not. Two more pregnancies ensued while using withdrawal as a birth-control method. Although the wife knows about douches and diaphragm, she refuses both. The former is too difficult and troublesome to use, the latter dangerous. She also fears sterilization, and after her last birth refused it, even though a physician advised it. With her current pregnancy, however, the doctor again suggested it, and she now plans to be sterilized, seeing this as the only effective method. Although the husband is willing, he says he lacks the financial means. However, the wife says that, if he does not have her sterilized, she will desert him and demand support.

Discussion: In the area of birth control this couple is dominated by the wife. This is simplified by the fact that the husband agrees in principle with her fertility ideals, although he does not hold them so strongly as she. It is probable that if it were not for the wife, birth control would not be used. Her resistance to other methods of birth control and her inability to secure a supply of condoms left withdrawal and sterilization as the only two means. The ineffectiveness of the former and the urging of the physician has led her to accept the latter, even though she has fears about its possible effects on health.

CONCLUSIONS

The case histories presented speak, largely, for themselves. However, to bring together the information in the former sections of the chapter, and to generalize from patterns running through the case histories not presented, a series of generalizations—or, more accurately, hypothesis—is given below.

1. Birth control is very commonly practiced. Nearly all the families in the sample who have had children in excess of their ideal number have practiced some method of birth control at some point in their marital histories.

2. The use of birth-control methods is erratic. A high proportion of those who practice birth control use the methods sporadically, change to other methods, or stop use entirely.

3. Tolerance to birth-control methods is low. Most methods are disliked or feared. It is partly for this reason that so many methods

are used erratically or discontinued, even though a family's ideal family size may be small. Moreover, any difficulties over supply (for example, temporary exhaustion of supplies at the health unit or new tasks which compete for time spent at the clinic) are enough to cause many families to discontinue use.

4. Strong concern over family size occurs late more typically than early. Since both men and women are eager to start their families early, especially to "get it over with as fast as possible," many families are unconcerned about fertility in the earlier years of marriage. When they do become concerned, they have little margin for error; but, because of their resistance against and lack of familiarity with birth-control measures, these are either avoided or used ineffectively. When concern sets in early, it is either on the part of one member only or it is of relatively weak intensity. These factors frequently vitiate the effectiveness of birth control. Consequently, both early and late users frequently resort to the adoption of drastic measures such as sterilization or discontinue the modern birth-control measures.

5. Sterilization is the most popular method of birth control, not only for the reasons stated above but also for its own peculiar merits. As one woman put it, "It is only once, sure, and then you forget about it and don't have to use those dirty things."

6. Women become concerned over family size earlier than men. Not only are their family ideals somewhat smaller than their husbands', but these are felt more intensely and at an earlier date. The difficulties of pregnancy, childbirth, and childrearing in the resourceless lower class are experienced by the mother. Male concern appears to occur later and is seldom so intense.

7. Fear of the physical effects of childbirth is a powerful stimulus to birth control and, in particular, to sterilization. The same fear of ill health, which underlies the rejection of mechanical and chemical contraceptives, prompts some women to "do anything" to prevent another childbirth. Sexual denial and sterilization are frequent outcomes.

8. Modesty is a powerful deterrent to information seeking for most women. Despite the easy access of health clinics, and the fre-

quent encouragement of friends and relatives, many women are too shy to enter the clinics.

9. Poor communication between spouses delays action on family limitation. The case histories are full of instances in which suspicion or modesty has prevented communication on family ideals or on the means for realizing these. However, there comes a point, even in the most traditional families, when pressure of numbers forces communication on ordinarily tabued topics.

10. The Public Health Units are the most frequent source of information on birth-control methods for our respondents, and the source of advice which is most likely to result in birth-control use. "Friends," who themselves are frequently attending birth-control clinics, are the second most frequently cited source of information, but in such cases the method is less frequently adopted. We may say that the Public Health physician is the most typical catalyst of birth-control use.

11. After a certain number of children, public pressure in the form of neighbors, relatives, and friends frequently precipitates birth-control use. Typically, these are married women who advise the wife because they "are sorry for her." It may be that after a woman has had the culturally approved number of children (three or four) the women of the community feel obligated to break tabus on sexual discussion and inform the young wife about birth control.

X

Summary and Recommendations

While possessing a number of Old World characteristics, in the past half century Puerto Rico has changed from a largely static agricultural society to a more industrialized one of rapid change; from the undeveloped to the developing kind of economy described in Chapter I. As late as 1920, more than six out of every ten workers were engaged in agriculture; in 1952, less than four of every ten were so employed.[1] The proportion living in cities has risen from 23 percent in 1910 to 40 percent in 1950. Emigration, which amounted to only 4,000 per year until 1945, has risen steadily since the war and has exceeded 50,000 per year since 1951.[2] Literacy, only 33 percent in 1910, rose to 76 percent in 1950. Conditions for social mobility have become increasingly favorable as Puerto Rico has moved from the traditional toward the more secular type of society.

The birth rate of the Commonwealth, on the other hand, has shown only slight and recent tendencies toward decline. This fact, in the light of the island's low death rate, has produced great problems in the way of population increase. The present work has been concerned with providing some of the explanations of the Commonwealth's high fertility.

In Chapter I we suggested that the birth rate in any culture is affected by the prevalence of checks on sexual relations and conception or birth. In Puerto Rico, checks on coital frequency are not of special significance. Chaperonage and the tabus on premarital intercourse for women are insurance against conception before

[1] A. Jaffe and L. de Ortiz, "The Human Resource—Puerto Rico's Working Force," mimeographed, San Juan, 1953.

[2] C. Senior, "Migration and Puerto Rico's Population Problem," *Annals of the American Academy of Political and Social Sciences*, Vol. 285, Jan. 1953.

marriage, but age at first union for females in the class under discussion is low enough to diminish the significance of this pattern. Tabued periods of intercourse within marriage normally occur only during periods when the chances of conception are negligible—post partum and menstrual. Distaste on the part of many women for sexual intercourse may be causing a fair degree of sexual denial, but the importance of this variable does not seem great, especially in the light of male dominance.

In the absence of such checks, the explanation for high fertility would at first glance seem simple, and the usual reasons would appear to suffice: (1) birth-control materials are not readily available to poorly educated, impoverished populations; (2) such populations are ignorant of birth-control methods; (3) such populations favor large families. Our investigations have indicated that none of these explanations is especially true for Puerto Rico.

Throughout the small homogeneous island which has relatively good systems of transportation and communication, a network of public health units and subunits has offered free birth-control materials and advice for over a decade. The dramatic attention given to birth control, sterilization, and overpopulation by the press, the Church, and, to a lesser extent, by politicians, has facilitated the spread of information. Thus we find that a high proportion of our sample is aware of modern methods and has access to free materials.

While birth-control means, especially sterilization, are utilized with greater frequency than might have been expected, the methods do not appear to be used with great effectiveness. Sterilization tends to occur late in the fertility history, and contraceptives are used erratically and carelessly and are often discontinued, with the result that their impact on fertility does not seem great. It should be recalled, however, that recent demographic data indicate that a substantial decline in fertility may be imminent.

But do Puerto Ricans *want* small families? In investigating what we have termed the fertility belief system of the lower-income group, it seems clear that in many respects they do. Both Hatt's large-scale objective survey and the present more intensive study have indicated that three children is seen by most Puerto Ricans as the ideal family size. Most of the population seem aware that adequate care and education for one's children cannot be provided if there are too many children. The belief that the number of one's children should be determined by Divine Providence, a belief widely held among peasant populations, is not typical of lower-class Puerto Ricans, who, more often than not, reject the Catholic position on birth control. Instead of female fears of barrenness, so often a part of the attitude structure of high-fertility groups, we have noted indifference to the idea of infecundity, while the idea that the number of children is an index of a man's virility seems overshadowed by the criterion of the number of children he can properly feed and clothe. What then stands in the way of a reduction in the birth rate? We can summarize a few major impediments under two broad classes—motivational and actional.

MOTIVATIONAL DETERRENTS

Despite the general compatibility of the fertility belief system with the small family we have noted that concern over family size tends to occur fairly late in the fertility history, often only after the family has been faced with severe economic pressures. The reasons for this late concern are at least partly due to marriage forms and to the character structure typical of the lower economic class.

Consensual union. While the consensual union in Puerto Rico evidences greater stability than common-law unions in other parts of the Caribbean, it is nevertheless less stable than marriage. Over a period of several unions, fertility may be lower because of the time which elapses between unions. However, within any one union, the realization of the fragile bond which unites the partners may have several consequences for fertility: (1) a lack of sense of responsibility for the care of one's children on the part of the male, since abandonment is an easy expedient if economic pressures become too great; (2) the desire or feeling of obligation to have children by each new partner (over a number of unions, this may in particular cases result in a higher total number than the individual would have wanted from one partner); (3) the use of children, more typically by the female partner, as "marital cement" to tie down the husband in the absence of legal bonds. The rapid production of children consolidates and in some sense legitimizes what might be little more than a temporary liaison.

About a quarter of all unions in Puerto Rico are consensual, and the persistence of the pattern indicates its utility. While marriage is generally viewed as more desirable than consensual union, the latter is not seriously condemned by the lower-class community and has a sufficient number of advantages to make it attractive. Because of the insulation of the sexes before marriage, men and women enter this status in considerable ignorance of one another. Divorce for this class is difficult and costly. The consensual union serves as a kind of trial marriage in which a mistake can be corrected without undue hardship. While a good number of such unions are subsequently legalized, the high degree of mutual suspicion and distrust which characterizes relations between the sexes even after marriage helps to keep most of them from being legalized.

Early age at marriage. Early marriage increases the period of exposure to pregnancy, and has an obvious effect on fertility. Moreover, in the light of the naiveté of the cloistered Puerto Rican female, and the apparent lack of realization of the responsibilities of marriage characteristic of the young-marrying females, early union may also help account for the lack of thought given to family limitation in the earlier years of marriage.

We have seen that while the community may be permissive as regards early marriage, it certainly does not encourage it—the ideal age for women being seen as twenty-one. But behavior is inconsistent with these ideals. We have suggested that rebellion against the parents may be a major factor in early age at marriage for the female.

During adolescence the girl tends to rebel against the general restrictions of the household—a complex we have termed cloister rebellion. Specifically, too, she rebels against the difficulties imposed upon her during courtship, when she is even more closely guarded than during childhood. Her cloistered existence, plus an occasional American movie, encourage a romantic view of marriage, which will free her from parental tyranny. The suitor commonly plays upon her feelings of repression and promises her freedom and a "new way of life." At the same time, for various reasons, the parents tend to disapprove of the courtship and often try to prevent it. This increases the girl's hostility toward the parents and intensifies the romantic aspect of the courtship, often with the assistance of such romantic techniques as intermediaries, secret notes, and clandestine meetings. The result is frequently a premature termination of the courtship and an elopement—characteristically into a consensual union.

The failure to romanticize marriage and a strong tie to the mother contribute in making the male decision to marry more mature. His emotional and personal needs seem adequately filled at home by his mother, while sexual needs are satisfied by means of prostitutes. He marries eventually, of course, to gain children and status in the community.

Machismo. The drive in males to manifest their virility we have termed *machismo.* The complex would not seem to have the importance, ascribed to it before the field investigation, of driving men to produce a limitless quantity of children. However, it may have other direct and indirect effects on fertility: (1) the anxiety to disprove sterility encourages a rapid first birth; (2) the anxiety over production of male offspring, to prove that one can "make males," may encourage higher fertility where female offspring occur earlier in birth order; (3) serial marriage and extramarital activity may be partly products of a need to demonstrate sexuality; (4) certain negative attitudes toward birth control seem related to this complex. For example, resistance to the condom in the way of preference for the "clean spur" (*espuela limpia*) might be interpreted as a product of a virility-manifesting drive. Moreover, anxiety over dominating sexual relations and conception may preclude giving permission to the wife to use female contraceptives.

A number of speculations have been advanced to explain the origins of the complex. In contrast with the girl, the boy's sexuality is encouraged so long as it is not directed at the virgins of the barrio. At the same time, the rearing of the male child is harsher and less consistent than that of the female. It was hypothesized that this creates a tendency toward mother dependency and the seeking of a mother figure in marriage. Unsatisfactory sexual relations with the wife then produce feelings of sexual inadequacy and the need to demonstrate virility through other channels.

ACTION DETERRENTS

Even assuming positive motivation, other factors serve as impediments to taking action in the area of fertility control.

Male dominance. In an equalitarian family set-up the desires of the wife have a much better chance of realization than in the husband-dominated household, where her opinions may count for little. Since husbands of the lower-income group appear to be less motivated to limit family size, more interested in sexual activity, and less exposed to birth-control clinics than their wives, fertility is likely to be higher than it would be if wives had greater authority.

Poor communication. Along with male dominance goes lack of communication between spouses as a barrier to action. Although both spouses may have small-family ideals, often they are not aware of the similarity of their opinions, a fact which delays action on the steps necessary to achieve these ideals. Second, knowledge of contraceptives possessed by one spouse is frequently not communicated to the other, another fact which lessens the likelihood that action will be taken.

We have suggested that the differential statuses of the sexes may contribute to this phenomenon. From childhood, males are considered to be so different from and better than females that adequate communication on intimate topics may subsequently be difficult. Even courtship, which frequently serves to bridge the differing worlds of the sexes in other cultures, does little to promote mutual understanding because of its rigid supervision by the girl's parents. In marriage, separate patterns of work and recreation, mutual suspicion of infidelity, and "respect" patterns serve to preserve the communications gap between the spouses. Sexual activity, moreover, is surrounded by communications tabus and is often characterized by sentiments of distaste, further impeding communication in the area of fertility control.

Female modesty. Modesty not only impedes communication between husband and wife but also keeps some women who are interested in birth control out of the clinics. Such women fear being seen there, asking for information, and being examined by a male physician. In several cases this was true despite the pressure of friends and relatives to attend the clinics.

The antecedents of this complex can be inferred from previous remarks. In Puerto Rican society, sex is regarded prudishly, and before marriage the girl is kept as much as possible in ignorance of it. The cultural ideal is the chaste, modest, and naive woman, who must be a virgin before marriage and behave like one subsequently.

Misinformation. Whereas most individuals in our sample are aware of at least one method of birth control, and of the supplies available in the Public Health Clinics, various prejudices against the specific methods keep many families from using them and cause others to discontinue use. The fear of contracting cancer from condoms, jellies, and diaphragms and the fear of not being able to extract the diaphragm are among those most frequently expressed.

A PARADIGM OF PUERTO RICAN FERTILITY

In attempting to explain Puerto Rican fertility, we have dwelled extensively on such matters as child rearing, the status of the sexes, sexual beliefs, and the forms of marriage. Often the complex described has no immediate relation to fertility but affects other variables which in turn bear more directly on fertility. Moreover, the particular pattern described often seemed to differ little, or only in degree, from comparable patterns in the continental United States. It is the sum of these various parts, however, which adds up to the island's fertility and which makes Puerto Rican culture distinctive. So that the essential parts of the pattern can better be viewed as a whole, a paradigm which summarizes many of the foregoing hypotheses and their interrelationships is provided below.

POSSIBLE DIRECTIONS FOR PROGRAMS OF POPULATION CONTROL

While the social scientist cannot establish the superiority of one value over another, he can assist in implementing given values. He can both indicate obstacles in the way of realization of existing

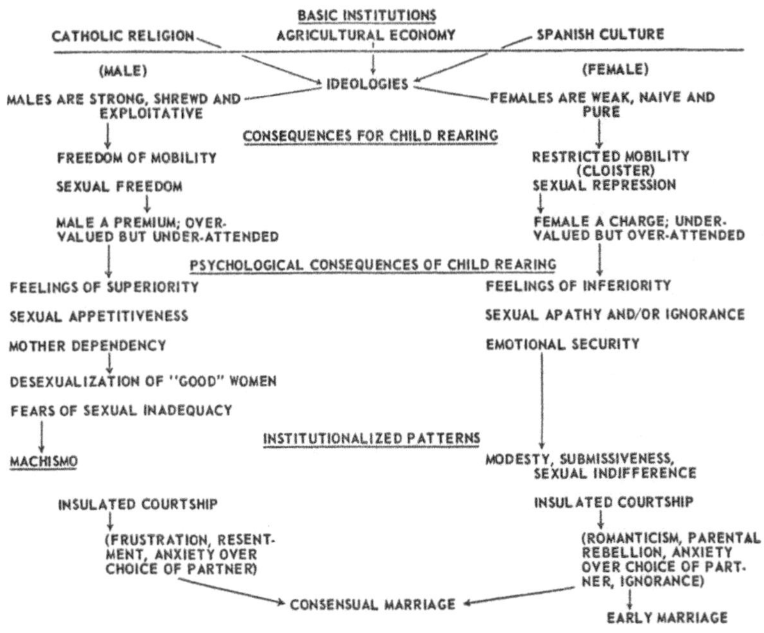

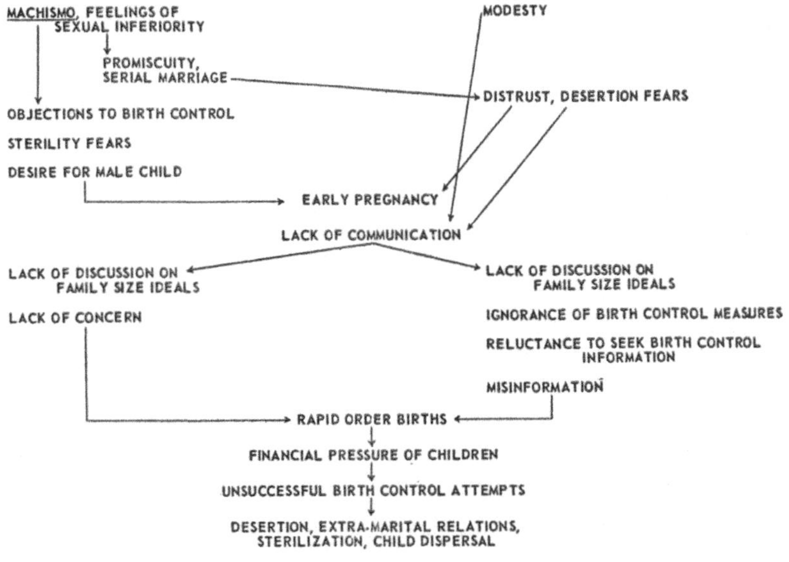

FIGURE III

A PARADIGM OF THE ANTECEDENTS AND CONSEQUENCES OF HIGH FERTILITY

values and suggest new and alternative means for their realization. In the present case we have found and reviewed a good deal of evidence which suggests that most of the people of Puerto Rico desire smaller families than they now have. We have also seen that the government of Puerto Rico is taking steps to assist the populace in the realization of such desires. Therefore, it would seem appropriate here to present an outline, based mainly on our research, of the way in which a more effective program of fertility control could be designed, if such were desired.

The reader should be reminded, however, that the data upon which most of the conclusions of this study are based, though systematically gathered and processed, consist of a small number of interviews in one area of Puerto Rico. Conclusions, then, must be considered as tentative and must await further research for verification.[8] The present section is written mainly for the considerable number of Puerto Ricans who feel that rapid population growth is one of the island's most pressing problems, one which demands new programming decisions in the immediate future. To such individuals and groups, it is hoped, the following section will be of some assistance.

We shall not be concerned here with such obvious but far-reaching programs as increasing education, employment of women, industrialization, and so forth, but rather limit ourselves to changes within the existing program of population control and to additional programs of relatively small dimensions.

CHANGES IN THE CURRENT PROGRAM

Of all possible programs, an expansion of sterilization facilities would be the one most likely to receive immediate widespread response. It may well be that sterilization is to be Puerto Rico's answer to the population problem, at least until social change has

[8] Such research is currently under way. For progress reports, see R. Hill, K. Back, and J. M. Stycos, "Family Structure and Fertility in Puerto Rico" (Social Science Research Center, University of Puerto Rico, Sept. 1954, mimeographed); K. Back, R. Hill, G. Arbona, and R. King, "Family Dynamics and Human Fertility—The Experimental Phase" (Social Science Research Center, University of Puerto Rico, July 1954, mimeographed); and R. Hill, K. Back, and J. M. Stycos, "Intra-Family Communication and Fertility Planning in Puerto Rico," *Rural Sociology,* forthcoming.

had a chance really to settle in, making possible the effective utilization of more flexible instruments of birth control. In light of the fact that concern over fertility tends to occur late, that tolerance of contraceptives is low, that modesty impedes discussion of methods associated with the sexual act, and that sterilization appears safe and easy to the Puerto Rican, this method may be the one which is most likely to bring the greatest degree of success in the shortest time. However, because of its irreversible nature, it would seem a more farsighted policy to step up action on contraceptives at the same time, with the expectation that at some point in the future the population might swing back to these less "permanent" techniques.

Another possible change would involve the improvement and expansion of the services of the prematernal health clinics. Although the 160 weekly clinics probably form the most extensive services of their kind in the world, a great deal of improvement is indicated. Some of the weak spots in the program are outlined below.[4]

Shortage of personnel. There is no full-time staff devoted to the prematernal program in any of the Public Health Units. The prematernal clinic is squeezed into a program including as many as nine other clinics. Clinics on venereal disease, prenatal and postpartum care, tuberculosis and crippled children are some of the weekly sessions which compete for the physicians' and nurses' time. Most prematernal clinics are open only half a day per week, and in some areas only one day per month.

Since the clinics are open so infrequently, many mothers are discouraged from attending. In many of the communities a woman will have to walk and climb miles to reach the clinic. If shopping time does not coincide with clinic time, the prospects of another such walk will hardly promote regular attendance. Additionally, modesty patterns create a resistance to attending clinics on a particular morning or afternoon of the week, since the town gossip will know for what reason the patient has entered the health station.

[4] The following section on limitations of the prematernal health program was originally printed in *The Annals of the American Academy of Political and Social Sciences,* Vol. CCLXXXV, Jan. 1953, as a part of an article entitled, "The Prospects of Birth Control in Puerto Rico," by the writer and Reuben Hill.

Apathy and autonomy. As a general rule, the principle of local autonomy for health units operates to maximize the motivation of physicians and their associates. In this instance the very flexibility of the centers brings about an emphasis on programs other than the prematernal clinics. The pressure of other clinics not only competes for time but also for the interest of the staff. Physicians tend to emphasize the clinics which deal with their areas of training and interest, and few men have been sufficiently trained in gynecology or obstetrics to be vitally interested in birth-control services. The prematernal clinics suffer in those centers where the medical staff prefers work with venereal disease, tuberculosis, or crippled children. This is seen in the criticism of the program that has been made by its officers:

1. A physician who is not particularly interested in the program will be careless about replenishing supplies of contraceptive materials. Since supplies are sent by the Health Department only upon request, an indifferent health officer can seriously hamper the program.
2. Whereas a physician interested in the program will refer many of his patients from other clinics to the prematernal clinic, an indifferent physician will treat only those who directly ask for advice and materials.
3. Visiting nurses are supposed to appraise the home situations both of patients and of nonpatients and recommend a visit to the clinic if a health reason indicates that this would be helpful to the family. Lack of sensitivity to the problem, however, frequently causes such nurses to concentrate on more routine matters.

Program ignores husband. An obvious shortcoming of the existing program is its failure to take into account the vital role played by the husband in family limitation. The centers concentrate their entire attention upon mothers. This situation has come about because the law requires the center to establish a health reason for providing contraceptive information and materials. Consequently the male, who is the real barrier to effective birth control, is not made part of the cooperative arrangement between the center and the family.

Disregard of modesty patterns. Although manned by native Puerto Ricans, the centers appear to ignore the deeply ingrained modesty patterns of Puerto Rican women. The program requires that every woman who applies or is referred to a prematernal clinic be given a vaginal examination by a physician, who then decides whether or not birth control is indicated. Since there are few female physicians on the island, these examinations are conducted by male physicians. There is abundant evidence that women avoid the Public Health Units precisely because they object to such examinations by male physicians. The husband often feels even more strongly than the wife about the impropriety of such examinations.

If the modesty impediment is to be overcome, female physicians need to be trained and placed in these clinics, and, wherever possible, nurses should be used to replace the male physicians. This can probably be done profitably in the fitting of the diaphragm, thus freeing the physician for other more technically medical duties.

Seeming passivity. The program presents a curious paradox. It is at once one of the most ambitious and widespread programs of birth control in the world, and yet it is basically neutral in the educational approach to people. Relatively little initiative is taken in getting people into the clinics. The staffs of the clinics see themselves as passive instruments to be used by those who desire to use the center's facilities. This seeming passivity is probably the program's most serious drawback at the present moment.

A new program. Clearly needed for maximum effectiveness is a broad program with several facets. Of foremost importance would be a public campaign to get more people into the prematernal clinics. The campaign might marshal all the available interpersonal and mass-media channels for disseminating information on birth control. Leaflets (especially to newlyweds), posters, mobile motion picture units, discussion groups with visual aids, and so forth, could be directed at the lower-income group in an effort to precipitate effective action. At the same time, agencies which have direct contact with the lower class might consider birth-control information as part of their program of education. The health education division of the Department of Health, the Agricultural Extension Service, and the Division of Community Education of the Department of Education are among the governmental divisions which might serve as central channels of dissemination. The content of the program would best be directed toward the intensifying of already positive attitudes and toward the weakening of negative attitudes. Authoritative rebuttal of the popular misconceptions about birth-control techniques alone could do a great deal. Since lower-class couples already have small-family ideals at marriage, it is merely a question of intensifying or catalyzing them, not so much of creating them. Recently married couples might be advised that the time to start family planning is in the present, not when it is too late. Women could be reminded that "starting soon" does not mean finishing soon, that rapid-order pregnancies are detrimental to health, and that a large family in present-day Puerto Rico tends to be more an economic liability than an asset. The latter arguments are known by most of the lower class and need merely be stressed and raised for discussion. These points should be emphasized before women attend clinics as well as while they attend them, to insure that birth-control practices will be initiated early and continued.

Along with the educational campaign could go wider distribution of birth-control materials with special attention given to contraceptives for the male. Since males will seldom attend a prematernal clinic, and many rural women find it difficult or unpleasant to attend, male contraceptives could be made available in country stores of the island, and, by means of government subsidy, could be available at a token cost.

Finally, an effort might be made to effect change in the more inaccessible areas of social life—family structure. Since communication between spouses was seen to be a major deterrent to birth-control practice, discussion groups on sex, marriage, child bearing, child rearing, and other related topics could be attempted, perhaps by such groups as the parent-teacher association. If less restrictive measures were taken with daughters, and if daughters possessed more information about sex and a greater awareness of the responsibilities of marriage, more careful choice of partners and later age at marriage might ensue. Premarital and marital counseling services could also work toward the same objectives.

CONCLUDING REMARKS

Both biology and culture join in making reproduction one of the strongest of human urges. A product of sexual drives, it is more directly sustained, supported, and encouraged by every society's social institutions—in particular, by that persistent complex of social relationships termed the family. In traditionally rooted societies, a large number of beliefs, attitudes, and patterns of social behavior within the family foster high rates of reproduction. If modern societies have significantly reduced their birth rate, this has occurred only after considerable changes in their social structures. Even then, these changes have taken many decades to affect the hard core of beliefs and practices surrounding reproduction. While it is true that the "reproductive revolution" was speeded by the development of modern methods of birth control, it is a reliable axiom that the widespread use of a particular invention, indeed often the invention itself, must be preceded by social changes which make the technique desirable and feasible.

This is nowhere clearer than in Puerto Rico, where excessive population growth imperils the whole society. While modern methods of birth control are freely available to all, and while drives toward reproduction have already been substantially weakened by social change, the birth rate remains largely unchanged. We have seen that there is such a broad network of family beliefs and practices directly and indirectly supporting high fertility that change in any one of its elements—even, for example, of such a presumably strategic belief as ideal family size—does not guarantee any substantial consequences for fertility. This analysis supplies no great hope to those who see an oral contraceptive as the panacea for the world's population problems. While such a discovery would certainly remove many of the current resistances to birth control, it is not the case that objection to particular methods is the major impediment to fertility control. Indeed, most of the current objections in Puerto Rico would also be directed at an oral contraceptive.

The present research suggests that investigation of the social institutions of a society, in particular of the family, is necessary for the understanding of its reproductive behavior. Moreover, only by a thorough understanding of these institutions can those in authority hope to shape an intelligent population policy.

Appendix A: Methodology

> Any person will talk freely to anybody whom he believes to be serious and trustworthy in character, and especially to one who has proven to be friendly to him.
>
> FROM AN INTERVIEWER'S NOTES

Every research project is confronted with decisions concerning the kind of data it will use and the way in which these will be collected. The extent and nature of pertinent prior research has a great deal to do with the eventual decisions.

PREVIOUS STUDIES

Previous studies on fertility in Puerto Rico are of various sorts. (1) Analyses of census data and vital statistics have been undertaken by Janer (1945), Tietze (1947), Perloff (1950), and Combs and Davis (1951). (2) Anthropological community studies by Rogler (1940), Siegel (1948), King (1948), Mintz, Manners, Padilla, and Wolf (1951) have dealt in part with family and reproductive patterns. (3) Studies of the attitudes and behavior of clinic patients with respect to birth control have been done by Beebe and Belaval (1942) and Cofresí (1951). (4) Large-scale interview studies with representative samples of the population were undertaken by Roberts and Stefani (1949) and Hatt (1952). The former touched only peripherally on family and fertility, while the latter study was devoted exclusively to attitudes and behavior pertinent to fertility.

While this is a fairly impressive backlog of research, it was felt that there was room for a more intensive investigation in the area of attitudes—a study which would probe deeper levels of motivation than was possible for the large-scale surveys, have wider scope than the clinical studies, and be more systematic in the collection of data on fertility than the community studies. For this and other reasons detailed below, it was felt that an interview form would have to be designed which would in some way meet several criteria: depth; scope and flexibility; comparability (i.e., the use of similar question wordings in covering similar content areas for all interviews); representativeness (i.e., a sample representative of a normal universe of lower-class Puerto Ricans).

The rationale behind the criterion of representativeness seems clear enough, and a later section is devoted to an explanation of how this problem was met. The other criteria, however, deserve further explanation.

Depth. The project was to be concerned with social-psychological dynamics of family life. Many of the subjects to be covered were thought to exist in the respondent's "preconscious" thinking. Consequently, some method which tapped various levels of consciousness and motivation seemed indicated.

Scope and Flexibility. The project was to be exploratory and preliminary to a larger and more quantitative study. This required that the questions cover a wide content range and that the instrument of exploration be as unstructured as possible in order to elicit both anticipated and unanticipated responses. The importance of the latter was all the greater because the study was to be performed in another culture, where responses were even less predictable than those in the writer's own.

Moreover, the project was to be concerned with intimate data on family life. Since rapport between a respondent and a stranger asking personal questions is difficult, a flexible method had to be designed which would allow the interviewer freedom to adapt his questions to the respondent's general frame of reference and emotional reactions from moment to moment during the interview. Thus, if the respondent grew uneasy or resistant in the face of a certain area of questioning, the interviewer might temporarily move to less delicate types of questions, lapse into casual conversation, or change his wording or general approach in order to avoid antagonizing the respondent.

Comparability. A number of broad hypotheses had been outlined prior to the field work. While it was felt that these hypotheses would not be validated or invalidated in an exploratory study, one of the functions of the project was to refine and to render likely or unlikely such hypotheses. This would facilitate their selection and validation in a more quantitative study. For this reason a certain degree of comparability of interviews was desired. This consideration precluded use of the purely clinical or the nondirective type of interview.

What form could incorporate all these elements? In summarizing the literature on interviewing, Hyman poses the problem of "the unpleasant choice between an interview situation uncontaminated with the interviewer's bias but also completely sterile, versus an interview situation potentially full of validity but with a high probability of bias."[1] As examples of two methodological poles, he mentions Kinsey,[2] whose interviewers were free to use their ingenuity in asking questions covering a specified range of topics; and Hamilton,[3] who had the interviewers sit at a precisely determined distance from the respondents and hand them cards with printed questions on them. In the former method, success depends almost completely upon the interviewer; in the latter, he is only a recorder of information. The closest parallels in Puerto Rico are the studies of King and Hatt. King had "intensive discussions" with forty-nine women in a small community where she lived for two months. Presumably no questionnaire or set method of questioning was used. Hatt, on the other hand, based his interviews on precisely worded questions from which the interviewers were not allowed to deviate. Our own choice lay between these two poles.

THE SEMISTRUCTURED INTERVIEW

The form finally devised lies between the clinical and the poll-type interview extremes but is considerably closer to the former than to the latter. It is a "focused interview"[4] in the sense that it focuses on fairly specific hypotheses, but in such a flexible fashion that it allows for unanticipated consequences. The interviewing however, does not concentrate on a particular event or experience as

[1] H. Hyman, "Interviewing as a Scientific Procedure," in D. Lerner and H. Lasswell, eds., *The Policy Sciences* (Stanford: Stanford University Press, 1951), p. 210.

[2] A. Kinsey, W. Pomeroy, and C. Martin, *Sexual Behavior in the Human Male* (Philadelphia: Saunders, 1948).

[3] G. Hamilton, *A Research in Marriage* (New York: Lear, 1948).

[4] See R. Merton, M. Fiske, and P. Kendall, "The Focussed Interview," (Bureau of Applied Social Research, Columbia University, 1952), mimeographed.

does the focused interview. Moreover, questions are more structured in the current method. Deviation from their form and order is permitted but used only when this seems necessary.

It differs from most interview forms in the structure and sequence of its questions. Both the interview as a whole and each major question within the interview become progressively focused. The total interview narrows from questions on extended family relations through ideal family roles and courtship and marriage behavior, until, in the fourth hour of interviewing, the focus is on the strategic dependent variables—fertility ideals and birth-control performance.[5]

Each question is broken down into progressively specific question parts, beginning with the greatest degree of spontaneity and range of response and ending with a minimum of range and spontaneity. The more specific questions have several advantages. First, they insure the coverage of particular hypotheses and the comparability of data. Second, they prevent the respondent from speaking completely in generalities and tie him down eventually to concrete responses. Third, they increase the "depth" of the general question. Fourth, they may suggest areas to the respondent which he had forgotten or neglected to mention. It is important to note, however, that such questions always *follow* careful routine probing after the general question, to allow for the greatest degree of spontaneity before pressing specific questions on the respondent.

In order better to illustrate this method, a sample question from the interview is reproduced. The format and logical structure are similar to most of the sixty-six major questions used in the interview. The interviewer writes the responses in the blank space at the left side of the page.

49,F (Global Question) Many people in Puerto Rico live together without being married. To what do you attribute this?

(First Order Probe) A. Are there any advantages for the couple in this type of marriage? What are they?

(Second Order Probes) 1. Does it give more freedom to the woman?

2. Does it give more freedom to the man or woman?

[5] See Appendix D for the full interview forms.

Not reproduced on the interview guide, but understood as a result of interviewer training, are the *exploratory probes,* which are employed wherever the respondent's comments seem to require further information. Such probes receive detailed classification below.

Probably the closest methodological parallel in the field of fertility is the study conducted in England by Mass Observation on attitudes toward family size.[6] As one source of data, one thousand interviews with married women were obtained. Similarity lies in the fact that many questions were broadly stated (as our global questions) and were asked in roughly the same fashion for the entire sample. However, there is no evidence that the global questions were followed up either by exploratory probing or by explicitly stated first or second order probes.

EXPLORATORY PROBING

The literature on interviewing has done little to systematize the types of probes we have termed exploratory. In the process of training personnel who had never heard of probing, it was necessary to classify the various types of exploratory probes so that they could better be communicated and more discriminately used.

The probes here outlined do not exhaust the types but are those which proved to be most fruitful in the present study.

Clarity and Completion Probes.[7] Clarity and completion probes are similar in the sense that both attempt to elicit additional information on a response which is inadequate. Clarity probes encourage the respondent to *explain* his responses and the reasoning behind them. Completion probes encourage him to *expand* them in order both to "round out" his response and to cover the range of his motivations. Examples of clarity probes are: "Why do you say that?" "Can you give me an example?" "I am not quite sure I see what you mean by that." Examples of completion probes are: "Can you tell me a little more about that?" "How interesting! Anything else?" The following illustration shows how a combination of clarity and

[6] *Britain and her Birth Rate* (London: John Murray, 1945).

[7] The distinction between probes of clarity and completion was suggested by Reuben Hill. The author had originally subsumed them both under the rubric of "generic type" probes.

completion probes and first and second order probes can elicit a great deal of unanticipated information.

(Global question: When should a couple have the first child?) At once, because that way you can see your children grown up sooner and you are still young to see them and help them in the future.

(Completion probe: Anything else?) Well, the sooner you start with children, the sooner you finish.

(First order probe: What about being afraid of being called barren? Could that have anything to do with it?) Yes, that is true because if they get pregnant too late, the man may say that she is pregnant of another man.

(First order probe: What about men wanting children soon?) They are crazy about having them soon. A father without children is no good. That is their happiness.

(Clarity probe: Why are they crazy to have them soon?) In order to prove they are fathers.

Reactive Probes. Reactive probes are aimed at eliciting the respondent's *feelings* on a theme which he or the interviewer has introduced. They are especially useful when the respondent is voicing an opinion more general than his own, an opinion which may or may not coincide with his own. In order to determine coincidence or discrepancy, his own reaction must be asked. Notice that in the following quotation the reactive probe elicited a vital piece of information—the fact that the husband did not believe in the reasons given by his wife for discontinuing birth control. This fact acts as a signal for the interviewer to discover the husband's *real* reason. The absence of this probe would have left the conclusion that birth control was not used because of fears of sickness.

My wife didn't want to use the condoms because she feared she might get sick. It seems to me that her friends told her that. (And what do you think about it?) They don't do harm to anybody.

In other cases the respondent will state a personal circumstance without stating his feeling toward it. Note that the initial reply to the question below might have misled the analyst into assuming that the woman was disgruntled at the state of affairs. The probe shows that precisely the contrary was true.

We women have only the liberties that our husbands grant us. (Do you think that's fair?) I think it is good because in that way there is more respect. . . . We women never think of anything that's good.

Channel Probes. Channel probes get at the source of a respondent's opinions. Examples are: "Where did you see that?" "Who told you that?" These are very useful not only for discovering the significant channels of communication but for unraveling the public from the private opinion. Moreover, they frequently *set up* responses which can then be subjected to reactive probes. The following illustration demonstrates a facile progression of completion, channel, and reactive probes.

A man should know when to have intercourse with his wife in order to avoid infection. (Do you know of any case where infection occurred?) I have heard that if one has contact with the wife when she is menstruating one may get infected. (Where did you hear that?) The people around here say it. (And what do you say?) I'm not sure, but I think that one should be careful.

Usually there is more than one source for a respondent's opinion. He will often offer one source for his opinions, forgetting or neglecting to mention others that may be reinforcing or even more important. One way to elicit such additional information is to ask a channel-completion probe such as, "Did you hear it *anywhere else?*" Frequently, however, this brings no response because it is so easy to say "no" (the respondent already having discharged his debt by giving one answer to the question) or because the respondent has forgotten other influences or does not consider them important enough to mention. It is frequently helpful, therefore, to *suggest* additional sources in a general manner. This is done quite effectively in the following illustration:

(Who has told you that?) Several old women. They say that if one denies her husband there will be no home, no union, and plenty of arguments. That's what they told me, and it's true. (Because of religion?) That's the law of God. I have read it in the Bible.

Hypothetical Probes. Hypothetical probes pose hypothetical situations for the respondent and elicit his reactions to them. Rather than being situations conceived *a priori* by the schedule designer, however, they grow out of the respondent's own verbalizations, the appropriate probe being injected smoothly by the interviewer at the appropriate time. Such probes depend to a great degree on the interviewer's ingenuity, of course, but there is at least one type of response which always lends itself easily to the hypothetical question —the implied alternative.

Implied alternatives are easily recognized in conditional clauses. In the case below, for example, the clause, "When she does not give a motive for it," is an open door to the hypothetical probe, "And if she does?" The probe changed the entire character of the initial response.

A good husband is one who cares for his wife, doesn't throw his money about, and doesn't let his wife go naked and hungry. He should not treat her badly nor beat her. All this particularly when she does not give a motive for it. (And if she gives a motive?) If she does, let him break a rib, because there are women who really deserve it.

Such probes often allow the interviewer to see through the respondent's public opinion and get at his real feelings. Moreover, they can be used to detect rationalizations and as a rough gauge of intensity of opinion. This type of hypothetical probe might be termed, "removing the cause." The respondent gives a reason (*Y*) why he believes *X* to be right or wrong. Suspecting rationalization or looking for a more general principle, the interviewer asks if *X* would be right or wrong if *Y* were no longer true.

This form can also be used where a clear alternative (as in the conditional-clause type) is not suggested. It simply takes the respondent's reason and hypothesizes its absence. The cases below show two different kinds of response.

(Why do you say that women shouldn't drink?) Because it's dangerous to their health. (If it were not dangerous, could they drink?) No, because if someone finds you drinking they might try to have fun with you.

(You told me there is danger in having little girls naked when boys are present. Is there any danger when boys are not present?) In that case little girls can be permitted to remain naked. . . . What could happen to them among themselves?

Another type of hypothetical probe, more difficult to codify, can be used in attempting to appraise intensity of feeling. It can be employed most profitably when a respondent appears to be speaking abstractly about X. In order to discover how strongly he holds his opinion, he may be asked what he would do or feel if X happened or applied to him personally. For example, parents usually talk about the disgrace of a girl marrying consensually. When asked what they would do if their daughter married in this fashion, however, many say they would be angry for a while and then forgive her, disclosing that the intensity of feeling is not so high as the original remarks of the respondent would seem to indicate. In the following illustration good probing brings out the relative weakness of the desire to have a small family.

One should have three children at the most, because they can be brought up in a different and better atmosphere. I have only three. I hope God doesn't send me more. (What would you do if God sent you more?) I would receive them with pleasure.

High-Pressure Probes. As Kinsey has pointed out, high-pressure techniques can be most effective when dealing with sexual matters. It is felt that considerable rapport is a prerequisite for this method. Once it is well established, should the interviewer feel confident that the respondent is mouthing a platitude or a socially acceptable response, he may put down his pencil and say in a friendly manner, "Is that really what *you* think?" In the following instance such a probe completely reversed the respondent's qualified acceptance of the large family.

If I were rich I would have many children. There would be food and clothing, and I could have a maid to help me. (Would you really like it, truly?) No, not truly. Children give too much trouble.

Other high-pressure probes revolve around pointing out contradictions to the respondent. Interviewers must be trained to be alert to contradictions and to handle them tactfully. In some cases, such as the first presented below, the respondent may not be aware of the contradiction; in others, as in the second case, they may be caught in a lie. It is in the latter cases, of course, that the greatest tact must be exercised in order not to antagonize the respondent.

If a man wants to take a daughter of mine by force, I should be man enough to prevent this. (How would you prevent it?) I'm ready to fight anyone who tried to dishonor my daughter. (How is it you ran away with your wife?) I wanted to marry her, but the family opposed me, so I had to take her away with me.

I have had them [condoms] in my pockets but have never used them. (Why not?) Because I didn't like them at all. (Why not?) Because I don't feel the same sensation. (Then you have used them?) Well yes, I used them once with a prostitute, but I don't like them.

APPRAISAL

It is felt that the interview form was successful in meeting the criteria of depth, scope, and flexibility. However, these were achieved to some degree at the expense of comparability. While a greater degree of comparability was achieved than is possible in using more nondirective methods, the semistructured interview still left much to be desired in this respect. To a certain extent this would seem to be a necessary consequence of meeting the other criteria. However, it is felt that another factor may have been the ambivalent feeling on the part of the Study Director toward the nature of the semistructured guide. At times flexibility and side-tracking from the routine questions were emphasized, at other times complete coverage of all items, including secondary and tertiary probes. It is obvious that the former type of interview is richer and more provocative qualitatively but causes considerable frustration in tabulation if accomplished at the expense of detailed coverage. The latter type, while ideal for tabulation purposes, sacrifices depth, spontaneity, and unanticipated responses.

Accenting complete coverage creates a mental set in the worker which discourages the freedom and spontaneity necessary in the truly qualitative interview. It enforces a kind of anxiety about covering each item which may blind or discourage the worker from detecting subtleties in the responses. Accenting the nondirective approach, on the other hand, poses operational barriers (time, oversight, and so forth) which tend to slight or to render trivial in the eyes of the interviewer the lower-level probes on the interview guide.

An improvement in format would help insure comparability. There is a tendency to consider second-order probes of little importance, for example, probably because they appear in such a subsidiary position in the format. Much valuable information was lost because important questions, for the sake of logical sequencing, were "buried" in second-order probes. In the future it would seem advisable to underscore all those first and second order probes which are important or for which comparable data are needed on all interviews.

Another improvement would lie in a more systematic appraisal of interviews as they come in. While all interviews were read as they were completed, the reading was done somewhat atomistically; that is, each was read with the object of evaluating the interviewer's technical proficiency at handling exploratory probes on the particular interview. Not until two thirds of the field work had been completed was a systematic appraisal aimed at general deficiencies accomplished. At that time a memorandum was addressed to the staff, embodying the criticisms, and was followed by a group discussion.

INTERVIEWING METHODS

Interviewing extensively on such delicate matters as sexual patterns and birth control presented definite methodological problems. First, how could this information be elicited from respondents in a culture where sexual discussion is tabued even more than it is in the United States? Second, how could one spouse be kept from biasing or even blocking the interview of the other spouse? Third, how could interviewing be accomplished without jeopardizing the cooperation of other respondents in the community? It was feared that, by means of the rapid grape vine and gossip channels typical of urban and rural Puerto Rico, respondents would almost certainly hear of the subject matter of the interview.

SEX TABUS

Women in Puerto Rico are carefully guarded from sexual activities and sexual expression. Men, while granted considerable freedom in this regard, are quite squeamish about discussing their own sexual behavior with strangers. Several steps were taken to overcome these tabus.

Interviewer Selection. Only males were to interview husbands, and only females were to interview wives. All interviewers had to be college graduates, married, of an outgoing personality type and sufficiently mature in appearance to inspire confidence.

Results were quite satisfactory. Two of the female interviewers had had previous research experience in Puerto Rico in anthropology or sociology. Another had had years of supervisory social-work experience, and the last was a medical social worker borrowed from the Department of Health. The male interviewers had no previous experience but were selected for their potentialities. The first had been a farmer before the war, after which he obtained a high-school and college education. The other owned a store in a small town. In both these cases it was felt that the combination of first-hand knowledge of lower-class Puerto Ricans and formal college training would serve as good background for depth interviewing.

Interviewer Training. Intensive training of the interviewers was the second step taken to insure the cooperation of respondents on sexual topics. These training methods are explained in detail in the following section.

Sequential Ordering of Questions. The questions proceeded from simple or objective questions to more detailed and open-ended ones, from relatively impersonal questions to intimate ones.

Staggering the Interview. The female interview was accomplished in two or three sittings rather than in one. This proved an effective device. In the first interview the field worker and respondent "got acquainted." Moreover, the respondent found the questions to be innocuous and developed confidence in her ability to respond satisfactorily. On completion of this initial session, the interviewer would praise the respondent, stay and chat a while, and casually remark that she would like to come back again, so interesting and detailed were the opinions of the subject. How this technique operated in practice is seen by the following account of an interviewing situation given by one of the female workers.

> The first time I saw the respondent I thought I wouldn't be able to get much information from her. In fact, I was afraid to start the interview in front of her mother, husband, and others present. On account of this, I didn't stay long the first day and only took the less personal

questions. But the second time she looked more willing to be interviewed. Then I had already taken coffee with her, and started a conversation on sea foods with her husband. . . . The third time I went, she had already suggested that we go to the bedroom where we could talk more freely. . . . There she informed me about different women her husband had had and that once she was about to kill one of them with her husband's revolver.

Usually the interviewer's second visit was anticipated with pleasure, and, not infrequently, respondents would dress up for the occasion and have lunch or some special dessert prepared. On the other hand, interviewers quickly became fond of or sympathetic toward respondents, brought them gifts, wrote letters, and paid extra visits. The staggered interview, it is felt, contributed greatly to the rapport and counterrapport developed by staff and subjects, for both realized after the first interview that they would meet once or twice again, thereby establishing a bond of interest not possible in the single, ephemeral interview.[8]

HUSBAND-WIFE BIAS

Since both husband and wife were to be interviewed, it was feared that the spouse who was first exposed to the intimate questions would cause trouble for the other. Specifically, if the husband heard that his wife had been asked such questions, he might refuse to cooperate himself or forbid his wife to speak to the interviewer again. Consequently, every attempt was made to have the second female interview coincide with the single, male interview. Since the first interview with the wife consisted of relatively impersonal questions, it was assumed that no reaction would be stirred up on the part of the husband.[9] Additionally, at the time of the first interview, an appointment was made at which both husband and wife could be interviewed simultaneously but separately. Thus, at the same time, the intimate questions would be asked both of husband and

[8] For reasons of economy and facility (many males had to be interviewed on holidays and evenings), males were interviewed only once. There appeared to be considerably more resistance to the intimate questions on the part of the men. To determine whether or not a staggered interview would help this situation would be an interesting project in its own right.

[9] There was apparently little danger that the husband would bias the response of his wife on specific items. See Chap. VI, footnote 13.

wife, and there would be no opportunity for either to jeopardize the interview of the other.

COMMUNITY RESISTANCE

As in most traditional societies, rumor and gossip are popular forms of entertainment and news getting in Puerto Rico's lower class. It was feared that the advent of a middle-class stranger, bearing explosive questions, would rapidly evoke so much controversy in the small town and barrio that closed doors would soon greet the interviewers. Both for this reason, and in order to get a greater geographical distribution of cases, only eight families were chosen from each rural and town area. The whole team of four female and two male interviewers worked simultaneously in the same area. Each female interviewer would administer two first interview halves and set appointments both for two second-half female interviews and the two corresponding husband interviews. Thus, in the second wave of interviewing, both male interviews and the intimate sections of the female interviews could be accomplished in a maximum of two days. Interviewers would then return to the office, translate their protocols, and simultaneously begin interviewing in the next area.

The greatest resistance was encountered in the city sample, where this method was not used.[10] In the city, men continually broke appointments, excused themselves in the middle of interviews and did not return, and so forth, creating real hardships for the male interviewer.[11] One case taken from the city shows how rumor laid the groundwork for community resistance.

When I reached the home of this respondent he was at his home. I explained him the aim of my visit. When I asked him if there was much talk about the project after I left, he replied, "You interviewed a man who lives on this street. That man told everybody around here about the questions of the study. He was very angry, but he didn't

[10] It was reasoned, erroneously, that gossip would not travel fast enough in the city to affect the interviewing.

[11] In one city case an interviewer described the occupational hazards: "It was pouring, and I could not leave the house. The man walked from one place to another. He started to sharpen a pair of scissors. Then he sharpened a kitchen knife. Later he moved a piece of pipe one and a half feet long from one place to another."

beat you up because you made no resistance to him. One day you came and he ran away. He said that that day he got on a bus and went out to the island, although he had no plans to go out.

"When you left his house, he came to the corner and talked with the man who has a store there. The storekeeper said, 'Let him come here. I know what I am going to tell him.' And all the men of this street were ready to put you out of the house. And there are men of this *barrio* who would even beat you up if you asked them intimate questions. And he did a bad thing, because now the people know that I was interviewed too. A friend of mine who lives nearby asked why I had answered such questions. I told him, 'I am a well-mannered man and I receive at home any person who visits me. Besides that, the lady who interviewed my wife and the gentleman who interviewed me are respectable persons. The study is not bad, on the contrary, it is a very good thing. And everybody should cooperate with the interviewers.'"

The combination of the "hit-and-run" technique and of skillful methods of rapport building was such that some respondents seemed to realize what they had been asked only after the interviewers had left. One or two felt they had been tricked into answering, others were fearful that they had given away too much information. In one village, rumor so distorted the questions of the study that a subsequent interviewing staff from another project encountered powerful resistance from respondents who refused to be questioned on "what type of underwear I wear." At any rate, few people had heard of the project before being called on, and what community reaction occurred did so too late to affect the study adversely.[12]

Among the 144 men and women contacted, only one refusal was encountered.[13] This refusal rate is sufficiently low to require further explanation. In addition to the techniques mentioned above

[12] In reinterviews conducted with 25 families several months after completion of the field work, only 9 respondents said they had heard nothing about the study from noninterviewed members of the community. On being told the nature of the study many noninterviewed members of the community were shocked and said they would not answer such questions. They were all reportedly assured by the persons interviewed that the study had been worthwhile and that the interviewer had been a responsible and "serious" person. These responses suggest not only that the interviewers did a good job of selling the study to informants but that considerable community resistance would have been encountered had the "hit-and-run" technique not been used.

[13] This individual, reputedly psychotic, jumped up after the first few questions and ran out of the house.

two other factors should be mentioned. (1) The lower classes in Puerto Rico are fairly humble before a person of a higher class. Many of them took it for granted that they would be expected to answer questions and did not stand on their "rights of privacy" as would many of the lower class in the United States. Indeed, most of the respondents were flattered to receive a visit from a person of the middle class, and were further flattered when that person would join them in coffee, sit on the floor if necessary, and sympathetically listen to their problems. As one respondent put it, "It is good to talk with people who know more than oneself." (2) The techniques of rapport building developed by the interviewers went beyond those of ordinary interviewers.

How can one account for the high degree of success achieved by personnel some of whom had never before administered a questionnaire and none of whom had worked with depth interviewing techniques? Part of the answer lies in the capacities and interests which the group fortunately possessed. Perhaps of equal importance, however, was the care and time taken in their training. Since, in the present study, the quality of the data is to a large degree a function of the quality of the interviewers, a detailed account of the training procedures is presented.

INTERVIEWER TRAINING[14]

One of the few researchers who has done a good deal of depth interviewing of the lower class on attitudes toward sex and birth control[15] has summarized her experience as follows:

> The interviewer needs to know something of people, to have an awareness of psychological mechanisms such as ambivalence, repression, and rationalization when he encounters them not in the text book but in the individual. Experience of this sort cannot be imparted in a short training course, however well directed it may be.[16]

[14] Much of this section was published as "Interviewer Training in Another Culture" in *Public Opinion Quarterly,* XVI, No. 2 (Summer 1952), 236–46.

[15] M. Woodside, *Sterilization in North Carolina: A Sociological and Psychological Study* (Chapel Hill: University of North Carolina Press, 1950).

[16] M. Woodside, "The Psychiatric Approach to Research Interviewing," in *Studies in Population: Proceedings of the Annual Meeting of the Population Association of America,* ed. by G. Mair (Princeton University Press, 1949), p. 167.

If these are not impossible standards for the ordinary interviewing team, they are at least imposing goals toward which to work. In addition, the process of training inexperienced individuals in the necessary skills for interviewing and of communicating the purpose and content of a study is a sufficiently difficult enterprise when dealing with members of ones' own culture. In a different culture, the difficulties are multiplied to an unknown degree.

Interviewer training consumed approximately three weeks. The first week was spent in assigned readings. The project design, the project hypotheses, and materials by sociologists and anthropologists on family and fertility in Puerto Rico composed the background reading materials. For interviewing techniques, the Training Guide on Techniques of Qualitative Interviewing, developed by Columbia University's Bureau of Applied Social Research, and Kinsey's chapters on methodology were employed. This was followed by a week of discussion on the content and techniques of the study. A third week was spent on trial interviews, with individual and group discussions held after their completion. The following remarks are an attempt to sum up what the author learned from his experience.

BASIC PROBLEMS

Interviewer training in quantitative studies ordinarily resembles the usual didactic method of the classroom, with the study director explaining what the interviewers are to do and then leaving the floor open for questions. Owing to the greater difficulty of depth interviewing and the small number of personnel involved, a less formal procedure is both desirable and feasible. In such a situation, interpersonal factors become more important. It is here that the study director must be most sensitive to cultural differences and adapt his techniques accordingly. For example, it goes without saying that the native language should be used if possible. It has been the classroom experience of the writer that even with individuals as bilingual as Puerto Ricans, discussion is immensely enhanced by permitting Spanish.[17] In the present case, interviewers

[17] Having little opportunity to exercise their English, most Puerto Ricans seem to lack confidence in speaking it to a continental. Others resent having to speak the language of the visitor rather than the visitor learning their language.

spoke in Spanish and the writer principally in English, a compromise which worked smoothly enough.

Ambivalence toward the Foreign Expert. In many underdeveloped countries today, the American is regarded ambivalently. As the technician and the representative from a rich and powerful nation, he is respected and envied; but, as an intruder often unsubtly telling the local population how things should be done he is feared and disliked. To this must be added another impediment to successful communication: the more rigid class and authority structures of most such countries. In combination, this means that the personnel may place a barrier between themselves and the trainer and react seemingly impassively to his comments. On the one hand, they may resent his presence and the presumption that he is better equipped than they to study their culture; on the other hand, they respect his technical knowledge and his superior position in the authority structure. The net effect may be busy pencils but muted tongues.

The trainer is put in a difficult position and must steer a delicate course. He must break down reserve while preserving respect. On the one hand, he may call on the typically Latin love of personal relationships. This means a spirit of camaraderie, and clear indications that the interviewer as a person is basically accepted and approved of. But, on the other hand, he can play the easy-going, democratic, back-slapping American only at the risk of impropriety.

In the present case, authority was emphasized principally in routine matters. For example, late-comers were reminded of the office hours, explanations were required from interviewers desiring time off, excessive talking was discouraged, and so forth. It was felt that this would preserve the role expectation of authority in an area where little harm could be done by such emphasis.[18] In the training

[18] These factors were probably stressed excessively. After reading this report, the writer's research assistant remarked that, while his generalizations about the Puerto Rican's acceptance of authority were correct, his own authority role was *overplayed* with reference to the demands enumerated above. She noted, however, that the group was divided in its resentment. Since the intricacy of the problem may thus be even greater than the writer anticipated, even more care in policy must be exercised, requiring a longer "feeling out" period before definite personnel policy is adopted.

sessions themselves, for the sake of a free exchange of ideas, authority, while not submerged, was relaxed.

In the first meeting, in order to begin the process of converting a crowd of seven into a group, each member introduced himself, his background, and how he happened to take his present position. The writer did the same, and then introduced the project, its history, its possible practical value to Puerto Rico, and its possible theoretical value to social science. The physical set-up involved a seminar table, with the writer at the head, and a blackboard to which he referred for a good share of the period. Following his remarks (about an hour), the group was called on for comments and questions. Only one person volunteered.

After this sobering experience, both physical structure and training procedure were considerably altered to allow greater informality. The director remained at his office desk, and the interviewers were grouped around. It was felt that the desk, while still a symbol of authority, was a more natural location than the head of a table, and that the absence of a blackboard would obviate the temptation of a classroom lecture. As a substitute for a discourse by the director, the interviewers were called on to explain the major hypotheses of the project as they understood them from their readings. From this point on, traditional training procedure was altered. The interviewers were asked to comment upon the validity of the hypotheses, citing their own experience as members of the culture. Discussion rapidly became heated as the interviewers disagreed with one another and vied for examples supporting or negating the hypotheses. The role of the director changed from lecturer to commentator.

This quickly gave the interviewers a sense of genuine participation. *They* became the experts telling the interested but naive foreigner about facets of their culture which he had never experienced. The respectful or resentful shell of reserve was broken down, and its place taken by a healthy give and take.

In response to a post-training questionnaire one interviewer was enthusiastic over the "unique" experience of contributing her ideas to a project:

> . . . the opportunity given to everyone of participating with his own knowledge and experience in the field *was unique* and helped very

much in the identification with the study in making it more and more *our project.*

Her own identification with the project was such that she later mentioned going to the field "to test *our* hypotheses."

Simultaneously, however, the role of the director as "theoretician," converting their words into significant hypotheses, plus his willingness to guide the discussion, presumably maintained the respect which might easily have been lost by an overly democratic or nondirective approach.[19]

A similar procedure was followed with respect to the interview guide. A rough translation into Spanish was provided for the interviewers, and in going over each item they were asked two basic questions: (1) What are we getting at by this question? (2) What is the wording which will best convey this to a lower-class respondent? Additionally, their own experiences were again elicited on the various subjects. The discussion on wording alone proved the worth of many heads, for the official translation was almost completely reworked.

Cultural Pitfalls. Continental social scientists are fond of reminding Puerto Ricans that theirs is a culture "in transition." Despite the fact that Puerto Rican personnel dress as continentals, speak English, and have many similar tastes, they have many traits more characteristic of individuals of less industrialized cultures. In the present case, three general characteristics are pertinent:[20] a tendency toward verbal inhibitions concerning sexual matters (at least on the part of Puerto Rican women); a sense of honor or dignity which makes the individual appear overly sensitive to criticism and

[19] The effort to compromise authoritarian and democratic procedure resulted in some confusion on the part of the interviewers, who did not always know whether to treat the writer as friend or boss. The clearest manifestation of this was in their naming procedure. Only two interviewers consistently used "Mr. Stycos." One called him "Mister" (a kind of compromise), another vacillated between "Joe" and "Mr. Stycos," and another abruptly changed from the former designation to the latter after a few weeks. The last interviewer, who customarily used "Joe," once stammered back and forth between the formal and informal designations, finally exclaiming in a frustrated tone: *"Ave María,* I don't know what to call you!"

[20] These same characteristics are of course present in the United States. It is the difference in their intensity in Puerto Rico which brings them to the foreground.

correspondingly receptive to praise; emphasis on personal relations.

Verbal tabus. Since a major part of the study was to be devoted to sexual matters, it was feared that the inhibitions and value judgments of Latin women would impede their ability to extract the maximum information from respondents. Previous experience as interviewer supervisor on the Hatt fertility study in Puerto Rico had led the writer to believe that lack of attention to this factor could have serious consequences. Hatt used a routine, lecture-and-manual method to train girls with no previous experience in interviewing on sex, and probably with little knowledge about reproduction and birth control. Perhaps as a result, data on coital frequency and birth control were so poor as to be considered unusable. To circumvent a repetition of this experience, various techniques were employed. A liberal attitude was a major criterion in selecting personnel. Only married, mature candidates were considered, and with each applicant the description of the study was skewed in the direction of its intimate side. If an applicant blanched, blushed, or manifested disapproved, she was not considered.

In the present case the writer's further precautions were probably largely unnecessary, since the women represented an unusually emancipated group, all having had experience in social work or anthropology. Yet from previous experience with such personnel, it was felt that no chances should be taken. Consequently, two additional measures helped insure a more open mind on sexual matters.

During training sessions, trainees were encouraged to talk freely of sexual matters, and as the more uninhibited would relate a sexual item, others would join in. By the end of training, the difference between *coitus reservatus* and *interruptus* and the Spanish folk terms used for these were discussed without any manifestations of embarrassment. One interviewer wrote:

> In the first conferences, although having the opportunity to express the ideas, I scarcely talked but listened to all that was said regarding relations and the intimate life of the family. I believe that was the whole group experience, but gradually we felt more at ease and could freely participate in the discussion of the subject.

While it is felt that the emotional problem with regard to sex was adequately handled, sex education itself was probably under-stressed. Occasionally, during the field work, interviewers disclosed pockets of ignorance on reproductive processes. In future studies, greater stress should be placed on sheer information.

Dignidad. Another carry-over from Spanish rural culture is the sometimes strong sense of ***dignidad*** possessed by men and women alike. It is a moral dimension in which worth is evaluated more in terms of the inherent qualities of the person than in terms of his productive capacity. Better suited to a more stable, agrarian society, the complex causes considerable conflicts in a more technological environment. Routine criticism or suggestions tend to be interpreted in personal terms, that is, as a reflection on the inherent worth of the worker. Even with such a highly selected group of interviewers, routine criticism was often greeted with anxiety, a strong feeling of inadequacy, and, occasionally, with resentment.

Consequently, to avoid a serious drop in morale, it was necessary continually to stress the fact that no one does a good depth interview until he has done a fair number of them; that criticism was intended to help the interviewer and not to reprimand him; that basically the interviewer was doing an excellent job. The praise, while entirely deserved, was more than the writer customarily feels necessary to give a technical staff. The atmosphere was a fragile one in which the entire staff (including clerical help) had to be handled with considerable delicacy to avoid damaging their sense of basic worth. Group meetings were often devoted as much to catharsis and ego rebuilding as to discussion of work problems.

If the responses of the interviewers to their training evaluation questionnaire can be considered reliable, the one area where cultural values were handled indelicately was that of pressure for output. The only adverse comments on the training referred to the excessive productive demands pressed upon the staff.

Personal loyalty. The writer first became alerted to the importance of personal loyalty during a study conducted in the Middle East by Columbia University's Bureau of Applied Social Research. The correspondence of the project's field director, William Millard, was filled with references to the crucial nature of the interviewer-director relationship. It was his belief that the key to successful training and work output in the Middle East was the development of a strong bond of personal loyalty between interviewers and director.

This proved true in Puerto Rico and probably holds for all underdeveloped countries where the pendulum is still somewhere between folk society and modern society. Faith in a personality rather than a cause, a blind devotion to one's family, kin, and town are all symptomatic of the folk culture and are still to a considerable extent characteristic of Latin America. It is not surprising then, that personnel will place great stress on "the man" who is their *jefe* (chief). Judging from written comments of the interviewers, much of their motivation stemmed from a sense of loyalty to the *jefe* as much as from interest in the study.

THE TEST SITUATION: TRAINING IN TECHNIQUES OF RAPPORT

It is difficult enough to train members of another culture in specific skills, but how can one instruct them in the techniques of rapport? That is, how can the naive foreigner tell natives of the culture how to gain the confidence of types of respondents about whom the trainer knows very little? It is perhaps here that the importance of the discussion method is greatest. The first step is for the interviewer-trainer to use his personnel as reflections of the culture. Thus he can assume that, if they possess such values as modesty, dignity, status, and a strong reliance upon interpersonal relationships, the same will be true of their respondents, at least if they are of the same class level. Thus, by learning how to establish rapport with his own personnel, he can feed back his experience to them, since they are presumably less sensitive to the subtleties of manipulated interpersonal relationships.

For example, it was quickly learned that the interviewer gave much more detailed information in the discussions if the trainer "played dumb" by insisting that as an "*Americano*" things had to be explained to him in greater detail. This technique in turn was taught to the interviewers, to be used whenever respondents felt they were detailing the obvious. "Yes, *we* know all that, but the Doctor is an American and wants to have it all explained in your own words" proved a very effective cultural twist to the stock answer to such complaints.

In the present case the interviewers could not be considered clear reflections of the population to be investigated. Since the respondents were to be selected from the poorest class in the population, there was no guarantee that they maintained the same value system as the educated and middle-class interviewers. Consequently, the interviewers had to be used as participant observers, guided by the trainer's questions. They were first told of the necessity of selling the study in the first five minutes of their interviews. Then they were asked, "Now, what values are most important to a lower-class Puerto Rican, the kind of values which you could emphasize to convince him quickly of the worth of the study and of your own worth?" In this way a great number of otherwise unanticipated rapport problems were discussed.

Following this academic discussion, a kind of psychodramatic technique was used. Interviewers were asked to simulate the first few minutes of the interviewing situation, with one interviewer playing herself and two others a lower-class husband and wife. Aggressive, docile, and negativistic respondent roles were worked out, as well as difficult situations such as the presence of visitors, children, and so forth. After each performance, the effectiveness of the interviewer's approach was discussed by the group. In this way both unconscious mannerisms[21] and outright errors of judgment were quickly picked up by the group and effectively communicated to the actor-interviewer.

Such peer criticism worked so well and took away so much of the pain of being criticized by "the boss" that it was later partially employed in evaluating trial interviews. Good and bad sections from trial interviews would be read and comments invited. Often the interviewer herself would eagerly suggest what she should have done, indicating that the method relieves much of the anxiety of the "school teacher" method of criticism.

RAPPORT TECHNIQUES IN PRACTICE

It should not be supposed that all rapport techniques were worked out in the training sessions. Indeed, probably the best methods were

[21] One girl, for example, nervously leafed through her interviewer guide while discussing the weather with a "respondent." It was suggested that this was akin to leveling a gun at someone while asking him about his health. The interviewer looked surprised and then pleased. "Why yes," she said, "I always do that during an interview, but I didn't realize it until just now."

devised by the interviewers in the field. "Making friends" with the respondents was the keynote of the interviewers' success. They went far beyond the customary procedures of winning sympathy for the study on the strength of its humanitarian and academic value and used all sorts of devices to gain the confidence and cooperation of respondents. The remarks of respondents throughout their interviews and reinterviews are eloquent testimonials to the job of "self-selling" performed by the interviewers. "I have never told this to another person" and "Only because we are so friendly do I tell you this" were typical remarks.

FOUR BASIC METHODS

What sort of techniques were used to build up a friendly relationship?

The Introduction. The initial impression was obviously important. Interviewers had decided while in training to introduce themselves as follows:

> I am from the University (known and highly respected by the lower class), doing a study of families of people like you. The scientists have studied the rich people too much and they want to learn more about the ordinary people. We think we can learn a lot about how to bring children up better and how husbands and wives can get along together better by hearing of your experiences. We come to your house only because your address was picked out of a hat, like the lottery. No one knows your name except me, and everything you tell me will be put together with what other people say. I have nothing to do with the government. Will you help me?

To what extent this form was followed is not known, but since the paragraph was a product of group discussion, it is probable that the interviewers stuck fairly closely to it. However, the information was apparently not given in one lump as above, but parceled out over a period of five to ten minutes of conversational chitchat prior to the interview.

Flattery. Interviewers were instructed to tell respondents that the scientists, previously having devoted their study to the upper classes, had finally realized that they had much to learn from the poor, and that they and the interviewer would be greatly indebted for as much information as the respondent could contribute. If this approach was not sufficient, more personal techniques were applied.

Below are two illustrations of a more personally tailored type of flattery.

On Question 35 I noticed he was scared giving the information. I think he was afraid not of giving the information but of my pencil. I told him that it was important to write down the information; that the study would not be complete without such information. Then I told him, "Ask me anything you want about my experiences with women. I am ready to give you any information, because I know you are a gentleman." That was enough to make him talk.

. . . The respondent showed disgust as if she weren't willing to be interviewed. The interviewer again explained the purpose of the interview, how other women had cooperated, and how valuable the information given by her would be to the study, inasmuch as she was a person who had gone to the Health Unit and had had dealings with nurses, doctors, and other mothers, and would help the study greatly. . . . She answered the rest of the questions willingly.

Identification. Wherever possible, interviewers would seek a link between themselves and the informants. This was a particularly effective method because of the class difference between the workers and the respondents. Some informants felt not only uneasiness in the presence of a member of a higher class but suspicion of exploitation.[22] For this reason, any way in which the identification of interviewer and respondent could be established made for trust and greater feeling of rapport. Since all the interviewers had children, these formed the most frequent common ground, but, as the illustrations below demonstrate, other links also proved effective.

[After an initial failure] I went back, prepared to make myself a real friend of hers. I gave her a cigarette every time I had one and started calling her *tu* (thou). I explained to her that I did this because I had found out she was more or less my age and for that reason I was going to call her *tu* from that day on. . . . After all these tricks I saw the woman changing. . . . She even threw her children out of the house so that we could talk freely about sex matters. We were good friends at the end of the interview.

At the bakery where he works I bought cheese and bread. . . . The next day I visited him, and he told me he was afraid of being interviewed. I told him that I, too, felt shy when I was living in the country

[22] A few respondents had previously been mulcted by "salesmen" and "promoters." Others feared the government might be planning to change their lives in some fashion.

but now it was different. It is a routine for me. He told me he was born in the country. We talked for some minutes about country life. . . . That was enough to win the man. I sold the project and made the interview.

I went to him and he told me, "The Government investigates even when one sleeps with his wife." . . . He continued arguing about politics, and I let him talk all he wanted. When he finished, I asked him, "May I come tomorrow to see what we can do?" He agreed. . . . The next Sunday I visited him. I had learned he was a veteran; that was the start. Then I explained the project, and he said he wanted to start immediately. I think . . . it was merely to cooperate with me and not with the study as a whole.

In cases of real resistance a we're-all-in-the-same-boat appeal was used in order to elicit the sympathy of the respondent. Interviewers complained that their jobs would be jeopardized if the respondent did not cooperate, that they were only doing their job, and so forth, putting the appeal on a personal rather than an abstract basis. In one case the interviewer had to resort to tears before cooperation was elicited, but subtler techniques were often as effective.

Overt Acts of Friendship. It has already been mentioned that interviewers frequently brought gifts on their second visit, exchanged correspondence, and helped respondents with personal problems. Such direct manifestations as these, most frequently occurring between the first and second interview, showed what no words alone could show—that interviewers were genuinely interested in respondents as people. Other methods were used which were effective in the initial interview. The most frequent of these was minor assistance in house work, particularly attending and feeding children.

[Speaking of a difficult respondent:] I could see she didn't know how to take care of the baby. I was so afraid she would let him fall, I got a little nervous and had to stop the interview, hold the baby in my arms, and put him to bed. When I left, she felt sorry and asked me to come back. She offered me lemonade every time I visited her.

She seemed very shy and uncommunicative. In fact, if it hadn't been for one of the kids I wouldn't have been able to do much there. We started talking about the child, why he was always crying, and she told me he had recently come from the hospital. So, whenever I went there I used to put him to sleep, give him his food, and take him on my lap. The boy seemed to like me, and because of this the mother and I got better acquainted.

[A woman who refused the initial interview.] The next day I went to ask her for some water and told her that I felt so tired that I decided to take a little rest there. I commented about how hard I had been working those days. The woman gave me coffee and asked me if I still had more interviews to do in the *barrio*. I told her that I was about to finish but that some respondents didn't talk so freely as she, and I had to spend a lot of time with them. At last the woman told me to see her that afternoon. Thank God, I won the case at last.

Appeal to a Higher Authority. Most country women are not accustomed to making important decisions on their own. To them, the advent of the stranger asking questions about one's family was unique and important enough to make them reluctant to decide whether or not the information should be given. One or two were so frightened that they ran to their husbands or parents. In such cases the interviewers were astute enough to realize that the important task was to convince the authority figure. The illustration below shows to what lengths this technique was occasionally carried.

She asked me to go to her parent's house, where she had to go to wash the clothes. I agreed with her and tried to make her understand that I wanted to talk to her but didn't want her to lose time of her work, that we could talk while she washed clothes. On the way to her house, she said that her father could talk more about the family than she. I wanted to take her out of her fear, so I commented that I would be glad to meet him. When we reached the house, there was her father talking to two neighbors. I had to explain the purpose of my visit and tried to sell the study as best I could. I knew that the respondent wanted her husband's or her father's approval before answering questions, so I decided to make the man understand the purpose of the study so that he could give his approval to his daughter.

The man was very communicative and expressed his approval of such an important thing. He asked his daughter to cooperate with me. So she took me to the brook where her mother and two sisters were washing the clothes. There, again, I had to explain the purpose of my visit, and the respondent's mother, who was an agreeable woman, became interested in the study, and she also asked her daughter to cooperate with it.

EFFECTS OF INTERVIEWING ON RESPONDENTS

In the reinterviews with 25 selected families, a question was asked to ascertain how the respondent had reacted to the interview and whether or not it had changed any of his or her views on the family. In several cases, the strong tabus on discussion of sexual matters between husbands and wives were broken down by the mere act of ventilating such ordinarily inarticulated subjects.

It was a new experience for me. I thought it was good because one would lose his fear and talk about [sexual matters] with other people. You know, talking about that was something bad before. Now it isn't bad for me . . . for I've seen you talk about it in such a natural way that I don't think it is bad at all.

Before I was interviewed I didn't dare to talk so much with anybody about sexual matters, and now I see it is so natural that I could easily talk about it with any person.

Now we talk about those things. Before, we almost never talked about that. (What do you mean by "before"?) Before you came here. We were not very accustomed to that. And we enjoy it very much [now].

In a few cases the influence of the interviewer went beyond the verbal and resulted in action. Despite the fact that interviewers were given strict instructions not to propagandize respondents,[23] the very discussion of intimate subjects was such a rare experience that it apparently activated latent or at least unexpressed sentiments.

The people are realizing that they are not able to support so many children, and everybody around here wants to have his wife sterilized. And since you came here we are more interested than ever.

Now I'm careful about the children, both the girls and the boys, and I don't let them be naked nor in the street till late. I also talked to my husband about avoiding children, and now we have agreed. We are using withdrawal. Meanwhile he is saving money to take me to the hospital to be sterilized.

I am making a campaign in the *barrio* so that the people try to avoid having so many children.

APPRAISAL

There seems little doubt that rapport was good. The only question here would seem to be, was it *too* good? In such a delicate area there might be certain advantages to avoiding intimacy and playing the

[23] If an interviewer was directly asked about various birth-control methods, however, she was allowed to explain them, *after the interview*.

stranger. Kinsey's intimacy-building methods prior to interviewing have been criticized,[24] and Mass Observation's experience in studies of sex and birth control in England was that "many people stopped at random on the street were eager to talk to perfect strangers whom they were not likely to see again."[25]

There is the additional possibility that the lower-class Latin, generally hospitable and highly respectful of educated visitors, might be overwilling to please and tell the interviewers what he believes they want to hear.

The hit-and-run method, in combination with the fact that only one or two sessions were held with each person, would to some degree lessen the possibility of excessive rapport. Moreover, the interviewers, themselves Puerto Ricans and at least one a former member of the rural lower class, might be expected to be somewhat sensitive to the over-obliging respondent—yet no such complaint was voiced in interviewer meetings. Unfortunately, however, there is no real way of gauging the effect of such factors in the present study. Since sex is more tabued in Puerto Rico than in the United States or England, the initial decision was to attempt to attain as high a degree of rapport as possible within the limitations. The possibility that this procedure defeated its own purpose cannot be tested but only noted. In future studies, greater use of such methods as cross checks in the interview would probably shed more light on this problem.

ANALYSIS

The present research and its analysis may be characterized as hybrid, falling somewhere between the two poles of quantitative and qualitative research. To clarify this, a few general characteristics of qualitative analysis are presented below, along with a description of how these criteria fit the present analysis.

[24] H. Hyman and P. Sheatsley, "The Kinsey Report and Survey Methodology," *International Journal of Opinion and Attitude Research,* II (1948), 183–95.

[25] L. England, "Little Kinsey: An Outline of Sex Attitudes in Britain," *Public Opinion Quarterly,* XIII (1949–50), 567–600, cited by H. Hyman, "Interviewing as a Scientific Procedure," in D. Lerner and H. Lasswell, eds., *The Policy Sciences* (Stanford: Stanford University Press, 1951), p. 213.

General Criteria for Qualitative Analysis	*Present Project*
". . . does not employ systematic operations for sampling, measurement, or control of variables."[26]	While the number of cases is small, these cases were systematically chosen. Moreover, while the method of data collection was relatively flexible (spontaneous probing, verbatim notes, noncategorical questions), it was sufficiently structured to guarantee a high degree of comparability of interviews, thus permitting fairly systematic analysis.
"Results are not reported in statistical tables but in descriptions, lists and verbal assertions."[27]	Results are reported both in statistical tables and in descriptions, lists and verbal assertions.
"Much 'qualitative' analysis is quasi-quantitative."[28]	A larger proportion of quasi-quantitative statements ("some," "many," "few," "a number," etc.) are found in the report than is usual in strictly quantitative studies, but these are outnumbered by tables and specific numerical reports such as, "a quarter of the respondents."
A higher ratio of non-content or interpretive statements than in strictly quantitative analysis, which is "more likely to focus first upon straight description of the content itself."[29]	The proportion of non-content statements is higher than in most quantitative studies, some going considerably "beyond the data."[30] However, these are outweighed by descriptive materials, and, more important, are labeled as speculation, the basis for which is as explicit as possible in the report.
Less formalized categories and more complex themes.[31]	There are a number of nonformal categories and complex themes in the report. The latter have been termed "matrix formulations" by Lazarsfeld and are descriptive concepts which sum up a great number of related behavioral or attitudinal items. Examples in the present report are the "cults of *machismo* and virginity." Again, however, these are outnumbered by more systematic and "quantifiable" content categories.

Thus, the present analysis has many similarities to both methods of analysis and cannot be classified as one or the other. We may proceed to more detailed information on analytical procedures. These may be divided conveniently into quantitative and qualitative methods.

QUANTITATIVE METHODS

That portion of the analysis which may be termed quantitative did not differ from the usual methods of survey or content analysis. Though coding difficulties were extensive because of the variability and complexity of the data, enough of the content was amenable to categorization, so that code books for male and female respondents could be drawn up. Coding was performed on large file cards, each of which could take eighty separate items, and tables were "run" by means of hand sorts.

Actually, the small number of cases in the sample raises the question, "Why bother to count?" Certainly any pretense at representativeness or a high degree of precision would be somewhat specious in the light of the few cases. Moreover, in some instances careful counting was not done. This was usually the case where responses on a given topic were spontaneous rather than the result of systematic questioning, or where the very presence of one type of response is sufficient to justify a hypothesis.[32] In general, however, careful counting was done, wherever this was possible and fruitful, for three reasons: there were enough cases so that counting was often essential in order to ascertain the ranking of variables; interrelationships of variables were made clearer by the cross-tabulation

[26] Allen Barton, "Outline of Examples for the Study of Qualitative Research" (Columbia University, offset, n.d.), p. 1.

[27] *Ibid,* p. 1.

[28] Bernard Berelson, *Content Analysis in Communication Research* (Glencoe: Free Press, 1952), p. 116.

[29] *Ibid,* p. 122.

[30] The justification for this is that, in an exploratory study, interpretive "hunches" can be as valuable for the follow-up study as purely descriptive materials.

[31] Berelson, *op. cit.,* pp. 125–28.

[32] See Berelson's discussion of the "presence-absence of particular content (rather than relative frequencies)" typical of qualitative analysis, *ibid,* pp. 119–21.

method, which, of course, depends upon counting procedures; the bases for hypotheses are made more explicit for the reader when counting procedures are used. This puts the reader in a position to judge whether or not the analyst's conclusions are warranted. Merton has succinctly described this function: "Although figures summarizing . . . case study materials are cited from time to time, these are merely heuristic, not demonstrative in character. They serve only to indicate the sources of interpretive hypotheses which await detailed, systematic inquiry."[33]

QUALITATIVE METHODS

The method of analysis which may be termed qualitative can be divided into two types, longitudinal and cross-sectional.

Longitudinal Method. By this method, one case is seen as a whole and, by a careful reading, developmental hypotheses in particular may be verified. If Case *X* is felt to stand for a general type, for example, it may be useful to trace back the history of his motivation in order to see what antecedents may be responsible for his present behavior. This method was used in connection with types of birth-control users. A model of the variables theoretically relevant to birth-control behavior was drawn up, and then case histories used to illustrate various types of combinations of the variables.

Cross-sectional Method. This method, together with the more quantitative ones, was the principal tool of analysis. First, all interviews were carefully read, notes taken, and hypotheses drawn up on the basis of the content assessment. Second, all items on the interview forms dealing with a particular hypothesis were scanned. In this way a clearer *Gestalt* of the particular factor under investigation was perceived. Third, 1,700 quotations were clipped from the interviews and formed a quotation file. Since quotations are used liberally throughout the report, this particular method of presentation requires a brief explanation.

Customarily, quotations are thought of as "window dressing," as colorful examples which "enliven the report." This is particularly true in quantitative studies in which the occasional quotation breaks

[33] Robert Merton, "Patterns of Influence," in Paul Lazarsfeld and Frank Stanton, eds., *Communication Research* (New York: Harper, 1949), p. 180.

the monotony of tables. In the present study the quotation serves a more important function. The quotation in the qualitative study is the writer's datum, just as the table is the datum of the quantitative study. Not to present quotations in a qualitative study is tantamount to leaving out the tables in a quantitative study. To do so is to throw the reader at the mercy of the writer's interpretation and honesty—a frequent problem in anthropological studies. With the quotations themselves exposed to view, the reader can decide for himself whether or not the interpretation seems sound.

There are, however, two basic problems in this type of analysis. First, the analogy between the quotation and the statistical table soon breaks down. While the latter is complete, the former is fragmentary and, by the same token, may be misleading. Every quotation or set of quotations represents only one cell in a table, not a whole table. The analyst may choose for quotation only his more articulate respondents, who are very likely to be different in class or education from those who go unquoted. He may tend to select the more spectacular illustrations and slight the humdrum but more characteristic. He may, on the other hand, present the major configurations and leave out the deviant cases, wherein may lie more fruitful leads. By picking and choosing which quotations he will present, the writer again has the reader at his mercy, albeit not to the same extent as the writer who presents no quotations.

The alternatives are either to present the total body of data along with the report or to sample systematically the quotations for selection. Both these methods are wasteful and unwieldy. Had the former method been used in the present study, about 2,500 pages would have to be added. The latter method is clumsy from a presentation point of view, but it is more feasible. Subsequent research should be directed at working out this technique.

THE FILE OF EXTRACTS

The interviews were read as they came in from the field, and notes were taken. As soon as the country interviews were completed (24 families), a file system was set up, designed to provide the illustrative material which forms a large part of this volume. Thirty categories were established covering the topics and hypotheses previously outlined, as well as new topics appearing as interviews were read.[24] Then all interviews were reread, and pertinent quotations clipped and affixed to file cards.. Each card contained a brief code for the identification, sex, and residence of the respondent, the question number to which the quote referred, and the category number. Cross-index cards were also included.

The important fact to note here is that the clipping was not done systematically. That is, not every reference to a given subject or hypothesis was clipped, but only those which were most illustrative (*positively or negatively*) of the hypothesis. Qualitative analysis was then done mainly from the card catalogue rather than from the interviews themselves. While the possibility of bias must of course be granted, it is felt that several factors mitigated its effects.

Interviews were always read first in their totality, and notes taken on the contents. These notes were used along with the quotations as a measure to prevent overgeneralization on any particular set of quotations. More important, however, is the fact that, wherever possible and pertinent, a hypothesis was checked by counting its manifestations in all of the interviews. These counts are reported in the text. Finally, a large number of extracts were made, a fact which to some degree would mitigate the bias inherent if only a small number were selected. Over 1,700 extracts, or an average of about a dozen quotations per respondent, were included in the file. Only two respondents in the sample received no representation in the file, and one respondent was represented by 35 quotations.

The first noticeable difference is between the sexes. Three fourths of the males were represented in the file from zero to ten times each, whereas only slightly over a quarter of the females were so infrequently included. The major factors explaining this difference are that the male interview was much shorter than the female, and that women were much more articulate than men.

The second point of difference concerns residence. With both males and females, but particularly with the former, country and town residents were represented much more frequently than were city respondents. One reason for this probably lies with the interviewing. Interviewers were best in the town areas. They had already

[24] See Appendix E.

TABLE 46

DISTRIBUTION OF FILE QUOTATIONS BY RESIDENCE OF RESPONDENTS

MALES

Number of File Quotations	*Country (percent)*	*Village (percent)*	*City (percent)*	*Total (percent)*
0–10	59	65	100	76
11–20	41	35	–	24
21 or more	–	–	–	–
	100	100	100	100
Number of respondents	(24)	(23)	(24)	(71)

FEMALES

Number of File Quotations	*Country (percent)*	*Village (percent)*	*City (percent)*	*Total (percent)*
0–10	30	14	42	28
11–20	54	62	42	53
21 or more	17	25	16	19
	101	101	100	100
Number of respondents	(24)	(24)	(24)	(72)

conquered their fears, had gained considerable experience, and were relieved at not having to walk for hours to reach a respondent. Consequently they were more at ease and more facile and imaginative in their probing. By the time the city sample was begun, however, the interviewers were fatigued from the field work, tired of the interview form, and perhaps overconfident about their ability to perform satisfactorily. Thus both quantity and quality of the responses declined in their interviews.

Something similar occurred to the analyst. By the time the city sample was read, diminishing returns were setting in—that is, the first 40 cases or so had provided enough qualitative material to cover the various hypotheses previously drawn up. Since the function of the file was mainly one of covering the range of responses and of selecting good examples for the generalizations made, after about half the sample had been taken further quotes added relatively little.

There is also the danger that the report itself may be biased by a tendency to select more frequently the comments of better educated or more sophisticated respondents. An analysis of the quotations contained in a mimeographed edition (reduced somewhat for publication) of the current volume disclosed that a small amount of bias was present, but in the unexpected direction—that is, there was a tendency for the more frequently quoted to come from the rural and less educated groups. We may conclude that the impressionistic method of quotation selection introduced no serious biases, although there may be some slanting toward more traditional groups in the population.

Appendix B: Respondent Characteristics

COUNTRY

Code	*Occupation*	*Age*	*Education (years)*	*Religion*	*Type of Union*	*Pregnancies in Present Union*
A3M	Taxi driver	31	9	Prot.	Rel.	—
A3F	Housewife	28	4	Prot.	Rel.	3
A5M	Foreman (sugar)	47	3	Cath.	Cons.	—
A5F	Housewife	35	1	Cath.	Cons.	9
A8M	Laborer (sugar)	27	4	Cath.	Civil	—
A8F	Housewife	25	7	Cath.	Civil	7
A9M	Laborer (sugar)	40	0	Cath.	Cons.	—
A9F	Housewife	25	1	None	Cons.	3
A10M	Laborer (coffee)	26	3	Prot.	Cons.	—
A10F	Housewife	24	3	Prot.	Cons.	2
A11M	Roadworker	34	4	Prot.	Civil	—
A11F	Housewife	28	6	Prot.	Civil	5
A12M	Farmer	24	4	Prot.	Cons.	—
A12F	Housewife	19	3	Prot.	Cons.	2
A13M	Farmer	33	1	Prot.	Cons.	—
A13F	Housewife	27	0	Prot.	Cons.	6
B1M	Laborer (minor crops)	39	3	Cath.	Cons.	—
B1F	Housewife	23	3	Cath.	Cons.	2
B3M	Laborer (sugar)	42	1	Cath.	Cons.	—
B3F	Housewife	35	5	Cath.	Cons.	14
B4M	Laborer (sugar)	47	5	Cath.	Rel.	—
B4F	Housewife	41	6	Cath.	Rel.	4
B5M	Unemployed laborer	53	5	Cath.	Cons.	—
B5F	Housewife	28	1	Cath.	Cons.	1
B6M	Merchant (minor crops)	23	2	Cath.	Cons.	—
B6F	Housewife	35	3	Cath.	Cons.	3
B7M	Farmer	45	4	Cath.	Civil	—
B7F	Housewife	45	3	Cath.	Civil	8
B8M	Laborer (minor crops)	46	6	Cath.	Civil	—
B8F	Housewife	36	0	Cath.	Civil	12
B9M	Farmer	50	5	Cath.	Civil	—
B9F	Housewife	41	3	Cath.	Civil	13
C1M	Peddler	54	0	Cath.	Civil	—
C1F	Housewife	42	3	Cath.	Civil	8
C2M	Laborer (factory)	33	9	Cath.	Cons.	—
C2F	Housewife	22	3	Cath.	Cons.	4
C3M	Unemployed laborer	24	5	Cath.	Cons.	—
C3F	Needleworker	23	4	No inf.	Cons.	2

COUNTRY

Code	Occupation	Age	Education (years)	Religion	Type of Union	Pregnancies in Present Union
C4M	Store clerk	31	8	Cath.	Rel.	–
C4F	Housewife	31	3	Cath.	Rel.	1
C6M	Owner (*cafetín*)	24	4	Cath.	Cons.	–
C6F	Housewife	26	3	Cath.	Cons.	3
C7M	Laborer (sugar)	40	4	Cath.	Rel.	–
C7F	Maid	25	2	Cath.	Rel.	6
C8M	Laborer (sugar)	32	5	Cath.	Cons.	–
C8F	Housewife	32	7	Cath.	Cons.	7
C10M	Chauffeur	54	0	Cath.	Civil	–
C10F	Housewife	50	4	Cath.	Civil	11

VILLAGE

Code	Occupation	Age	Education (years)	Religion	Type of Union	Pregnancies in Present Union
X2M	Laborer (sugar)	44	0	Cath.	Civil	–
X2F	Housewife	45	8	Cath.	Civil	7
X3M	Mechanic (sugar)	50	9	Other	Cons.	–
X3F	Housewife	41	9	Other	Cons.	7
X5M	Mechanic	43	6	Cath.	Cons.	–
X5F	Housewife	54	0	Cath.	Cons.	1
X6M	Laborer (sugar)	34	8	Cath.	Cons.	–
X6F	Housewife	40	0	Cath.	Cons.	0
X7M	Mechanic (sugar)	42	3	Prot.	Rel.	–
X7F	Janitress	32	3	Cath.	Rel.	7
X8M	Grocery store clerk	33	9	Prot.	Civil	–
X8F	Housewife	33	6	Prot.	Civil	5
X9M	Unemployed laborer	63	0	Cath.	Cons.	–
X9F	Janitress	43	0	Cath.	Cons.	6
X10M	Carpenter	43	8	Cath.	Civil	–
X10F	Maid	36	1	Spiritualist	Civil	8
Y1M	Student	27	12	Cath.	Civil	–
Y1F	Housewife	27	8	Prot.	Civil	2
Y2M	Laborer (sugar)	35	8	Cath.	Civil	–
Y2F	Housewife	27	0	None	Civil	6
Y3M	Unemployed croupier	36	6	Cath.	Civil	–
Y3F	Housewife	32	6	Cath.	Civil	3
Y4M	Laborer (sugar cane)	32	3	Prot.	Rel.	–
Y4F	Housewife	26	4	Cath.	Rel.	3
Y5M	Carpenter	51	5	Cath.	Civil	–
Y5F	Janitress	38	5	Prot.	Civil	11
Y6M	Foreman (sugar)	42	5	Cath.	Civil	–
Y6F	Housewife	40	2	Cath.	Civil	4
Y7M	Laborer (sugar)	46	2	Cath.	Cons.	–
Y7F	Housewife	36	2	Other	Cons.	1
Y8M	Laborer (sugar)	32	9	Cath.	Rel.	–
Y8F	Housewife	27	8	Prot.	Rel.	5

VILLAGE

Code	Occupation	Age	Education (years)	Religion	Type of Union	Pregnancies in Present Union
Z1M	Laborer (sugar)	37	2	Prot.	Rel.	—
Z1F	Housewife	23	6	Prot.	Rel.	3
Z3M	Peddler	62	4	Prot.	Rel.	—
Z3F	Housewife	42	3	Prot.	Rel.	2
Z4M	Barber	36	10	Cath.	Civil	—
Z4F	Housewife	30	4	Cath.	Civil	3
Z5M	Not interviewed	—	—	—	—	—
Z5F	Housewife	21	3	Prot.	Rel.	1
Z6M	Laborer (factory)	65	0	Cath.	Cons.	—
Z6F	Housewife	40	3	Cath.	Cons.	1
Z7M	Laborer (factory)	29	9	Prot.	Civil	—
Z7F	Housewife	24	6	Prot.	Civil	3
Z8M	Unemployed laborer	33	8	Prot.	Civil	—
Z8F	Housewife	31	3	Prot.	Civil	4
Z9M	University student	32	13	Cath.	Rel.	—
Z9F	Housewife	22	14	Cath.	Rel.	2

CITY

Code	Occupation	Age	Education (years)	Religion	Type of Union	Pregnancies in Present Union
H1M	Mechanic (foundry)	31	1	Cath.	Cons.	—
H1F	Housewife	25	7	Cath.	Cons.	9
H2M	Mechanic (sugar)	37	13	Cath.	Civil	—
H2F	Housewife	21	4	Cath.	Civil	4
H4M	Truck driver	28	8	Cath.	Rel.	—
H4F	Housewife	24	7	Cath.	Rel.	4
H5M	Peddler	33	3	Cath.	Civil	—
H5F	Housewife	28	5	Cath.	Civil	6
H6M	Laborer (laundry)	40	5	Cath.	Cons.	—
H6F	Housewife	34	0	Cath.	Cons.	1
H7M	Laborer	31	4	Cath.	Cons.	—
H7F	Housewife	19	2	Cath.	Cons.	3
H9M	Bank messenger	27	5	Prot.	Cons.	—
H9F	Maid	31	0	Cath.	Cons.	2
H10M	Waiter	34	3	Cath.	Rel.	—
H10F	Housewife	32	3	Cath.	Rel.	2
H11M	Electrician	28	6	Cath.	Rel.	—
H11F	Housewife	23	0	Cath.	Rel.	6
H12M	Bakery shop clerk	24	4	Cath.	Cons.	—
H12F	Housewife	28	4	Cath.	Cons.	2
H13M	Messenger (laundry)	22	4	Cath.	Cons.	—
H13F	Housewife	27	7	Cath.	Cons.	4
H14M	Helper (navy base)	30	3	Cath.	Rel.	—
H14F	Housewife	17	5	Cath.	Rel.	2
H15M	Truck driver	30	5	Cath.	Cons.	—
H15F	Housewife	21	3	Cath.	Cons.	3
H16M	Electrician	29	7	Cath.	Cons.	—

CITY

Code	Occupation	Age	Education (years)	Religion	Type of Union	Pregnancies in Present Union
H16F	Housewife	28	7	Cath.	Cons.	4
H17M	Peddler	33	2	Cath.	Civil	—
H17F	Housewife	28	4	Cath.	Civil	6
H18M	Longshoreman	36	4	Cath.	Cons.	—
H18F	Housewife	39	4	Cath.	Cons.	3
H19M	Longshoreman	42	0	Cath.	Cons.	—
H19F	Housewife	38	3	Cath.	Cons.	6
H20M	Peddler	40	7	Prot.	Cons.	—
H20F	Housewife	34	8	Prot.	Cons.	2
H21M	Soldier	31	7	Cath.	Civil	—
H21F	Housewife	21	8	Cath.	Civil	2
H23M	Fisherman	31	5	Cath.	Cons.	—
H23F	Housewife	22	6	Cath.	Cons.	3
H24M	Laborer (Gas Co.)	37	3	Cath.	Cons.	—
H24F	Housewife	32	1	Cath.	Cons.	3
H31M	Chauffeur	36	2	Cath.	Cons.	—
H31F	Housewife	38	0	Cath.	Cons.	2
H39M	Lottery ticket seller	34	4	Spiritualist	Civil	—
H39F	Housewife	39	4	Cath.	Civil	6
H45M	Peddler	38	3	Cath.	Rel.	—
H45F	Housewife	26	6	Cath.	Rel.	4

Appendix C: The Construction of Indices

INDEX OF GENERAL COMMUNICATION

This index was derived from cross runs of the following four questions, all taken from the female interview:

Q.28C1: Is there anything in your husband's life that he doesn't discuss with you?

Q.28C2: Is there anything in your life that you don't discuss with him?

Q.28B: What things do you and your husband do together?

Q.28C: What sort of things do you talk about frequently?

1. Questions 28C1 and 28C2 were cross-tabulated as shown in Table 47.

TABLE 47

DEGREE OF DISCUSSION BETWEEN SPOUSES[a]

WIFE DISCUSSES WITH HUSBAND	HUSBAND DISCUSSES WITH WIFE			
	Everything	*Not Outside Life*	*Not Other Women*	*Nothing*
Everything	*A*	*B*	*A*	*B*
Something but not everything	*A*	*B*	*C*	*B*
Nothing	—	*C*	—	*B*

[a] Twenty respondents gave no information on either or both of these questions. In such cases, other pertinent items on their interview forms were read, and the respondents placed in categories *A*, *B*, or *C*, according to the reader's judgment.

2. A rating of "High Communication" was given to those respondents satisfying any two of the following criteria:

   a. Respondent falls into a category labeled *A* in Table 47.
   b. Q.28B: Wife and husband engage in outside activities together, i.e., go to movies, take rides, take children to the park, etc.
   c. Q.28C: Wife and husband discuss their hopes and future plans.

3. A rating of "Low Communication" was given to those respondents satisfying any one of the following criteria:

   a. Respondent falls into a category labeled *B* in Table 47.
   b. Q.28B: Wife and husband do nothing together except eat and sleep.
   c. Q.28C: Wife and husband discuss nothing.

4. A rating of "Medium Communication" was given to all remaining respondents.

INDEX OF DOMINANCE RELATIONS

This index was derived from the responses to Q.20,F. Four areas demonstrative of dominance relations between husband and wife were delineated: (1) large-item buying; (2) small-item buying; (3) solution of disagreements; (4) domains. Each of these areas was scored according to a three-point scale, as follows:

Large-item buying (houses, furniture, radios):

1. No participation by wife. Husband decides what is to be purchased and makes actual purchase alone.
2. Wife participates in suggesting possible purchases and in purchasing. The decision as to whether a particular purchase shall be made, however, rests with the husband.
3. Wife participates in the decision to purchase.

Small-item buying (small household items, personal clothing for wife and children):

Scored as above.

Solution of disagreements:

1. In cases of disagreement between husband and wife, there is no discussion of the problem. Wife never answers her husband, his decisions being final.
2. While there is evidence of some mutual discussion, the husband makes the final decision.
3. Both partners, or the wife alone, make the final decision.

Domains (the areas over which each partner exercises control):

1. Wife assumes no responsibility for decisions on household matters. She executes her husband's orders.
2. Household decisions made jointly or by the wife alone. All business[1] matters, however, are exclusively the husband's concern.
3. Wife helps her husband make business decisions.

The sum of each respondent's scores was recorded, and the resulting frequency distribution was divided into three groups containing roughly equal numbers. The lowest-scoring third was classified as "Traditional," the highest third as "Least Traditional," and the intermediate group as "Less Traditional." Those cases for which information was available for only one of the four areas were scored by means of subjective appraisal of other responses.

[1] "Business" is broadly defined. Not only does it refer to the husband's work but in a good percentage of instances it includes the buying of groceries.

Appendix D: Interview Forms

SOCIAL SCIENCE RESEARCH CENTER
UNIVERSITY OF PUERTO RICO

FAMILY LIFE PROJECT
Female Interview

Interviewer: Duration of Interviews:
Informant Number: Date:

1. Description of the house (type of construction, number of bedrooms and beds)
2. Occupation of male head of the family
3. Total number of persons living in the house
4. Persons living in the house who are not the Informant's children

	Relationship to Informant	*Age*	*Sex*
(1)			
(2)			
(3)			
(4)			
(5)			
(6)			

5. Financial condition
6. Source of income (list all persons contributing to the family income, including remittances from relatives and friends)

	Kinship	*Type of Assistance*	*Residence*
(1)			
(2)			
(3)			

7. Highest grade attained in school
8. Age 9. Color 10. Religion
11. Place of birth: Country Small town Large town City Foreign country
12. How many different places have you lived in? (List places and length of time)
13. Marital unions:

	First	*Second*	*Third*
A. Age at which union began			
B. Age at which union ended			
C. Type of union			

D. Reason for separation
E. Number of pregnancies

14. *Pregnancies (List) Dead Living at Home Living Elsewhere*

15. Whom do you consider to be your closest relatives? (List)
Kinship Maternal Paternal Grade of Kin

15*a*. Which of these relatives live near you? (Draw a circle)

16. For which do you feel more attachment, for your father's or for your mother's side of the family? Why?

17. It is said that in American families in general, parents and their children live alone without relatives. What do you think about that?
   A. (If the informant does not approve:) In general, why is it good to have relatives?
      1. What do your relatives do for you? What do you do for them?
         a. Do you lend each other money? What do you think of that?
         b. Do you sometimes help them in anything? Do they help you?
         c. And your parents? Do you help them in any way?
         d. And your children? Do they help you in any way?
   B. In what way do you keep in touch with your family?
      1. How many times a (week) (month) (year) do you go to visit relatives? How often do they come to visit you?
      2. Do you ever send your children to visit them? For what purpose? And they, do they send their children to see you? For what purpose? How many times a (month) (year) (week)? For how long?

18. As for relatives who do not live in this (town) (barrio), what sort of relationship do you have with them?
   A. Have your relations with them changed since you moved? How? Would you prefer to be nearer them or do you like to continue living as you are now?
   B. Do you visit them sometimes? Do they visit you? Why is that? Can you give some examples?
   C. Do you write each other? How often?
   D. Do they ever send their children to visit you or stay with you for a while? For what reason? Do you send your children?

19. There is a saying that goes: "Who is your brother? Your closest neighbor." What do you think of that?
   A. To whom do you feel closer, your neighbors or your relatives? Why?
      1. With whom do you exchange more visits, with your relatives or neighbors?

20. Who decides, in general, matters of importance, you or your

husband? (In business matters; in household matters.) Can you give me some examples? What do you think of that? Do you consider it natural, right, or do you believe some other way would be better?

A. When something important is to be purchased, how do you decide if it should be bought or not? (From the moment one of you is interested in buying it until the moment the decision is made whether to buy or not.) Give an example.

B. Was it the same in your parents' home? Who made the decisions there, your father or your mother?

1. (If the situation was different:) Which way do you think is better?

C. Do you recall any instance in which you and your husband were not in accord on an important decision? Tell me what happened, how you felt, and how the matter ended.

21. Who takes the greater part in bringing up the children?

A. And your husband, does he have anything to do with them? What, for instance?

1. Do you think this is all right? Or do you believe (you) (your husband) should take a greater part in it?

B. When the children want to do something, whom do they ask for permission? For instance?

C. You and your husband, are you in agreement on how children should be brought up? Do you recall any instances in which you did not agree? For example?

D. And your husband, in whom does he show more interest, the girls or the boys? Why? And you? In what way?

22. How should children be brought up? The way their parents were brought up or some other way? Why?

A. Are you rearing, or do you plan to rear, your children differently from the way you were brought up? What way?

1. Do you intend to be more, less, or just as strict as your parents were with you when your boy friend was courting you? Why?

23. In what way should little girls be brought up differently from little boys? Why?

A. At what age should little girls be dressed? And little boys? (If there is a difference:) Why the difference?

1. Some people say they do not clothe little boys because they are prettier than the girls. What do you think of that?

2. They also say they dress little girls up for the sake of modesty. What do you think? And why not little boys?

3. Is there any danger in having them [girls] naked? For example? And for the boys, is there any danger?

24. What is your idea of a good boy?
    A. What are some examples of what a good boy would do?
    B. Has a son got obligations toward his parents after leaving the home? What, for instance?
        1. Should children look after their parents in their old age, or should the parents look after themselves?
    C. When a son gets married, whom should he help more, his parents or his parents-in-law?
        1. Is it really done that way? Give an example.
    D. And the daughter, whom should she help more?
    E. Who gives more help to the parents after their marriage, the daughter or the son?
25. Is there any difference between what a good boy would do and what a good girl would do? What?
26. When you were a child, how did you get along with your parents?
    A. For whom did your father have more affection, the boys or the girls? In what way? Why do you think that was?
    B. And what about your mother, for whom did she have more affection?
    C. What about you? For whom did you have more affection, for your mother or father? Why?
27. What is your idea of a good father?
    A. What are some examples of what a good father does?
28. What is your idea of a good husband?
    A. What are some examples of what a good husband does?
29. And your husband, how would you rate him as a (husband) (father)?
    A. Would you say he is:

	Husband	*Father*
1. Extraordinarily good		
2. Very good		
3. Fair		
4. Bad		
5. Very bad		

    B. What things do you and your husband do together?
    C. What sort of things do you talk about most frequently?
        1. Is there anything in his life that he does not discuss with you?
        2. Is there anything in your life that you do not discuss with him?
30. What is your idea of a good wife?
    A. Give me some examples of things a good wife does.
31. What is your idea of a good mother?
    A. Give me some examples of things a good mother does.

32. What is your idea of a happy family?
    A. How is your family, in this regard?
    B. What sort of things do you and your children do together?
    C. What is the best way of settling family disagreements?
33. Do you like to tell your children about your family of old and about the things you used to do?
    A. Which is the relative farthest removed about whom you talk to your children?
    B. Who is the oldest relative you know of?
34. What are your ideas of how a young girl should behave with men before marriage? And with her sweetheart?
    A. With regard to her virginity?
        1. Would you say it is very important, more or less important, or not very important for a girl to be a virgin before she marries? Why?
        2. Do you believe the majority of girls around here are virgins before marriage? (Try to find an example of a girl who was not, and the reaction of the informant and that of the community.)
    B. What should a young girl know about sexual matters before marriage? How should she go about finding out? Where?
    C. What do you think of love? Is this an important factor in the choice of a mate? Tell me what you understand by love. (Try to differentiate between affection and love.)
    D. Which is more important for a woman, that she be married to a good man, or to one she is very much in love with?
35. At what age do you think a girl ought to get married? Why?
    A. Why not before?
    B. Why not later?
36. Why did you get married at age *X*?
    A. (If respondent's age at marriage is different from the one she considers ideal:) I see you married (before) (after) the age you think ideal. Why?
        1. Did you fall in love?
        2. Were your girl friends getting married?
        3. Did you want to leave home?
    B. Do you think it would have been better if you had married at the ideal age? Why?
        1. Would you have liked to stay a (longer) (shorter) time at your parents' home? What was there that you (liked) (disliked) so much?
        2. As to having children, would you have liked to have had them (earlier) (later)?

37. Now, can you tell me something about your first marriage? Tell me more of how you came to be married?
    A. How long had you known your husband before you married him? How long a courtship did you have? How often did you see him? How did you see each other? Where?
    B. Which were the qualities that you liked best in your husband?
    C. Did your parents approve or disapprove of your courtship? What influence did they have on your decision?
38. Where did you go to live after your marriage? Why?
    A. Did you live with or near to your parents or your parents-in-law? Why did you live (not live) with or near them?
    B. As to your children, do you think they will live with or near you after they are married? Would you like to have them live near you or would you prefer them to live farther away? Why?
39. Many women tell us that they expected better things from marriage. How would you say yours has turned out?
    A. Has it turned out as well as you expected? In what way? (Compare with what she previously mentioned as having expected from marriage.)
40. Coming back to your marriage, tell me, in general, what did you expect from marriage? Why did you expect that?
    A. Children?
    B. Economic security?
    C. Companionship?
    D. Sexual relations?
41. Of what aspect of marriage were you afraid?
    A. Housework?
    B. Pregnancy?
    C. A domineering husband?
    D. Sexual relations?
42. Some people tell us that they did not know what to expect of marriage because they knew very little of men in general. Now that you have been married for some time, would you say you knew much, little, or nothing about men before you married? What did you know? Why did you know so (much) (little)?
    A. Did you have male friends before you married? How did you see each other?
    B. (If no mention of sex is made:) As to having children, what did you know about that? How is it that you (knew) (did not know) about it? How did you learn it? Where?
        1. As to birth control? Sexual relations?
        2. Did you discuss sexual matters with anyone? With whom? What in particular?

43. What are the most important differences between men and women?
    A. In their way of thinking?
    B. In their feelings and emotions?
    C. In their behavior?
    D. In their (goodness) (purity)?
44. Speaking of sexual matters, who do you think derives more pleasure from sexual relations, the man or the woman? Why? Do you have any examples to give me?
    A. (If the answer is "the man":) Doesn't the woman have any pleasure? Do you think this is right?
45. In your own case, what would you say about your husband? Would you say he gets more pleasure than you do from sexual relations? For instance? What do you think of that?
    A. Does this worry you? Does this cause any problems? What do you do to solve them?
    B. Do you discuss sexual matters with your husband at any time? What, for instance?
    C. There are times when he wants sexual relations and you do not? What do you do? Why? What does he say?
46. What do you recall from your wedding night?
47. Who do you think has more rights in Puerto Rico, men or the women? In what sense? What do you think of that?
    A. As to sexual relations?
        1. Before marriage.
        2. After marriage.
48. We were discussing women's rights a while ago. Have you any rights?
    A. In what respect does your husband have more rights than you? Why? What do you think of it?
        1. What things does he forbid you? E.g., cosmetics, going out alone, dancing with other men.
49. Many people in Puerto Rico live together without being married. To what do you attribute this?
    A. Are there any advantages for the couple in that type of marriage? What are they?
        1. Does it give the woman more freedom? What sort of freedom?
        2. Does it give the man more freedom? What sort of freedom? Is the freedom greater for the woman or for the man?
        3. Who gets more advantages out of this type of union, the woman or the man? Why?
50. (If the marriage is consensual:) People give many reasons for not being married by the Law or by the Church. What were your reasons?

A. You and your husband, did you feel the same about that kind of marriage, or was one of you more interested than the other in marrying that way? (If the latter is the case:) What was that difference of opinion due to? How come (your) (your husband's) opinion was finally decisive?
B. That decision you both made, was it affected by the expense of a civil or church wedding?
C. What did your parents think of this kind of marriage?
D. Before you got married, what advantages did you expect from this type of union?
E. Now you have been married a certain length of time, do you still consider that those advantages exist? For instance?
F. Do you now see any advantages you were not aware of before?
G. If you had to start all over again, would you do the same? Why? Why not?

51. How soon after marriage do you think a couple should have the first child? Why?
   A. Why so soon?
      1. Are people in agreement with that? Why?
      2. Do you believe it is healthier for the woman? Why?
      3. Some women fear they might be called *machorras,* barren. Has that got anything to do with having children early in marriage?
      4. What about the husbands?
52. Tell me, when did you have your first baby? (If it varies from the ideal:) Why did you have it (before) (later) than your ideal?
53. How many years apart should couples have children? Why?
54. What is the ideal number of children for a family to have? Why?
   A. Why not more?
   B. Why not less?
55. You yourself, for instance, how many children do you want? (If the number wanted or the number the informant already has varies from the ideal:) Why do you (want) (have) more children than you believe ideal? (If the ideal number is more than three:) Why do you want so many?
   A. What are the advantages of a large family?
      1. Help in old age? (If in the affirmative:) What do you expect them to do for you? Do you believe they'll do it?
      2. Are you proud of having so many children? What makes you feel proud?
      3. Are your children an entertainment for you? In what way?
   B. (If the number is less than the ideal:) Why do you have fewer children than what you think ideal?
      1. What do you believe are the disadvantages of a large family?

(a) Is it a lot of work to bring them up?
(b) Are children a source of danger for the mother's health?
(c) Are they a source of danger for the other children?

C. (If she wants few:) And if you had money? Why?

56. What kind of family would you like to have: one with more girls than boys, more boys than girls, or an equal number of each? Why?
   A. And your husband? Why?
   B. Is the mother more important for the daughters or the sons? Why?
57. And the men, in general, do they like to have many or few children?
58. And your husband, does he wish to have more than, less than, or the same number of children as you? (If the same:) Have you ever discussed it with each other? What are his reasons for agreeing with you?
   A. (If the number he wishes varies:) Why does he wish for (more) (less) than you? Have you ever discussed it? What does he say? Who will have the say-so, he or you? Why?
   B. Many men in Puerto Rico want more children than their wives do. Why do you think this is so?
59. Have you ever used a birth-control method? (If in the affirmative, proceed with Q.60.) (If in the negative:) Why? (If the informant prefers small families:) If you prefer small families, why don't you practice birth control?
   A. Do you know any of the birth-control methods? (If affirmative:) Which ones? Why don't you use them?
      1. Do you know where you can obtain birth control methods?
      2. Are you ashamed to ask for them? What makes you feel this way?
      3. Are you ashamed of using them? What makes you feel this way?
      4. Do you think they are harmful? In what way?
      5. Does religion have anything to do with your decision? In what way?
      6. What does your husband think of this?
   B. (If answer to "A" is negative:) Have you ever heard of rubbers, jelly, diaphragm, sponge, douche? What about withdrawal? What about an operation on the woman? What about rhythm? And abstinence? (If the answer is in the affirmative:) How is it that you have never used them?
   C. (If the informant has never used these methods:) What would have to happen to make you use some birth-control method?

60. (If the informant has used a contraceptive method:) When did you decide for the first time to limit the number of children you wished to have? What was the cause of such a decision?
   A. When did you first decide you did not wish to have any more children? Why?
   B. What did you know about methods to avoid children before you heard about method *X*?
   C. When, under what circumstances, did you first hear some reference to method *X*?
   D. What did you like best about that method?
   E. Did you discuss it with your husband? What did he think of it? (If the husband was the one who suggested the contraceptive method:) What did you think of the idea when he suggested it? Do you ever discuss these matters with your husband?
61. After using method *X*, what did you like best about it? What made you dislike it? And your husband?
62. (If the informant no longer uses method *X* but uses method *Y*:) What made you change from *X* to *Y*? (Repeat the series of questions above.)
63. (If the informant no longer uses any method at all:) What made you stop using method *X*? Why didn't you try some other method?
64. What would have to happen to cause you to use any of these methods again?
65. What changes have you noticed in the way in which families live nowadays as compared to the days when you were brought up? What are these changes due to? What do you think of them?
   A. With regard to relations between parents and children?
   B. With regard to relations between girls and boys?
   C. With regard to relations between husband and wife?
66. (For women who work:) Does it cause you problems in your home to work outside?
   A. What does your husband think of your work?

SOCIAL SCIENCE RESEARCH CENTER
UNIVERSITY OF PUERTO RICO

FAMILY LIFE PROJECT

Male Interview

Interviewer: Duration of Interviews:
Informant Number: Date:

1. Highest grade attained in school
2. Age 3. Color 4. Religion

5. Place of birth: Country Small town Large town City Foreign country
6. How many different places have you lived in? (List places and length of time)
7. Number of marital unions

	First	*Second*	*Third*
A. Age at which union began			
B. Age at which union ended			
C. Type of union			
D. Reason for separation			
E. Number of pregnancies			

8. How many *compadres*[1] do you have? (List)
   A. *Relationship Occupation Residence When Chosen Reason for Choice*
   B. Which one of these is your favorite *compadre*? Why?
   C. Toward which of these do you feel the least attachment? Why?
9. Is it important for a man to have *compadres*? Why?
   A. What do they do for you?
      1. Do they help you with your work? In what way? How often?
      2. Do they lend you money?
10. In your estimation, what are the most important qualities in a man?
    A. What about being a "complete man?" Is that important for a man? Why?
       1. Of the following qualities, which do you consider to be the most important for a man? Next in importance? (List the qualities mentioned by the informant, including *machismo,* placing them in order of importance.)
       2. Speaking of being a "complete man": how does a man show it? How does he prove it?
          a. What about his fertility? What about his virility?
          b. How can a father teach his sons to become "complete men?"
          c. What about your sons?
11. How does a man gain the respect of other men around here?
    A. What about having a large family? Would that help? In what way?
12. Of what things should a man be proud?
    A. With regard to the family name? (Should a man be proud of his family name, or isn't that important?) Give an example.
       1. What do you understand by a good name?
13. How many years of schooling would you like your sons to have? Why?

[1] *Compadres* are the godfathers of one's children.

14. How many years of schooling would you like for your daughters? Why?
15. Why do you want them to have (the same) (a different) education?
16. What kind of work would you like for your sons? Why?
    A. Do you expect to be able to help them in some way? How?
17. Would you like your daughters to work? What kind of work?
18. Should sons be brought up differently from daughters? In what way? Why?
    A. Is the father more important for the daughters or for the sons? Why?
    B. At what age should boys and girls be dressed?
19. What kind of family would you like to have, one with more girls than boys, more boys than girls, or an equal number of each? Why?
    A. When your wife is going to have a baby, what do you hope for, a boy or a girl? Why?
20. What is your idea of a good son?
    A. What are some examples of what a good son would do?
        1. Does a son have obligations toward his parents after having left home? What, for instance?
            a. In your case, do you expect your sons to fulfil those obligations?
21. What is your idea of a good daughter?
    A. What are some examples of what a good daughter would do?
22. What is your idea of a good wife?
    A. What are some of the things a good wife would do?
        1. Should the wife be humble with her husband? In what way, for example?
        2. What about sexual matters, is that important? What obligations do women have toward their husbands? Why?
    B. And your wife, how would you describe her? Would you say she is:
        1. Extraordinarily good?
        2. Very good?
        3. Fair?
        4. Bad?
        5. Very bad?
23. What are the most important differences between men and women?
    A. In their way of thinking?
    B. In their feelings and emotions?
    C. In their behavior?
    D. In their (goodness) (purity)?

24. And in sexual matters, what are the differences?
    A. Who do you think derives more pleasure from sexual relations, the woman or the man? Why? For example?
        1. (If the answer is, "The man":) And, in general, doesn't the woman have any pleasure? What do you think of that?
25. Who do you think has more rights, women or men? In what way? What do you think of that?
    A. As to sexual relations before marriage? After marriage?
26. How should young men behave towards young girls before marriage? And with their girl friends? And with the fiancée?
    A. What should a young man know about women before getting married? Why?
        1. Where should he look for that information?
    B. What experience should a young man have before getting married? Why?
        1. (Where) (With whom) should he get that experience?
27. And the girls, how should they behave with the young men before they marry?
    A. What should they know?
    B. What experience should they have with men?
    C. Why is it that the woman's experience should be different from that of the man?
28. Tell me something about yourself before you got married. What did you know of women? What experience had you had?
    A. When did you have your first sexual experience with a woman? How did you feel? Were you proud? Ashamed? Did you talk about this with anyone? What did you talk about?
    B. How many experiences of this kind did you have before you married the first time? Tell me something about that.
    C. Try to remember before your first sexual experience. What did you know about women before this? Where did you learn it?
    D. What about birth-control methods? Did you know anything about them? Where did you learn about this? Did you ever use any method before you got married? What do you think about them?
29. What is the best age for a man to get married? Why that age?
    A. Why not before?
    B. Why not later?
30. (If the respondent's age at his first marriage was earlier or later than the one he considers ideal:) Why did you get married (earlier) (later) than the age you consider best?
31. How soon after marriage do you think a couple should have the first child? Why?

A. Why so soon?
 1. Is a man anxious to have his first child? Why?

32. Now, tell me about your first marital union. Was this experience quite different from the one(s) you had before you married?
 A. What were you looking for in a wife?
  1. As to sexual relations? Was that important?
  2. As to sexual relations, did you find your wife different from the women you knew before you married?
  3. And your feelings toward her, were they different?

33. What is the ideal number of children for a family to have? Why this number? How many children would you like to have? (If the number wanted or the number the informant already has varies from the ideal:) Why do you (want) (have) more children than what you believe ideal?
 A. What are the advantages of a large family?
  1. Help in old age?
   a. (Are you) (Would you be) proud of having a large family? What makes you proud?
 B. (If the number is less than the ideal:) What are the disadvantages of a large family?

34. Have you ever used any birth-control methods in any of your marriages? (If the answer is "No":) Why?
 A. Do you know any of the birth-control methods? (If the answer is "No," proceed with B) (If the answer is "Yes":) Which ones? Why don't you use any of these methods?
  1. Do you know where to get them?
  2. Do you believe they give less pleasure?
  3. Do you associate them with something wrong, e.g., with prostitutes? (If the answer is "Yes" to 2 or 3:) Then why don't you let your wife use some method?
 B. Have you heard talk of condoms, jelly, diaphragm, douches? An operation on the wife? Withdrawal? Sexual abstinence? Rhythm? What do you think of them? How is it that you have never resorted to any of them?
 C. What would have to happen to make you use some birth-control method?

35. (If the informant has used a contraceptive method:) When did you decide for the first time to limit the number of children you wished to have?
 A. What made you decide to limit the number of children?
 B. What made you decide to use that particular method in preference to some other?

36. After you used that method, how did you like it?
    A. What do you think made you (like) (dislike) it?
    B. How long did you use it?
    C. How often did you use it?
    D. Why don't you use it always?
37. (If the informant no longer uses method *X* but changed to *Y*:) What made you change from *X* to *Y*? (Repeat the series of questions above.)
38. (If the informant no longer uses any method:) Why did you stop using *X*?
39. Why don't you try some other method?
40. What would have to happen to cause you to use any of these methods again?
41. Data on all other unions (consensual, concubinal, or legal)
42. What is the greatest worry with which men like you are faced?
    A. What can you do about it?
    B. With what attitude should a man face such problems?
43. What are your hopes for the future?

Appendix E: Categories for File Index of Selected Quotations

1. Premarital insulation
2. Premarital exploration
3. Premarital anxieties, expectations, promises
4. Virginity
5. Courtship
6. Early marriage, elopement, and consensual marriage
7. Wedding night
8. Infidelity and sexual-transgression anxiety
9. Inter-sex hostility
10. Small-family mindedness
11. Large-family mindedness
12. Expressions of *machismo* and *machorrismo*
13. Sexual denial, enjoyment, acquiescence
14. Child rearing, general
15. Differential dressing of children
16. Differential training and education of children
17. Sex of offspring, preference for
18. Parent-child bonds

18a. Care for the aged

19. Aspiration for children
20. Contraception
21. Modesty
22. Role conceptions of men and women
23. Dominance relationships
24. Decision making
25. Postmarital insulation of female
26. Double standard in sexual relationships
27. Changing patterns
28. Self aspirations
29. Lack of communication
30. *Compadrazgo*
31. Desexualization
32. Interviewing
33. Miscellaneous

List of Works Cited

Aptekar, Herbert. Infanticide, Abortion and Contraception in Savage Society. New York: William Goodwin, 1931.

Back, K., R. Hill, G. Arbona, and R. King. "Family Dynamics and Human Fertility—The Experimental Phase." Social Science Research Center, University of Puerto Rico, July 1954, mimeographed.

Balfour, M. "Problems in Health Promotion in the Far East," in Modernization Programs in Relation to Human Resources and Population Problems. New York: Milbank Memorial Fund, 1950.

Barton, Allen. "Outline of Examples for the Study of Qualitative Research." Offset, Columbia University, n.d.

Beebe, Gilbert, and José Belaval. "Fertility and Contraception in Puerto Rico," *Puerto Rico Journal of Public Health and Tropical Medicine,* Vol. VII (September 1942).

Belaval, J., E. Cofresí, and J. Janer. "Opinión de la clase médica de Puerto Rico sobre el uso de la esterilización y los contraceptivos." Mimeographed report, July 1953.

Benedeck, Therese. "The Emotional Structure of the Family," in Ruth Anshen, ed., The Family: Its Function and Destiny. New York: Harper, 1949.

Berelson, Bernard. Content Analysis in Communication Research. Glencoe: Free Press, 1952.

Bromley, Dorothy Dunbar. Birth Control: Its Use and Misuse. New York: Harper, 1934.

Bunce, A. "Economic and Cultural Bases of Family Size in Korea," in Approaches to Problems of High Fertility in Agrarian Societies. New York: Milbank Memorial Fund, 1952.

Cantril, H., and M. Strunk. Public Opinion 1935-1946. Princeton: Princeton University Press, 1951.

Casanova, Ana Adela. "Estudio general de diez núcleos familiares del barrio 'Chicambá' de Ponce." Unpublished term paper, School of Social Work, University of Puerto Rico, 1951.

Census of Population 1950, Preliminary Report. Washington , D. C.: Bureau of the Census.

Chandrasekharan, C. "Cultural Patterns in Relation to Family Planning in India," Third International Conference on Planned Parenthood, Report of Proceedings. Bombay: Family Planning Association of India, 1952.

Clare, Jeanne E., and Clyde V. Kiser. "Social and Psychological Factors Affecting Fertility: Preference for Children of Given Sex in Relation to Fertility," *Milbank Memorial Fund Quarterly,* XXIX (October 1951), 440-92.

Código Civil de Puerto Rico. San Juan: Government Printing Office.

Cofresí, Emilio. Realidad poblacional de Puerto Rico. San Juan: Imprenta Venezuela, 1951.

Combs, J. W., and Kingsley Davis. "The Pattern of Puerto Rican Fertility," *Population Studies,* Vol. IV (March 1951).

Connell, K. The Population of Ireland, 1750-1845. Oxford: Clarendon Press, 1950.

Cruz Apellaniz, Angelina. "Estudio de los problemas de conducta evidenciados en niños procedentes de hogares donde faltan los padres." Unpublished thesis, School of Social Work, University of Puerto Rico, 1935.

Davis, Kingsley. "Changing Modes of Marriage: Contemporary Family Types," in Becker and Hill, eds., Marriage and the Family. Boston: Heath, 1942.

______ "Human Fertility in India," *American Journal of Sociology,* Vol. LII, No. 3 (November 1946).

______ "Puerto Rico: A Crowded Island," *Annals of the American Academy of Political and Social Science,* Vol. CCLXXXV (January 1953).

______ "Romantic Love and Courtship," in Davis, Bredemeier, and Levy, eds., Modern American Society. New York: Rinehart, 1949.

______ "Statistical Perspective on Marriage and Divorce," *Annals of the American Academy of Political and Social Science,* Vol. CCLXXII (November 1950).

Día, El (Ponce), February 12, 15, 16, 1949.

Diario, El (San Juan), March 3, 29, 1949.

Duval, Evelyn M. "Conceptions of Parenthood," *American Journal of Sociology,* LII (November 1946), 193-204.

Ellis, Havelock. Studies in the Psychology of Sex. New York: Random House, 1942.

England, L. "Little Kinsey: An Outline of Sex Attitudes in Britain," *Public Opinion Quarterly,* XIII (1949-50), 567-600.

Ford, Clellan S. "Control of Conception in Cross-Cultural Perspective," *World Population Problems and Birth Control, Annals of the New York Academy of Sciences,* Vol. LIV (May 1952).

Ford, C., and F. Beach. Patterns of Sexual Behavior. New York: Harper, 1951.

Fromm-Reichmann, Frieda. "Notes on the Mother Role in the Family Group," *Bulletin of the Menninger Clinic,* IV (September 1940), 132-48.

Gregory de Torres, Sara. "Elopement in the Lower Classes in Puerto Rico." Unpublished term paper, University of Puerto Rico, 1951.

Hagood, M. J. Mothers of the South. Chapel Hill: University of North Carolina Press, 1939.

Hamilton, G. A Research in Marriage. New York: Lear, 1948.

Hatt, Paul K. Backgrounds of Human Fertility in Puerto Rico: A Sociological Survey. Princeton: Princeton University Press, 1952.

Henriques, F. "West Indian Family Organization," *American Journal of Sociology,* Vol. LV, No. 1 (July 1949).

Hill, R., K. Back, and J. M. Stycos. "Family Structure and Fertility in Puerto Rico." Social Science Research Center, University of Puerto Rico, September 1954, mimeographed.

Himes, Norman E. Medical History of Contraception. London: George Allen and Unwin, 1936.

Hyman, H. "Interviewing as a Scientific Procedure," in D. Lerner and H. Lasswell, eds., The Policy Sciences. Stanford: Stanford University Press, 1951.

Hyman, H., and P. Sheatsley. "The Kinsey Report and Survey Methodology," *International Journal of Opinion and Attitude Research,* II (1948), 183-95.

Imparcial, El (San Juan), February 15, 1949; August 25, September 19, 1951; October 1, 1952.

Jacobs, A. C. "Common Law Marriage," in Encyclopedia of the Social Sciences.

Jaffe, A., and L. de Ortíz. "The Human Resource—Puerto Rico's Working Force." Mimeographed, San Juan, 1953.

Janer, José. "Population Growth in Puerto Rico and Its Relation to Time Changes in Vital Statistics," *Human Biology,* XVII (December 1945), 267-313.

Kerr, M. Personality and Conflict in Jamaica. Liverpool: University Press, 1952.

King, M. "Cultural Aspects of Birth Control in Puerto Rico," *Human Biology,* Vol. XX, No. 1 (February 1948).

Kinsey, A., W. Pomeroy, and C. Martin. Sexual Behavior in the Human Male. Philadelphia: Saunders, 1948.

Landy, David. "Childrearing Patterns in a Puerto Rican Lower Class Community." Unpublished manuscript, University of Puerto Rico, 1952.

Lang, Olga. Chinese Family and Society. New Haven: Yale University Press, 1946.

Levy, Marion. The Family Revolution in Modern China. London: Oxford University Press, 1949.

Lewis, Oscar. "Husbands and Wives in a Mexican Village: A Study of Role Conflict," *American Anthropologist,* Vol. LI (October 1949).

Mass Observation. Britain and Her Birth Rate. London: John Murray, 1945.

May, Geoffrey. Social Control of Sex Expression. London: George Allen and Unwin, 1930.

Merton, Robert. "Patterns of Influence," in Paul Lazarsfeld, and Frank Stanton, eds., Communications Research 1948-1949. New York: Harper, 1949.

Merton, R., M. Fiske, and P. Kendall. "The Focused Interview." Mimeographed, Bureau of Applied Social Research, Columbia University, 1952.

Mihanovich, C. S., G. J. Schnepp, and J. L. Thomas. Marriage and the Family. Milwaukee: Bruce Publishing Co., 1952.

Milagrosa, La (San Juan), October 25, 1950.

Mintz, Sidney. "Cañamelar: The Contemporary Culture of a Rural Puerto Rican Proletariat." Unpublished Ph.D. dissertation, Columbia University, 1951.

Moore, Wilbert. "Attitudes of Mexican Factory Workers toward Fertility Control," in Approaches to Problems of High Fertility in Agrarian Societies. New York: Milbank Memorial Fund, 1952.

Mundo, El (San Juan), March 17, October 3, 1949; September 7, 11, October 15, 24, 1951.

Muñoz Morales, Luis. Reseña histórica y anotaciones al Código Civil de Puerto Rico. Santurce: Imprenta Soltera, 1947.

Murdock, G. Social Structure. New York: Macmillan, 1949.

Myrdal, A. "Population Trends in Densely Populated Areas," *Proceedings of the American Philosophical Society*, Vol. VC, No. 1 (February 1951).

Notestein, F. "Summary of the Demographic Background of Problems of Underdeveloped Areas," *Milbank Memorial Fund Quarterly*, Vol. XXVI, No. 3 (July 1948).

——— "The Facts of Life," in Ruth Anshen, ed., The Family: Its Function and Destiny. New York: Harper, 1949.

Padilla, Elena. "Nocora: An Agrarian Reform Sugar Community in Puerto Rico." Unpublished Ph.D. dissertation, Columbia University, 1951.

Parke, Robert. "Internal Migration in Puerto Rico." Unpublished Master's essay, Columbia University, 1952.

Petrullo, Vincenzo. Puerto Rican Paradox. Philadelphia: University of Pennsylvania, 1947.

"Post-War Divorce Rates Here and Abroad," *Statistical Bulletin*, June, 1952.

"Quarter's Polls, The," *Public Opinion Quarterly*, Vol. XI, No. 3 (Fall 1947); Vol. II, No. 4 (Winter 1947).

Reed, R. "The Interrelationship of Marital Adjustment, Fertility Control, and Size of Family," in P. Whelpton and C. Kiser, eds., Social and Psychological Factors Affecting Fertility. New York: Milbank Memorial Fund, 1950.

Riesman, David. The Lonely Crowd. New Haven: Yale University Press, 1950.

Roberts, Lydia J., and Rosa Luisa Stefani. Patterns of Living in Puerto Rican Families. Río Piedras: University of Puerto Rico, 1949.

Rogler, Charles. Comerío—A Study of a Puerto Rican Town. University of Kansas, 1940.

Rosario, José. The Development of the Puerto Rican Jíbaro and His Present Attitude toward Society. San Juan, 1935.

——— A Study of Illegitimacy and Dependent Children in Puerto Rico. San Juan: Imprenta Venezuela, 1936.

Royal Commission on Population Report. London: H. M. Stationery Office, 1949.

Ryan, B. "Institutional Factors in Sinhalese Fertility," *Milbank Memorial Fund Quarterly,* Vol. XXX, No. 4 (October 1952).

Sánchez Hidalgo, Efraín. "El sentimiento de inferioridad en la mujer puertorriqueña," *Revista de la Asociación de Maestros,* XI (December 1952), 170-71.

Senior, Clarence. "Puerto Rican Emigration." Mimeographed, University of Puerto Rico, 1947.

——— "Disequilibrium between Population and Resources: The Case of Puerto Rico," Proceedings of the Inter-American Conference on the Conservation of Renewable Natural Resources, 1948.

——— "An Approach to Research in Overcoming Cultural Barriers to Family Limitation," in G. Mair, ed., Studies in Population. Princeton: Princeton University Press, 1949. Proceedings of the Annual Meeting of the Population Association of America.

——— "Migration and Puerto Rico's Population Problem," *Annals of the American Academy of Political and Social Sciences,* Vol. CCLXXXV (January 1953).

Sereno, Renzo. "Cryptomelanism: A Study of Color Relations and Personal Insecurity in Puerto Rico," *Psychiatry,* Vol. X (August 1947).

Siegel, Morris. "Lajas: A Puerto Rican Town." Unpublished manuscript, University of Puerto Rico, 1948.

Sovani, N. "The Problem of Fertility Control in India: Cultural Factors and Development of Policy," in Approaches to Problems of High Fertility in Agrarian Societies. New York: Milbank Memorial Fund, 1952.

Statistical Yearbook of Puerto Rico, 1949-50; 1950-51. San Juan: Departamento de Instrucción.

Steward, Julian. "Cultural Patterns of Puerto Rico," *Annals of the American Academy of Political and Social Science,* Vol. CCLXXXV (January 1953).

Stone, Abraham, and Norman Himes. Planned Parenthood: A Practical Guide to Birth Control Methods. New York: Viking Press, 1951.

Stycos, J. Mayone. "Patterns of Communication in a Rural Greek Village," *Public Opinion Quarterly,* Vol. XVI (Spring 1952).

_______ "Interviewer Training in Another Culture," *Public Opinion Quarterly,* Vol. XVI (Summer 1952).

_______ "Family and Fertility in Puerto Rico," *American Sociological Review,* XVII (October 1952), 572-80.

_______ "Female Sterilization in Puerto Rico," *Eugenics Quarterly,* I, No. 2 (June 1954), 3-9.

_______ "The Pattern of Birth Control in Puerto Rico," *Eugenics Quarterly,* I, No. 3 (September 1954), 176-81.

Stycos, J. Mayone, and R. Hill. "The Prospects of Birth Control in Puerto Rico," *Annals of the American Academy of Political and Social Sciences,* Vol. CCLXXXV (January 1953).

Taeuber, Irene. "The Reproductive Mores of the Asian Peasant," in G. Mair, ed., Studies in Population. Princeton: Princeton University Press, 1949. Proceedings of the Annual Meeting of the Population Association of America.

Taylor, Milton. "Neo-Malthusianism in Puerto Rico," *Review of Social Economy,* Vol. X (March 1952).

Thompson, Clara. "The Role of Women in This Culture," *Psychiatry,* Vol. IV (February 1941).

_______ "Penis Envy in Women," *Psychiatry,* Vol. VI (May 1943).

Tietze, Christopher. "Human Fertility in Puerto Rico," *American Journal of Sociology,* LIII (July 1947), 34-40.

Torres Rioseco, Arturo. "The Family in Latin America," in Ruth Anshen, ed., The Family: Its Function and Destiny. New York: Harper, 1949.

Ungern-Sternberg, Roderich von. The Causes of the Decline in Birth-Rate within the European Sphere of Civilization. Tr. by Hilda H. Wullen. Cold Spring Harbor, Long Island, N. Y.: Eugenics Research Association Monograph Series, No. 4, 1931.

Vance, Rupert. "The Demographic Gap: Dilemma of Modernization Programs," in Approaches to Problems of High Fertility in Agrarian Societies. New York: Milbank Memorial Fund, 1952.

Van de Velde, H. Ideal Marriage: Its Physiology and Technique. London: William Heineman, 1926.

Verbo (Río Piedras), Vol. III, No. 2 (January 1952).

West, J. Plainville, U.S.A. New York: Columbia University Press, 1945.

Whelpton, P., and C. Kiser. "Developing the Schedules, and Choosing the Type of Couples and the Area to be Studied," in P. Whelpton and C. Kiser, eds., Social and Psychological Factors Affecting Fertility. New York: Milbank Memorial Fund, 1950.

Willems, E. "Structure of the Brazilian Family," *Social Forces,* Vol. XXXI, No. 4 (May 1953).

Winch, R. "Further Data and Observations on the Oedipus Hypothesis," *American Sociological Review,* Vol. XVI, No. 6 (December 1951).

Wolf, Eric. "Culture Change and Culture Stability in a Puerto Rican Coffee Community." Unpublished Ph.D. dissertation, Columbia University, 1951.

Wolf, K. "Growing up and Its Price in Three Puerto Rican Subcultures," *Psychiatry,* Vol. XV, No. 4 (November 1952).

Woodside, M. "The Psychiatric Approach to Research Interviewing," in G. Mair, ed., Studies in Population. Princeton: Princeton University Press, 1949. Proceedings of the Annual Meeting of the Population Association of America.

——— Sterilization in North Carolina: A Sociological and Psychological Study. Chapel Hill: University of North Carolina Press, 1950.

Index